Alecio,
Mis mejores deseos por una vida llena de dicha, felicidad y salud en unión de tu familia
Werner Hoeger.
6 de abril de 1986.

Lifetime Physical Fitness and Wellness

A Personalized Program

Werner W. K. Hoeger
University of Texas, Permian Basin

MP
Morton Publishing Company
925 W. Kenyon Ave., Unit 4
Englewood, Colorado 80110

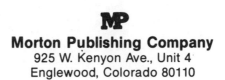

Printed in the United States of America

ISBN: 0-89582-152-4

Preface

The current American way of life no longer provides the human body with sufficient physical exercise to maintain adequate health. Furthermore, many present lifestyle patterns are such a serious threat to our health that they actually increase the deterioration rate of the human body and often lead to premature illness and mortality.

Although people in the United States are firm believers in the benefits of physical activity, adequate nutrition, and positive lifestyle patterns as a means to promote better health, most do not reap these benefits because they simply do not know how to implement a sound physical fitness and wellness program that will indeed yield the desired results.

Scientific evidence has clearly shown that improving the quality and most likely the longevity of our lives is a matter of personal choice. The biggest challenge that we are faced with at the end of this century is to teach individuals how to take control of their personal health habits to insure a better, healthier, happier, and more productive life. The information presented in this book has been written with this objective in mind, providing you with the opportunity to initiate your own positive health and lifestyle program.

As you work through the different chapters in the book, you will be able to develop and regularly update your own lifetime program to improve the various components of physical fitness and personal wellness. The emphasis throughout the different chapters is on teaching you how to take control of your own personal health and lifestyle habits, so that you can make a constant and deliberate effort to stay healthy and realize your highest potential for well-being.

This book is dedicated to my wife and children. Without my wife's input, assistance, constant support, and my children's patience and encouragement, this book could not have been written.

ACKNOWLEDGMENTS

The author wishes to express his gratitude to Dr. Lois S. Hale, Dr. David R. Hopkins, and Dr. Raymond M. Zurawski for their valuable contributions and support; to Richard K. Riley for his input and suggestions in the preparation of the final manuscript; to Gayla J. Carbajal for the long and late hours spent typing the manuscript; to Travis Woodward, Sandy L. Collins, and Tony Marquis for their help with the photography in this book; and to everyone else whose contributions made this work possible.

Table of Contents

CHAPTER ONE

Introduction to Lifetime Physical Fitness and Wellness

Movement and physical activity are basic functions for which the human organism was created. However, advances in modern technology have almost completely eliminated the need for physical activity in most everyone's daily life. Exercise is no longer a natural part of our existence. We now live in an automated society, where most of the activities that used to require strenuous physical exertion can be accomplished by machines with the simple pull of a handle or push of a button. The available scientific evidence shows that physical inactivity and a sedentary lifestyle have become a serious threat to our health and significantly increase the deterioration rate of the human body.

With the new developments in technology, two additional factors have significantly changed our lives and have had a negative effect on human health: nutrition and environment. Fatty foods, sweets, alcohol, tobacco use, and pollution in general have detrimental effects on people.

At the beginning of the century, the most common health problems in the United States were such infectious diseases as tuberculosis, diphtheria, influenza, kidney disease, polio, and other diseases of infancy. Progress in the field of medicine allowed for the elimination of these diseases, but as the American lifestyle changed, a parallel increase was seen in chronic diseases such as hypertension, atherosclerosis, coronary disease, strokes, diabetes, cancer, emphysema, and cirrhosis of the liver.

As the incidence of chronic diseases increased, it became obvious that prevention was the best medicine when dealing with these new health problems. Some research now indicates that over 53 percent of all disease is self-controlled and that 83 percent of all deaths in the United States prior to the age of sixty-five are preventable. The leading causes of death in the country today are basically lifestyle related (Table 1.1). About 70 percent of all deaths are caused by cardiovascular disease (includes heart disease and cerebrovascular diseases) and cancer. Approximately 80 percent of these could be prevented through a positive lifestyle program. Accidents are the fourth cause of death. While not all accidents are preventable, many are. A significant number of fatal accidents are related to alcohol and lack of use of seat belts. The fifth cause of death, chronic and obstructive pulmonary disease, is largely related to tobacco use.

Table 1.1. Leading Causes of Death in the United States: 1983

1. Heart disease
2. Cancer
3. Cerebrovascular diseases
4. Accidents
5. Chronic and obstructive pulmonary disease

From the National Center for Health Statistics

CARDIOVASCULAR DISEASE

The most prevalent degenerative diseases in the United States are those of the cardiovascular system. Approximately 50 percent of all deaths in the country result from cardiovascular disease. According to the American Heart Association, heart and blood vessel disease costs were in excess of $72.1 billion in 1985. Heart attacks alone cost American industry 132 million workdays annually, including $12.4 billion in lost productivity because of physical and emotional disability. The 1982 estimates by the American Heart Association showed that:

- 43,500,000 Americans were affected by cardiovascular disease
- 37,990,000 had high blood pressure (one in four adults)
- 4,670,000 were afflicted by coronary heart disease
- 2,040,000 had rheumatic heart disease
- 1,900,000 suffered strokes
- 1,500,000 suffered heart attacks with over a half a million dying as a direct result of them

It must be noted that about 50 percent of the time, the first symptom of coronary heart disease is a heart attack itself, and 40 percent of the people who suffer a first heart attack die within the first twenty-four hours. In one out of every five cardiovascular deaths, sudden death is the initial symptom. Over 100,000 of those that die are men in their most productive years between the ages of forty and sixty-five. Additionally, the American Heart Association estimates that over $700 million a year are spent in replacing employees who are recovering from heart attacks. Oddly enough, most coronary heart disease risk factors are reversible and can be controlled by the individuals themselves through appropriate lifestyle modifications.

Even though cardiovascular disease is still the leading cause of death in the country, the mortality rates for this disease have been decreasing in the last two decades. It is estimated that in 1983, 165,000 lives were saved that were expected to die as a direct result of heart and blood vessel disease. This reduction is attributed primarily to prevention programs dealing with risk factor management and to better health care.

CANCER

Cancer is defined as an uncontrolled growth and spread of abnormal cells in the body. Some cells grow into a mass of tissue called a tumor, which can be either benign or malignant. A malignant tumor would be considered a "cancer." If the spread of cells is not controlled, death ensues. Approximately 20 percent of all deaths in the United States are due to cancer. About 462,000 people died of this disease in 1985, and an estimated 910,000 new cases were expected the same year. Table 1.2 shows the 1985 estimated figures by the American Cancer Society for major sites of cancer, excluding nonmelanoma skin cancer and carcinoma in situ.

Table 1.2.
Estimated New Cases and Deaths for Major Sites of Cancer: 1985

Site	New Cases	Deaths
Lung	144,000	126,000
Colon-Rectum	138,000	60,000
Breast (Women)	119,000	38,000
Prostate	86,000	26,000
Pancreas	25,000	24,000
Urinary	60,000	20,000
Leukemia	25,000	17,000
Ovary	19,000	12,000
Uterus	52,000[a]	10,000
Oral	29,000	10,000
Skin	19,000[b]	7,000

From 1985 Cancer Facts and Figures. American Cancer Society, 1985.

[a]New cases total over 100,000 if carcinoma in situ is included
[b]Estimates are over 400,000 if new cases of nonmelanoma are included

Scientific evidence and testing procedures for the early detection of cancer are continuously changing and improving. Cancer is now viewed as the most curable of all chronic diseases. Over 5 million Americans with a history of cancer are now alive, and close to 3 million of them are considered cured. Evidence now indicates that as much as 80 percent of all human cancer can be prevented through positive lifestyle modifications, including a diet low in fat and high in fiber, abstinence from cigarette smoking, and moderate use of alcohol. The basic guidelines for cancer prevention are outlined in Chapter 8.

WHAT IS PHYSICAL FITNESS?

Physical fitness has been defined in many different ways. A physician may define it as the absence of disease. The American Medical Association has defined it as the general capacity to adapt and respond favorably to physical effort. The President's Council on Physical Fitness and Sports has indicated that physical fitness is the measure of the body's strength, stamina, and flexibility. A more appropriate definition is that individuals are physically fit when they can meet the ordinary as well as the unusual demands of daily life safely and effectively without being overly fatigued, and still have energy left for leisure and recreational activities.

Physical fitness can be classified into two categories: health-related fitness and motor skill-related fitness. Most authorities agree that from a health point of view, total physical fitness involves four basic components that are separate parameters, but are all interrelated. These components are cardiovascular endurance, muscular strength and endurance, muscular flexibility, and body composition (ideal body weight and fat percentage). In order to improve the overall fitness level, an individual has to participate in separate programs to improve each one of the four basic components. However, after the initial fitness boom swept across the country in the 1970s, it became clear that just improving the four components of physical fitness alone would not always decrease the risk for disease and insure better health. As a result, a new concept developed in the 1980s that goes beyond the basic components of fitness. This new concept is referred to as "wellness," which will be discussed later on in this chapter.

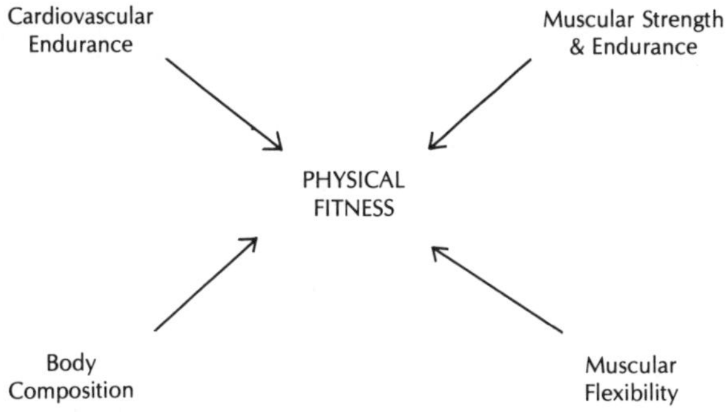

Figure 1.1. *Health-Related Components of Physical Fitness*

The motor skill-related aspects of fitness are of greater significance in athletics. In addition to the previous four components, motor skill-related fitness includes speed and power, coordination, agility, reaction time, and balance. While these components are important in achieving success in athletics, they are not crucial for the development of better health. Therefore, in this book only the health-related components of fitness will be discussed.

THE WELLNESS CONCEPT

Wellness can be defined as the constant and deliberate effort to stay healthy and achieve the highest potential for total well-being. The concept of wellness incorporates many other components other than those associated with physical fitness, such as proper nutrition, smoking cessation, stress management, alcohol and drug control, and regular physical examinations (*see* Figure 1.2). The difference between physical fitness and wellness is clearly illustrated in the wellness continuum shown in Figure 1.3. An individual who is running three miles per day, lifting weights regularly, participating in stretching exercises, and watching his body weight can easily be classified in the good or excellent category for each one of the fitness components. However, if this same individual suffers from high blood pressure, smokes, consumes alcohol, and/or eats fatty foods, the individual is probably developing several risk factors for cardiovascular disease and may not be aware of it (a risk factor is defined as an asymptomatic state that a person has that may lead to disease).

One of the best examples in recent years was the tragic death in 1984 of Jim Fixx, author of *The Complete Book of Running.* At the time of his death, Fixx was fifty-two years old. He had been running between sixty and eighty miles per week and had felt that anyone in his condition could not die from heart disease. At age thirty-six, Jim Fixx had been smoking two packs of cigarettes per day, weighed about 215 pounds, did not engage in regular cardiovascular exercise, and had a family history of heart disease. His father had experienced a first heart attack at age thirty-five and later died at age forty-three. Perhaps in an effort to decrease his risk of heart disease, Fixx began to increase his fitness level. He started to jog, lost fifty pounds, and quit cigarette smoking. His exercise program did not make him immune to heart disease, but it probably delayed the onset of the fatal heart attack. Additionally, Jim Fixx declined several times to have an exercise electrocardiogram (EKG) test done, which would have most likely revealed his heart condition. This unfortunate death is a clear example that just improving basic components of physical fitness is not always a risk-free guarantee for everyone, but that all wellness components should be taken into consideration for a happier and healthier life.

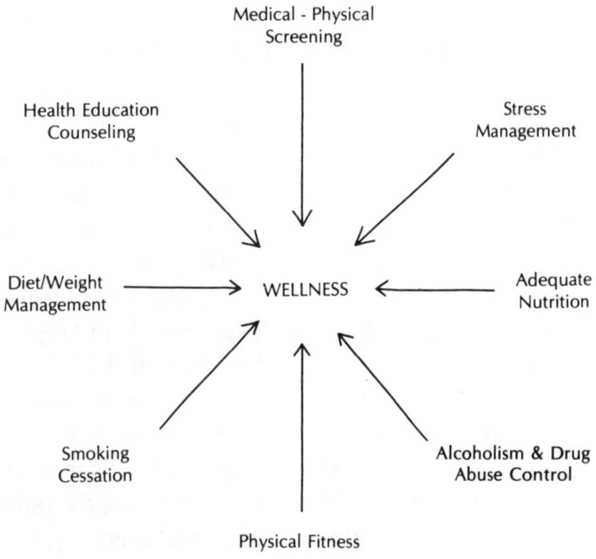

Figure 1.2. *Wellness Components*

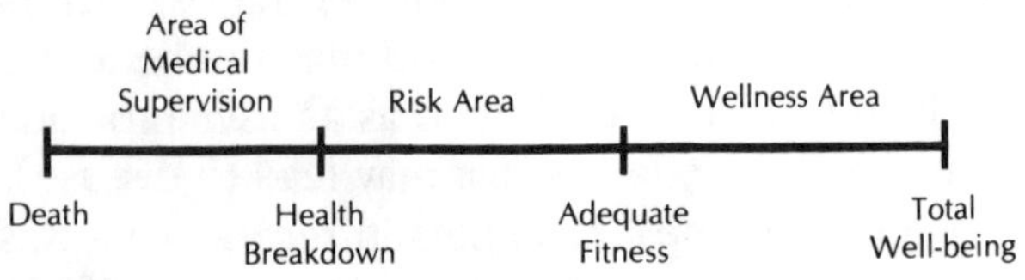

Figure 1.3. *Wellness Continuum*

RELATIONSHIP BETWEEN FITNESS/WELLNESS AND HEALTH

A most inspiring story illustrating what fitness can do for the person's health was reported in the March 1983 issue of *Runner's World.* George Snell from Sandy, Utah, was forty-five years old at Christmas 1981 and weighed approximately 400 pounds. His blood pressure was 220/80, he became blind because of diabetes that he did not know he had, and his blood glucose level was 487. Snell started a walking/jogging program in January 1982. After only eight months, he had lost close to 200 pounds, his eyesight had returned, his glucose level was down to 67, and he was taken off medication. That same year in October, less than ten months after initiating his personal exercise program, he completed his first marathon, a running course of 26.2 miles.

While there are many benefits to be enjoyed as a result of participating in a regular physical fitness and wellness program, the greatest benefit of all is that individuals enjoy a better quality of life. Even though there are some indications that they will also live a longer life, statistically this is difficult to prove because of the many different factors that can have an effect on our health and well-being. Tables 1.3 and 1.4 are examples of scientific research that has shown an inverse relationship between exercise and premature mortality rates. However, when it comes to quality of life, there is no question that physically fit individuals who lead a positive lifestyle live a better and healthier life. These people can enjoy life to its fullest potential, with a lot fewer health problems than inactive individuals who may also

Table 1.3.
Cause-Specific Death Rates[a] per 10,000 Man-Years of Observation Among 16,936 Harvard Alumni, 1962-1978, by Physical Activity Index

Cause of Death (n = 1,413)	% of Total Deaths	Physical Activity Index, Kcal/week		
		<500	500-1,999	2,000+
Cardiovascular Diseases	45.3	39.5	30.8	21.4
Cancer	31.6	25.7	19.2	19.0
Accidents	5.5	3.6	3.9	3.0
Suicides	4.8	5.1	3.2	2.9
Respiratory Diseases	4.3	6.0	3.2	1.5

From Paffenbarger, R. S., R. T. Hyde, A. L. Wing, and C. H. Steinmetz. "A Natural History of Athleticism and Cardiovascular Health. *JAMA* 252(4): 491-495, 1984. Copyright 1985, American Medical Association.

[a]Adjusted for differences in age, cigarette smoking, and hypertension.

Table 1.4.
Deaths from Coronary Heart Disease per 100 Men and Women by Amount of Physical Exertion

		Degree of Exercise			
Sex	**Age**	**None**	**Slight**	**Moderate**	**Heavy**
Men	40-49	1.46	1.17	1.12	1.00
	50-59	1.43	1.17	1.06	1.00
	60-69	1.91	1.64	1.19	1.00
	70-79	2.91	2.03	1.45	1.00
Women	40-49	—	1.29	1.07	1.00
	50-59	—	1.21	1.06	1.00
	60-69	2.01	1.86	1.11	1.00
	70-79	3.15	2.30	1.33	1.00

From Hammond, E. C., and L. Garfinkel. "Coronary Heart Disease, Stroke, and Aortic Aneurysm." *Archives of Environmental Health* 19(8):174, 1979. A publication of the Helen Dwight Reid Educational Foundation. (Table based on data of more than 1 million men and women studied over a period of six years).

Table 1.5.
Benefits Derived from a Comprehensive Fitness and Wellness Program

1. Improves and strengthens the cardiovascular system (improved oxygen supply to all parts of the body, including the heart, the muscles, and the brain)
2. Maintains better muscle tone, muscular strength, and endurance
3. Improves muscle flexibility
4. Helps maintain ideal body weight
5. Improves posture and physical appearance
6. Decreases risk for chronic diseases and illness (heart disease, cancer, strokes, high blood pressure, pulmonary disease, arthritis, etc.)
7. Decreases mortality rates from chronic diseases
8. Decreases risk and mortality rates from accidents
9. Relieves tension and helps in coping with stresses of life
10. Increases levels of energy and job productivity
11. Slows down the aging process
12. Improves self-image, morale, and aids in fighting depression
13. Motivates toward positive lifestyle changes (better diet and nutrition, smoking cessation, alcohol and drug abuse control)
14. Decreases recovery time following physical exertion
15. Speeds up recovery following injury and/or disease
16. Eases the process of childbearing and childbirth
17. Regulates and improves overall body functions
18. Improves quality of life, makes people feel and live better

be indulging in negative lifestyle patterns. While it is difficult to compile an all-inclusive list of the benefits of physical fitness and wellness, Table 1.5 provides a summary of many of these benefits.

HEALTH CARE COSTS VERSUS PHYSICAL ACTIVITY AND WELLNESS PROGRAMS

As the need for physical exertion steadily decreased in the last century the nation's health expenditures dramatically increased (see Figure 1.4). Total medical expenditures in the United States in 1950 were $12 billion. In 1960 this figure

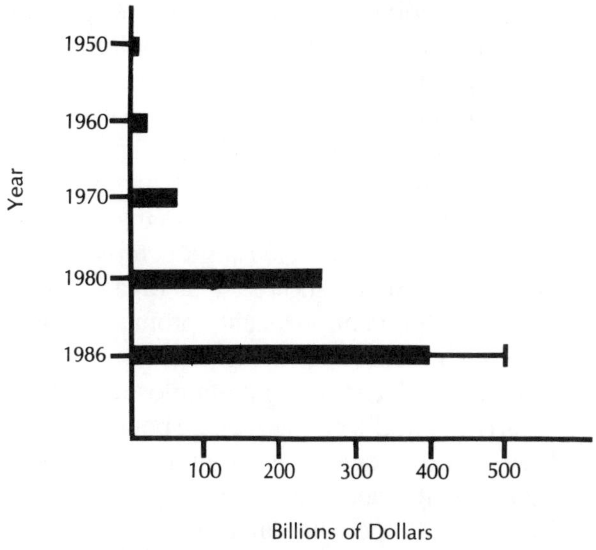

Figure 1.4. *U.S. Health Care Cost Increments in the Last Four Decades*

reached $26.9 billion, by 1970 it increased to $75 billion, and by 1980 health care costs accounted for $243.4 billion. At the present rate this figure is estimated to be about $500 billion in 1986, which is in excess of 10 percent of the Gross National Product. Over half of this cost is being absorbed by American business and industry.

A clear example of the benefits derived from fitness and wellness is seen among many corporations in our country that are now offering health promotion programs to their employees. Many companies are now finding out that it costs less to keep an employee healthy than treating him once he's sick. The following list of facts and figures points out the need, as well as economical and health benefits to organizations providing wellness programs:

1. The cost of insurance premiums to American industry continues to increase each year. For example, the cost of insurance premiums for 15,000 employees of the Kimberly-Clark Corporation in 1977 was $14.3 million. This figure had increased by 75 percent in only four years. At the Ford Motor Company, health benefits are the most expensive fringe benefit, increasing in cost from $450 million in 1977 to $600 million in 1979. Similarly, since 1975 General Motors has been spending more for health benefits than for steel used in building automobiles.
2. The backache syndrome, usually the result of physical degeneration (inelastic and weak muscles), cost American industry over $1 billion annually in lost productivity and services alone. An additional $225 million are spent in workmen's compensation. The Adolph Coors Company in Golden, Colorado, which initiated a wellness program in 1981 for employees and their families, reported savings of more than $319,000 in 1983 alone through a preventive and rehabilitative back injury program.
3. A 1981 survey of the 1,500 largest employers in the United States showed that organizations that offer prevention/health promotion programs to their employees had an average annual health care cost per employee of $806. This compared with the average per employee cost of $1,015 for all companies, representing a $209 savings per employee per year (an approximate 20 percent difference).
4. The Prudential Insurance Company of Houston conducted a study of its 1,300 employees. Those who participated for at least one year in the company's fitness program averaged 3.5 days of disability, as compared to 8.6 days for nonparticipants. The study estimated the direct savings from salary paid out during sickness at $204 per employee, and three to four times that amount in indirect costs due to replacements, productivity loss, overtime, etc.
5. The Mesa Petroleum Company in Amarillo, Texas, has been offering an on-site fitness program since 1979 to its 350 employees and their family members (64 percent of the employees use the fitness center on a regular basis). A 1982 survey showed an average of $434 per person in medical costs for the nonparticipating group in the company, while the participating group averaged only $173 per person per year. This represents a yearly reduction of $200,000 in medical expenses. Sick-leave time was also significantly less for the physically active group — twenty-seven hours per year as compared to forty-four for the inactive group.

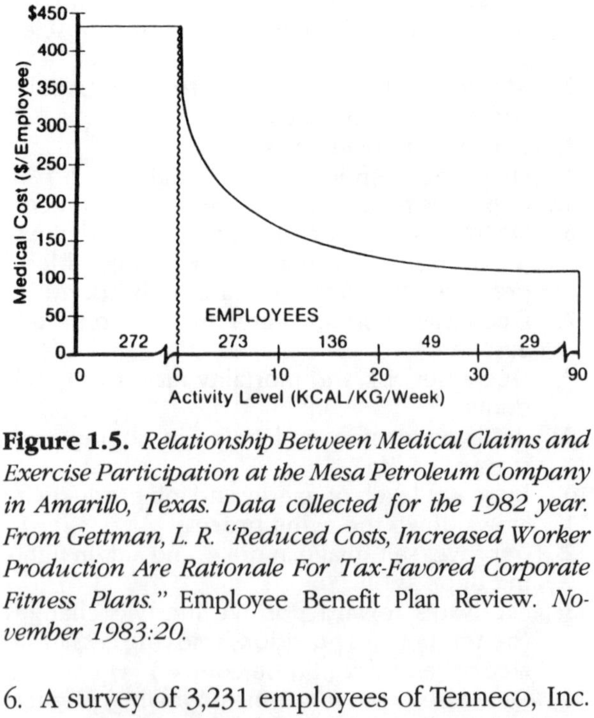

Figure 1.5. *Relationship Between Medical Claims and Exercise Participation at the Mesa Petroleum Company in Amarillo, Texas. Data collected for the 1982 year. From Gettman, L. R. "Reduced Costs, Increased Worker Production Are Rationale For Tax-Favored Corporate Fitness Plans."* Employee Benefit Plan Review. *November 1983:20.*

6. A survey of 3,231 employees of Tenneco, Inc. in Houston found that job productivity is related to fitness. Individuals with high ratings of job performance also rated high in exercise participation.
7. In 1980, the New York Telephone Company spent $2.84 million on wellness and prevention programs for 80,000 of their employees. However, as a direct result of the program, the

company saved $5.54 million in employee absence and treatment costs. This represented a health care cost reduction of $69.25 per employee.

8. An independent research project of the Canadian government in 1981 documented an $84 per employee savings in health care costs for Canada Life Assurance Company in the first year of its wellness program. An additional $210 per employee savings in absenteeism and turnover was also calculated. The results were obtained by comparing figures with the North American Life Company, which offered no fitness or lifestyle programs.

In addition to the above benefits, many corporations are now using fitness and wellness as an incentive to attract, hire, and retain their employees. Organizations devote resources to these programs because they know they can expect less absenteeism, hospitalization, disability, job turnover rates, premature death, and health costs, as well as increased morale and job productivity. Many companies are now taking a hard look at the fitness level of potential employees and are seriously using this information in their screening process. Some organizations even refuse to hire smokers and/or overweight individuals. On the other hand, many executives feel that an on-site health promotion program is the best fringe benefit that they can enjoy at their company. Young executives are also looking for such organizations, not only for the added health benefits, but because an attitude of concern and care by corporate officials is shown.

A PERSONALIZED APPROACH

With such impressive information now available on the benefits of fitness and wellness, it is clear that improving the quality and possibly longevity of our lives is a matter of personal choice. A better and healthier life is something that every person needs to strive to attain for himself. The biggest challenge for the 1980s and 1990s is to teach individuals how to take control of their personal health habits by practicing positive lifestyle activities that will decrease the risk of illness and help achieve total well-being.

As a result of the fitness and wellness movements in the past two decades, most people in the country now see a need to participate in such programs to improve and maintain adequate health. However, many people are still not participating because they are unaware of the basic principles for safe and effective exercise participation. Others are exercising erroneously and therefore do not reap the full benefits of their program.

Since physical fitness and wellness needs vary significantly from one individual to the other, exercise and wellness prescriptions have to be individualized in order to obtain optimal results. The information presented in this book has been developed to provide the reader with the necessary information to write his/her own program to improve the various components of physical fitness and to promote preventive health care and personal wellness. In the ensuing chapters you will learn how to:

1. Assess and improve your current level of cardiovascular endurance, muscular strength and endurance, muscular flexibility, and body composition.
2. Conduct your own nutritional analysis, write a diet and weight control program, and follow the recommendations for adequate nutrition.
3. Assess your levels of tension and stress and conduct a stress management program.
4. Quit cigarette smoking if you are presently doing so.
5. Determine your potential risk for cardiovascular disease and cancer, and implement the guidelines for a risk reduction program.

YOUR PERSONAL FITNESS AND WELLNESS PROFILE

As you work through the next few chapters, you will be able to develop your personal profile. When you obtain the information pertaining to each component of fitness and wellness, enter your results on the profile found in Appendix A, Figure A.1. Once the results for each component have been established, either with the help of your instructor, or using your own judgment, set the target goals to achieve over the next ten to fourteen weeks. During the first two or three weeks, pay particular attention to the components of physical fitness. You should first determine the fitness components of the profile so that you may proceed with your exercise program and allow sufficient time to retest each fitness component within eight to twelve weeks of the initial assessment.

A WORD OF CAUTION BEFORE YOU START

In 1984 and 1985, several tragic deaths occurred while some prominent national figures had been exercising. These unfortunate events raised some questions as to the safety involved in exercise participation. Therefore, before you start to engage in any sort of exercise, fill out the questionnaire given in Figure 1.7. If your answer to any of the questions is positive, you should consult a physician before participating in a fitness program. Physical activity is contraindicated under some of the conditions listed in this questionnaire, and others may require an exercise EKG test. In the event that you have any questions regarding your current health status, consult your doctor before initiating, continuing, or increasing your level of physical activity.

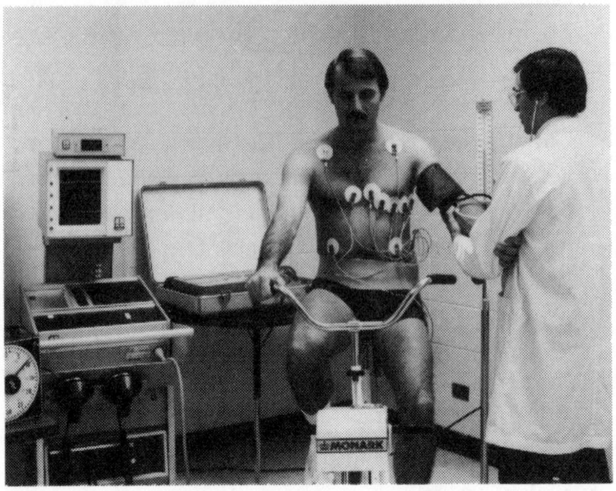

Figure 1.6. *Exercise Tolerance Test with Twelve-lead Electrocardiographic Monitoring (Courtesy of The University of Texas of The Permian Basin Wellness Center, Odessa, Texas)*

References

1. Allsen, P. E., J. M. Harrison, and B. Vance. *Fitness for Life: An Individualized Approach.* Dubuque, IA: Wm. C. Brown, 1984.
2. American Cancer Society. *1985 Cancer Facts and Figures.* New York: The Society, 1985.
3. American College of Sports Medicine. *Guidelines for Graded Exercise Testing and Exercise Prescription.* Philadelphia: Lea and Febiger, 1980.
4. American Heart Association. *Heart Facts.* Dallas, TX: The Association, 1985.
5. Cooper, K. H. *The Aerobics Program for Total Well-Being.* New York: Mount Evans and Co., 1982.
6. Fielding, J. E. "Preventive Medicine and the Bottom Line." *Journal of Occupational Medicine* 21(2):79-82, 1979.
7. Fitness Monitoring Inc. "Health Care Cost Containment: Can You Afford to Sit on the Sidelines Any Longer?" Lake Geneva, WI: The Author, 1982.
8. Gettman, L. R. "Reduced Costs, Increased Production Are Rationale for Tax-Favored Corporate Fitness Plans." *Employee Benefit Plan Review* 20-22, November 1983.
9. Hammond, E. C., and L. Garfinkel. "Coronary Heart Disease, Stroke, and Aortic Aneurysm." *"Archives of Environmental Health* 19(8):174, 1979.
10. Herbert, H. R., L. Montgomery, and H. P. Wetzler. *Planning a Fitness Program for Industry.* Washington, D.C.: President's Council on Physical Fitness and Sports, 1983. Contained in Federal Fit Kit.
11. Hockley, R. V. *Physical Fitness: The Pathway to Healthful Living.* St. Louis: Times Mirror/Mosby College Publishing, 1985.
12. Hoeger, W. W. K. *Ejercicio, Salud y Vida [Exercise, Health and Life].* Caracas, Venezuela: Editorial Arte, 1980.
13. Marcotte, B., and J. H. Price. "The Status of Health Promotion Programs at the Work Site, A Review." *Health Education* 4-8, July/August, 1983.
14. Paffenbarger, R. S., R. T. Hyde, A. L. Wing, and C. H. Steinmetz. "A Natural History of Athleticism and Cardiovascular Health." *JAMA* 252:491-495, 1984.
15. Parkinson, R., and Associates. *Managing Health Promotion in the Workplace.* Palo Alto, CA: Mayfield Publishing Company, 1982.
16. *Physical Fitness in Business and Industry.* Washington, D.C.: President's Council on Physical Fitness and Sports, 1972.
17. Sorochan, W. D. *Promoting Your Health.* New York: John Wiley & Sons, Inc., 1981.
18. Staff. 1983 Runner's World National Achievement Awards. *Runner's World* 44-47, March 1983.
19. Staff. "New Fitness Data Verifies: Employees Who Exercise Are Also More Productive." *Athletic Business* 8(12):24-30, 1984.
20. Van Camp, S. P. "The Fixx Tragedy: A Cardiologist's Perspective." *Physician and Sports Medicine* 12(9): 153-155, 1984.
21. Wiley, J. A., and T. C. Camacho. "Lifestyle and Future Health: Evidence from the Alameda County Study." *Preventive Medicine* 9:1-21, 1980.
22. Williams, M. H. *Lifetime Physical Fitness: A Personal Choice.* Dubuque, IA: Wm. C. Brown, 1985.

Figure 1.7. *Health History Questionnaire*[a]

1. Have you ever or now have any of the following conditions:

A.	Elevated blood pressure	___Yes	___No
B.	Elevated blood lipids (cholesterol and triglycerides)	___Yes	___No
C.	Chest pain at rest or during exertion	___Yes	___No
D.	Uneven, irregular, or skipped heartbeats	___Yes	___No
E.	A racing or fluttering heart	___Yes	___No
F.	An abnormal resting or stress electrocardiogram	___Yes	___No
G.	Coronary artery disease	___Yes	___No
H.	A myocardial infarction (heart attack)	___Yes	___No
I.	A blood embolism	___Yes	___No
J.	Thrombophlebitis	___Yes	___No
K.	Rheumatic fever	___Yes	___No
L.	Congestive heart failure	___Yes	___No
M.	Diabetes	___Yes	___No
N.	Smoke cigarettes	___Yes	___No
O.	Family history of coronary artery disease, syncope, or sudden death before age sixty	___Yes	___No
P.	Any other heart problem that makes exercise unsafe	___Yes	___No

2. Do you suffer from any of the following conditions:

A.	Arthritis, rheumatism, or gout	___Yes	___No
B.	Chronic low back pain	___Yes	___No
C.	Any other joint, bone, or muscle problem	___Yes	___No
D.	Any respiratory problems	___Yes	___No
E.	Obesity (more than 30 percent overweight)	___Yes	___No
F.	Any physical disability that could interfere with safe exercise participation	___Yes	___No

3.	Are you taking any prescription drug?	___Yes	___No
4.	Are you thirty-five years or older?	___Yes	___No
5.	Do you have any other concern regarding your ability to safely participate in an exercise program?	___Yes	___No

[a] If your answer to any of the above is positive, consult your physician before you initiate an exercise program.

Student's Signature: ______________________________ Date: ______________

CHAPTER TWO

Cardiovascular Endurance Assessment and Prescription Techniques

Cardiovascular endurance has been defined as the ability of the heart, lungs, and blood vessels to deliver adequate amounts of oxygen and nutrients to the cells to meet the demands of prolonged physical activity. As a person breathes, part of the oxygen contained in ambient air is taken up in the lungs and transported in the blood to the heart. The heart is then responsible to pump the oxygenated blood to all organs and tissues of the body. At the cellular level, oxygen is used to convert food substrates, primarily carbohydrates and fats, into energy necessary to conduct body functions and maintain a constant internal equilibrium.

During physical exertion, a greater amount of energy is needed to carry out the work. As a result, the heart, lungs, and blood vessels have to deliver more oxygen to the tissues in order to supply the required energy to accomplish the task. During prolonged physical activity, an individual with a high level of cardiovascular endurance is able to deliver the required amounts of oxygen to the tissues with relative ease. The cardiovascular system of a person with a low level of endurance has to work much harder. The heart has to pump more often to supply the same amount of oxygen to the tissues and therefore will fatigue faster. Hence, a higher capacity to deliver oxygen indicates a more efficient cardiovascular system.

Cardiovascular endurance activities are also frequently referred to as "aerobic" exercises. The word "aerobic" means "with oxygen." Hence, whenever an activity is carried out where oxygen is utilized to produce energy, it is considered an aerobic exercise. Examples of cardiovascular or aerobic exercises are walking, jogging, swimming, cycling, cross-country skiing, rope skipping, aerobic dancing, etc. On the other hand, "anaerobic" activities are carried out "without oxygen." The intensity of anaerobic exercise is so high that oxygen is not utilized to produce energy. Since energy production is very limited in the absence of oxygen, these activities can only be carried out for short periods of time. The higher the intensity, the shorter the duration. Such activities as the 100, 200, and 400 meters in track and field, the 100 meters in swimming, gymnastics, routines, and weight training are good examples of anaerobic activities. Only aerobic activities will help increase cardiovascular endurance. Anaerobic activities will not significantly contribute toward the development of the cardiovascular system.

IMPORTANCE OF CARDIOVASCULAR ENDURANCE

A sound cardiovascular endurance program greatly contributes toward the enhancement and maintenance of good health. Although there are four components of physical fitness, cardiovascular endurance is the single most important factor. Certain amounts of muscular strength and flexibility are necessary in daily activities to lead a normal life. However, a person can get away without large amounts of strength and flexibility but cannot do without a good cardiovascular system. Aerobic exercise is especially important in the prevention of coronary artery disease. A poorly conditioned heart that has to pump more often just to keep a person alive is subject to more wear-and-tear than a well-conditioned heart. In situations where strenuous demands are placed on the heart, such as doing yardwork, lifting heavy objects or weights, or running to catch a train, the unconditioned heart may not be able to sustain the strain. Additionally, regular participation in cardiovascular endurance activities helps you achieve and maintain ideal body weight, the fourth component of physical fitness.

BENEFITS OF CARDIOVASCULAR ENDURANCE TRAINING

Every individual who initiates a cardiovascular or aerobic exercise program can expect several physiological changes as a result of training. Some of these benefits are:

1. A decrease in resting heart rate and an increase in cardiac muscle strength. During resting conditions, the heart ejects between five and six quarts of blood per minute. This amount of blood is sufficient to meet the energy demands in the resting state. As any other muscle, the heart responds to training by increasing in strength and size. As the heart gets stronger, the muscle can produce a more forceful contraction that causes a greater ejection of blood with each beat (stroke volume), yielding a decreased heart rate. This reduction in heart rate also allows the heart to rest longer between beats.

   Resting heart rates are frequently decreased by ten to twenty beats per minute (bpm) after only six to eight weeks of training. A reduction of twenty bpm would save the heart about 10,483,200 beats per year. The average heart beats between seventy and eighty bpm. However, in highly trained athletes, resting heart rates are commonly found around 40 bpm.

2. A lower heart rate at given work loads. When compared with untrained individuals, a trained person has a lower heart-rate response to a given task. This is due to the increased efficiency of the cardiovascular system. Individuals are also surprised to find that following several weeks of training, a given work load (let's say a ten-minute mile) elicits a much lower heart rate as compared to the initial response when training first started.

3. A decrease in recovery time. Trained individuals enjoy a quicker recovery to resting values following an exercise bout. A fit system is able to restore at a greater speed any internal equilibrium that was disrupted during exercise.

4. An increase in the number and size of the mitochondria. All energy necessary for cell function is produced in the mitochondria. As the size and number increase, so does the potential to produce energy for muscular work.

5. An increase in the number of functional capillaries. These smaller vessels allow for the exchange of oxygen and carbon dioxide between the blood and the cells. As more vessels open up, a greater amount of gas exchange can take place, therefore decreasing the onset of fatigue during prolonged exercise. This increase in capillaries also speeds up the rate at which waste products of cell metabolism can be removed. Increased capillarization is also seen in the heart, which enhances the oxygen delivery capacity to the heart muscle itself.

6. An increase in the functional capacity of the lungs. This is reflected through a decrease in air flow resistance to and from the lungs, an increase in the amount of air that can be inspired in a single maximal ventilation, and an increase in the diffusing capacity of the lungs, which facilitates the exchange of oxygen and carbon dioxide.

7. An increase in the oxygen-carrying capacity of the blood. As a result of training, there is an increase in the red blood cell count, which contains hemoglobin that is responsible for transporting oxygen in the blood.

8. A higher oxygen uptake. The amount of oxygen that the body is able to utilize during physical activity is significantly increased. This allows the individual to exercise longer and at a higher rate before becoming fatigued.

9. A decrease in blood lipids. A regular aerobic exercise program will cause a reduction in blood fats such as cholesterol and triglycerides, both of which have been linked to the formation of the atherosclerotic plaque that obstructs the arteries. This reduction decreases the risk of cardiovascular disease.

CARDIOVASCULAR ENDURANCE ASSESSMENT

Cardiovascular endurance, cardiovascular fitness, or aerobic capacity is best determined by the maximal amount of oxygen that the human body is able to utilize per minute of physical activity. This value is commonly expressed in liters per minute (L/min) and milliliters per kilogram per minute (ml/kg/min). The latter is most frequently used because it takes into consideration total body mass (weight). When comparing two people with the same absolute value, the individual with the smaller body mass will have a higher relative value, indicating that a greater amount of oxygen is available to each kilogram (2.2 pounds) of body weight.

The most precise way to determine maximal oxygen uptake is through direct gas analysis. This is frequently done by using a metabolic cart through which the amount of oxygen consumption can be directly established. However, this technique is very sophisticated, and the test requires very costly equipment and technical expertise. As a result, several simple techniques have been developed that will accurately estimate maximal oxygen uptake and only require limited equipment.

CARDIOVASCULAR FITNESS TESTS

In this chapter three common techniques used in assessing cardiovascular fitness will be explained. You will need to select only one of these three tests to determine your current cardiovascular fitness level.

While most healthy individuals are able to perform any of these tests, before you choose one of them, read the following introduction and possible contraindications to each test. Make sure that you have carefully filled out the questionnaire in Figure 1.7 in Chapter 1. If medical clearance is necessary, check with a physician before you take any of the tests. Your choice of test should also be based on the physical facilities and equipment available to you. After selecting a test, you may go directly to the description of the test procedures and prepare to take your test. You also need to keep in mind that these are three different testing protocols and that each test will not necessarily yield the same results. Therefore, you should always use the same test when conducting pre- and post-assessments in order to make valid comparisons.

1. **The 1.5-mile run test.** This test is most frequently used to predict cardiovascular fitness according to the time it takes to run/walk a 1.5-mile course. Maximal oxygen uptake can then be predicted based on the time it takes to cover the distance.

   The only equipment necessary to conduct this test is a stopwatch and a track or premeasured 1.5-mile course. It is perhaps the easiest test to administer, but caution should be taken when conducting the test. Since the objective of the test is to cover the distance in the shortest period of time, it is considered to be a maximal exercise test. The use of this test should be limited to conditioned individuals who have been cleared for exercise. It is contraindicated for unconditioned beginners (you should have at least six weeks of aerobic training), symptomatic individuals, and those with known cardiovascular disease and/or heart disease risk factors.

2. **The step test.** A step test requires little time and equipment and can be administered to most everyone, since submaximal work loads are used to assess cardiovascular fitness. The

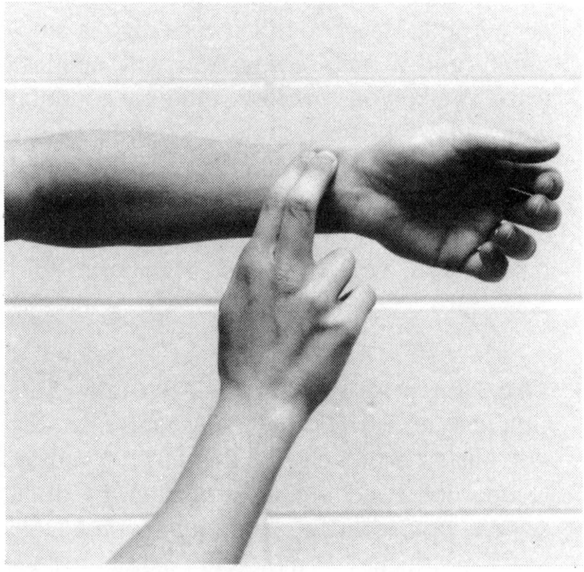

Figure 2.1. *Pulse taken at the radial artery.*

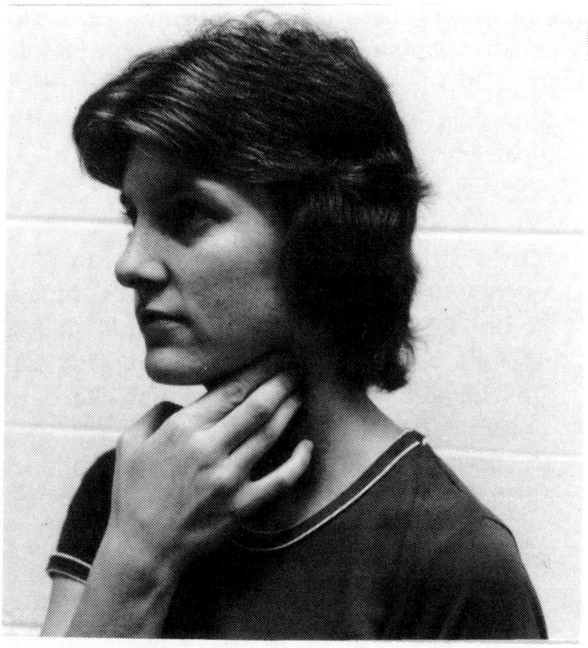

Figure 2.2. *Pulse taken at the carotid artery.*

submaximal work load and little time to administer. Since the person does not have to support his/her own body weight during the test, it becomes especially useful in testing overweight individuals and those with joint problems in the lower extremities.

The bicycle ergometer to be used on this test should allow for the regulation of work loads (see test procedures for the Astrand-Rhyming test). Besides the bicycle ergometer, a stopwatch and an additional technician are needed to perform the test. The duration of the test is six minutes, and the heart rate is taken every minute. At the end of the test, the heart rate should be between 120 and 170 bpm. Good judgment is essential when administering the test to older people. Low work loads should be used, because if the higher heart rates are reached (150 to 170 bpm), these individuals are probably working near or at their maximal capacity, making it an unsafe test to perform without adequate medical clearance and/or supervision.

only exceptions are significantly overweight individuals and those with joint problems in the lower extremities. With this test, recovery heart rates are used to estimate maximal oxygen uptake through the use of predicting equations.

The actual step test only takes three minutes. A fifteen-second recovery heart rate is taken between five and twenty seconds following the test. The equipment required is a bench or gymnasium bleacher 16¼ inches high, a stopwatch, and a metronome. You will need to learn to take your own heart rate by counting your pulse. This can be done on the wrist by placing two or three fingers over the radial artery (on the side of the thumb) or over the carotid artery in the neck just below the jaw next to your voice box (See Figures 2.1 and 2.2).

3. **The Astrand-Rhyming test.** Because of its simplicity and practicality, the Astrand-Rhyming test has become one of the most common techniques used when estimating maximal oxygen uptake in the laboratory setting. The test is conducted on a bicycle ergometer, and, similar to the step test, it only requires a

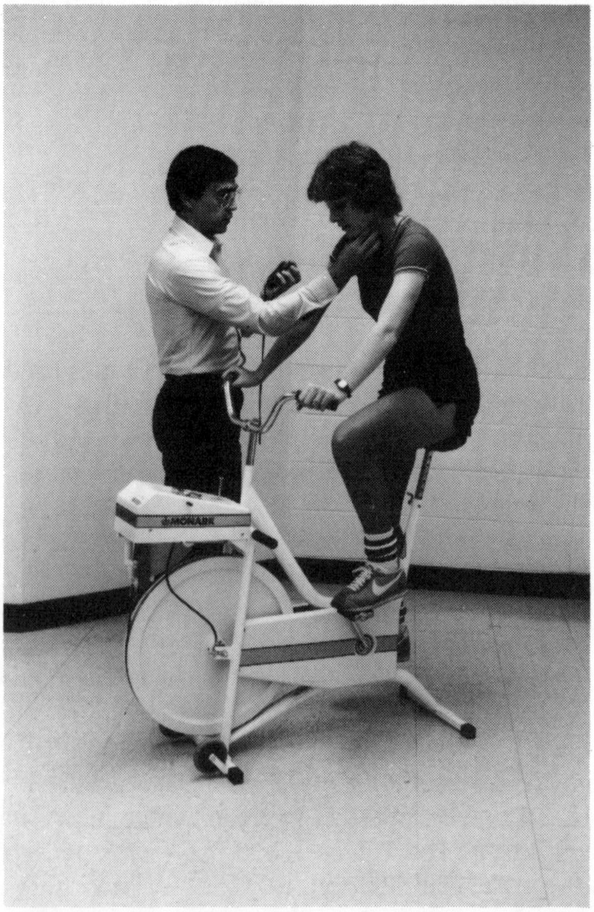

Figure 2.3. *Monitoring heart rate on the carotid artery during the Astrand-Rhyming test.*

Figure 2.4. *Procedures for The 1.5-Mile Run Test to Assess Maximal Oxygen Uptake.*

1. Make sure that you qualify for this test. This test is contraindicated for unconditioned beginners, individuals with symptoms of heart disease, and those with known heart disease and/or risk factors.
2. Select the testing site. Find a school track (each lap is one-fourth of a mile) or a premeasured 1.5-mile course.
3. Have a stopwatch available to determine your time.
4. Conduct a few warm-up exercises prior to the test. Do some stretching exercises, some walking, and slow jogging.
5. Initiate the test and try to cover the distance in the fastest time possible (walking or jogging). Time yourself during the run to see how fast you have covered the distance. If any unusual symptoms arise during the test, do not continue. Stop immediately and retake the test after another six weeks of aerobic training.
6. At the end of the test, cool down by walking or jogging slowly for another three to five minutes. Do not sit or lie down after the test.
7. According to your performance time, look up your estimated maximal oxygen uptake in Table 2.1.
8. Example. A twenty-year-old female runs the 1.5-mile course in twelve minutes and forty seconds. Table 2.1 shows a maximal oxygen uptake on 39.8 ml/kg/min for a time of 12:40. According to Table 2.6, this maximal oxygen uptake would place her in the good cardiovascular fitness category.
9. Use the following form to record your own test results (extra spaces are provided for future tests):

Name: ______________________________

A. Date: ________ ________ ________ ________

B. Time: ________ ________ ________ ________

C. Max. VO_2: ________ ________ ________ ________

Table 2.1.
Estimated Maximal Oxygen Uptake (Max VO_2) in ml/kg/min for the 1.5-Mile Run Test

Time	Max VO_2	Time	Max VO_2	Time	Max VO_2	Time	Max VO_2	Time	Max VO_2
6:10	80.0	8:50	59.1	11:30	44.4	14:10	35.5	16:50	29.1
6:20	79.0	9:00	58.1	11:40	43.7	14:20	35.1	17:00	28.9
6:30	77.9	9:10	56.9	11:50	43.2	14:30	34.7	17:10	28.5
6:40	76.7	9:20	55.9	12:00	42.3	14:40	34.3	17:20	28.3
6:50	75.5	9:30	54.7	12:10	41.7	14:50	34.0	17:30	28.0
7:00	74.0	9:40	53.5	12:20	41.0	15:00	33.6	17:40	27.7
7:10	72.6	9:50	52.3	12:30	40.4	15:10	33.1	17:50	27.4
7:20	71.3	10:00	51.1	12:40	39.8	15:20	32.7	18:00	27.1
7:30	69.9	10:10	50.4	12:50	39.2	15:30	32.2	18:10	26.8
7:40	68.3	10:20	49.5	13:00	38.6	15:40	31.8	18:20	26.6
7:50	66.8	10:30	48.6	13:10	38.1	15:50	31.4	18:30	26.3
8:00	65.2	10:40	48.0	13:20	37.8	16:00	30.9	18:40	26.0
8:10	63.9	10:50	47.4	13:30	37.2	16:10	30.5	18:50	25.7
8:20	62.5	11:00	46.6	13:40	36.8	16:20	30.2	19:00	25.4
8:30	61.2	11:10	45.8	13:50	36.3	16:30	29.8		
8:40	60.2	11:20	45.1	14:00	35.9	16:40	29.5		

Adapted from: Cooper, K. H. "A Means of Assessing Maximal Oxygen Intake." *JAMA* 203:201-204, 1968. Pollock, M. L., et al. *Health and Fitness Through Physical Activity.* New York: John Wiley and Sons, 1978. Wilmore, J. H. *Training for Sport and Activity.* Boston: Allyn and Bacon, Inc., 1982.

Figure 2.5. *Procedures for the Step Test. A Submaximal Cardiovascular Endurance Test to Assess Maximal Oxygen Uptake.*

1. The test is conducted with a bench or gymnasium bleachers 16¼ inches high.
2. The stepping cycle is performed to a four-step cadence (up-up-down-down). Men should perform twenty-four complete step-ups per minute, regulated with a metronome set at ninety-six beats per minute. Women perform twenty-two step-ups per minute, or eighty-eight beats per minute on the metronome.
3. Allow a brief practice period of five to ten seconds to familiarize yourself with the stepping cadence.
4. Begin the test and perform the step-ups for exactly three minutes.
5. Upon completion of the three minutes, remain standing and take your heart rate for a fifteen-second interval from five to twenty seconds into recovery. Convert recovery heart rate to beats per minute (multiply fifteen-second heart rate by four).
6. Maximal oxygen uptake in ml/kg/min is estimated according to the following equations:
   Men: maximal oxygen uptake = 111.33 – (0.42 × recovery heart rate in bpm)
   Women: maximal oxygen uptake = 65.81 – (0.1847 × recovery heart rate in bpm)
7. Example. The recovery fifteen-second heart rate for a male subject following the three-minute step test is found to be thirty-nine beats. Maximal oxygen uptake is estimated as follows:
   Fifteen-second heart rate = 39 beats
   Minute heart rate = 39 × 4 = 156 bpm
   Maximal oxygen uptake = 111.33 – (0.42 × 156) = 45.81 ml/kg/min
8. Maximal oxygen uptake can also be obtained according to recovery heart rates in Table 2.2.
9. To record your own test results, use the following form (additional spaces are provided for future tests):

   Name: ______________________ Sex: __________

   A. Date: ________ ________ ________ ________

   B. Heart Rate (bpm): ________ ________ ________ ________

   C. Max. VO_2: ________ ________ ________ ________

From McArdle, W. D., et el. *Exercise Physiology: Energy, Nutrition, and Human Performance.* Philadelphia: Lea & Febiger, 1981.

Table 2.2.
Predicted Maximal Oxygen Uptake (Max VO_2) for the Three-Minute Step Test in ml/kg/min.

15-Sec HR	HR-bpm	Max VO_2 Men	Max VO_2 Women
30	120	60.9	43.6
31	124	59.3	42.9
32	128	57.6	42.2
33	132	55.9	41.4
34	136	54.2	40.7
35	140	52.5	40.0
36	144	50.9	39.2
37	148	49.2	38.5
38	152	47.5	37.7
39	156	45.8	37.0
40	160	44.1	36.3
41	164	42.5	35.5
42	168	40.8	34.8
43	172	39.1	34.0
44	176	37.4	33.3
45	180	35.7	32.6
46	184	34.1	31.8
47	188	32.4	31.1
48	192	30.7	30.3
49	196	29.0	29.6
50	200	27.3	28.9

Figure 2.6. *Procedures for the Astrand-Rhyming Test. A Submaximal Cardiovascular Endurance Test to Estimate Maximal Oxygen Uptake.*

1. Adjust the bike seat so that the knees are almost completely extended as the foot goes through the bottom of the pedaling cycle.
2. During the test, the speed should be kept constant at fifty revolutions per minute. Test duration is six mintues.
3. Select the appropriate work load for the bike based on age, health, and estimated fitness level. For unconditioned individuals: women, use 300 kpm (kilopounds per meter) or 450 kpm; men, 300 kpm or 600 kpm. Conditioned adults: women, 450 kpm or 600 kpm; men, 600 kpm or 900 kpm.[a]
4. Ride the bike for six minutes and check the heart rate every minute, during the last ten seconds of each minute. Heart rate should be determined by recording the time it takes to count thirty pulse beats, and then coverting to beats per minute using Table 2.3.
5. Average the final two heart rates (fifth and sixth minutes). If these two heart rates are not within five beats per minute of each other, continue the test for another few minutes until this is accomplished. If the heart rate continues to climb significantly after the sixth minute, stop the test and rest for fifteen to twenty minutes. You may then retest, preferably at a lower work load. The final average heart rate should also fall between the ranges given for each work load in Table 2.4 (e.g., men: 300 kpm = 120 to 140 beats per minute; 600 kpm = 120 to 170 beats per minute).
6. Based on the average heart rate of the final two minutes and your work load, look up the maximal oxygen uptake in Table 2.4 (e.g., men: 600 kpm and average heart rate = 145, maximal oxygen uptake = 2.4 liters/minute).
7. Correct maximal oxygen uptake using the correction factors found in Table 2.5 (e.g., maximal oxygen uptake = 2.4 and age thirty-five, correction factor = .870. Multiply 2.4 × .870 and final corrected maximal oxygen uptake = 2.09 liters/minute).
8. To obtain maximal oxygen uptake in ml/kg/min, multiply the maximal oxygen uptake by 1,000 (to convert liters to milliliters) and divide by body weight in kilograms (to obtain kilograms, multiply your body weight in pounds by .454).
9. Example: Corrected maximal oxygen uptake = 2.09 liters/minute
   Body weight = 132 pounds or 60 kilograms (132 × .454 = 60)

   Maximal oxygen uptake in ml/kg/min = 2.09 × 1,000 = 2,090
   2,090 divided by 60 = 34.8 ml/kg/min
10. To record your own test results, use the following form (extra spaces are provided for future tests):

Name: ______________________ Sex: __________

A. Date:	____	____	____	____
B. Weight in lbs.	____	____	____	____
C. Weight in kg. (B × .454)	____	____	____	____
D. Work load (kpm)	____	____	____	____
E. Fifth min. HR (bpm)	____	____	____	____
F. Sixth min. HR (bpm)	____	____	____	____
G. Avg. HR (E and F)	____	____	____	____
H. Max. VO_2 in L/min (Table 2.4)	____	____	____	____
I. Corr. factor (Table 2.5)	____	____	____	____
J. Corrected Max. VO_2 (H × I)	____	____	____	____
K. Max. VO_2 in ml/kg/min (J × 1000, divided by C)	____	____	____	____

[a]On the Monarch bicycle ergometer when riding at a speed of fifty revolutions per minute, a load of 1 kp = 300 kpm, 1.5 kp = 450, 2 kp = 600 kpm, and so forth, with increases of 150 kpm to each ½ kp.

Table 2.3.
Conversion of the Time for 30 Pulse Beats to Pulse Rate Per Minute

Sec.	bpm	Sec.	bpm	Sec.	bpm
22.0	82	17.3	104	12.6	143
21.9	82	17.2	105	12.5	144
21.8	83	17.1	105	12.4	145
21.7	83	17.0	106	12.3	146
21.6	83	16.9	107	12.2	148
21.5	84	16.8	107	12.1	149
21.4	84	16.7	108	12.0	150
21.3	85	16.6	108	11.9	151
21.2	85	16.5	109	11.8	153
21.1	85	16.4	110	11.7	154
21.0	86	16.3	110	11.6	155
20.9	86	16.2	111	11.5	157
20.8	87	16.1	112	11.4	158
20.7	87	16.0	113	11.3	159
20.6	87	15.9	113	11.2	161
20.5	88	15.8	114	11.1	162
20.4	88	15.7	115	11.0	164
20.3	89	15.6	115	10.9	165
20.2	89	15.5	116	10.8	167
20.1	90	15.4	117	10.7	168
20.0	90	15.3	118	10.6	170
19.9	90	15.2	118	10.5	171
19.8	91	15.1	119	10.4	173
19.7	91	15.0	120	10.3	175
19.6	92	14.9	121	10.2	176
19.5	92	14.8	122	10.1	178
19.4	93	14.7	122	10.0	180
19.3	93	14.6	123	9.9	182
19.2	94	14.5	124	9.8	184
19.1	94	14.4	125	9.7	186
19.0	95	14.3	126	9.6	188
18.9	95	14.2	127	9.5	189
18.8	96	14.1	128	9.4	191
18.7	96	14.0	129	9.3	194
18.6	97	13.9	129	9.2	196
18.5	97	13.8	130	9.1	198
18.4	98	13.7	131	9.0	200
18.3	98	13.6	132	8.9	202
18.2	99	13.5	133	8.8	205
18.1	99	13.4	134	8.7	207
18.0	100	13.3	135	8.6	209
17.9	101	13.2	136	8.5	212
17.8	101	13.1	137	8.4	214
17.7	102	13.0	138	8.3	217
17.6	102	12.9	140	8.2	220
17.5	103	12.8	141	8.1	222
17.4	103	12.7	142	8.0	225

Table 2.4.
Maximal Oxygen Uptake Estimates in Liters/Minute

	Work Load (kpm/min)									
	Men					Women				
Heart Rate	**300**	**600**	**900**	**1200**	**1500**	**300**	**450**	**600**	**750**	**900**
120	2.2	3.4	4.8			2.6	3.4	4.1	4.8	
121	2.2	3.4	4.7			2.5	3.3	4.0	4.8	
122	2.2	3.4	4.6			2.5	3.2	3.9	4.7	
123	2.1	3.4	4.6			2.4	3.1	3.9	4.6	
124	2.1	3.3	4.5	6.0		2.4	3.1	3.8	4.5	
125	2.0	3.2	4.4	5.9		2.3	3.0	3.7	4.4	
126	2.0	3.2	4.4	5.8		2.3	3.0	3.6	4.3	
127	2.0	3.1	4.3	5.7		2.2	2.9	3.5	4.2	
128	2.0	3.1	4.2	5.6		2.2	2.8	3.5	4.2	4.8
129	1.9	3.0	4.2	5.6		2.2	2.8	3.4	4.1	4.8
130	1.9	3.0	4.1	5.5		2.1	2.7	3.4	4.0	4.7
131	1.9	2.9	4.0	5.4		2.1	2.7	3.4	4.0	4.6
132	1.8	2.9	4.0	5.3		2.0	2.7	3.3	3.9	4.5
133	1.8	2.8	3.9	5.3		2.0	2.6	3.2	3.8	4.4
134	1.8	2.8	3.9	5.2		2.0	2.6	3.2	3.8	4.4
135	1.7	2.8	3.8	5.1		2.0	2.6	3.1	3.7	4.3
136	1.7	2.7	3.8	5.0		1.9	2.5	3.1	3.6	4.2
137	1.7	2.7	3.7	5.0		1.9	2.5	3.0	3.6	4.2
138	1.6	2.7	3.7	4.9		1.8	2.4	3.0	3.5	4.1
139	1.6	2.6	3.6	4.8		1.8	2.4	2.9	3.5	4.0
140	1.6	2.6	3.6	4.8	6.0	1.8	2.4	2.8	3.4	4.0
141		2.6	3.5	4.7	5.9	1.8	2.3	2.8	3.4	3.9
142		2.5	3.5	4.6	5.8	1.7	2.3	2.8	3.3	3.9
143		2.5	3.4	4.6	5.7	1.7	2.2	2.7	3.3	3.8
144		2.5	3.4	4.5	5.7	1.7	2.2	2.7	3.2	3.8
145		2.4	3.4	4.5	5.6	1.6	2.2	2.7	3.2	3.7
146		2.4	3.3	4.4	5.6	1.6	2.2	2.6	3.2	3.7
147		2.4	3.3	4.4	5.5	1.6	2.1	2.6	3.1	3.6
148		2.4	3.2	4.3	5.4	1.6	2.1	2.6	3.1	3.6
149		2.3	3.2	4.3	5.4		2.1	2.6	3.0	3.5
150		2.3	3.2	4.2	5.3		2.0	2.5	3.0	3.5
151		2.3	3.1	4.2	5.2		2.0	2.5	3.0	3.4
152		2.3	3.1	4.1	5.2		2.0	2.5	2.9	3.4
153		2.2	3.0	4.1	5.1		2.0	2.4	2.9	3.3
154		2.2	3.0	4.0	5.1		2.0	2.4	2.8	3.3
155		2.2	3.0	4.0	5.0		1.9	2.4	2.8	3.2
156		2.2	2.9	4.0	5.0		1.9	2.3	2.8	3.2
157		2.1	2.9	3.9	4.9		1.9	2.3	2.7	3.2
158		2.1	2.9	3.9	4.9		1.8	2.3	2.7	3.1
159		2.1	2.8	3.8	4.8		1.8	2.2	2.7	3.1
160		2.1	2.8	3.8	4.8		1.8	2.2	2.6	3.0
161		2.0	2.8	3.7	4.7		1.8	2.2	2.6	3.0
162		2.0	2.8	3.7	4.6		1.8	2.2	2.6	3.0
163		2.0	2.8	3.7	4.6		1.7	2.2	2.6	2.9
164		2.0	2.7	3.6	4.5		1.7	2.1	2.5	2.9
165		2.0	2.7	3.6	4.5		1.7	2.1	2.5	2.9
166		1.9	2.7	3.6	4.5		1.7	2.1	2.5	2.8
167		1.9	2.6	3.5	4.4		1.6	2.1	2.4	2.8
168		1.9	2.6	3.5	4.4		1.6	2.0	2.4	2.8
169		1.9	2.6	3.5	4.3		1.6	2.0	2.4	2.8
170		1.8	2.6	3.4	4.3		1.6	2.0	2.4	2.7

From Astrand, I. *Acta Physiologica Scandinavica* 49(1960). Supplementum 169:45-60.

Table 2.5.
Age-Based Correction Factors for Maximal Oxygen Uptake

Age	Correction Factor	Age	Correction Factor
14	1.11	40	.830
15	1.10	41	.820
16	1.09	42	.810
17	1.08	43	.800
18	1.07	44	.790
19	1.06	45	.780
20	1.05	46	.774
21	1.04	47	.768
22	1.03	48	.762
23	1.02	49	.756
24	1.01	50	.750
25	1.00	51	.742
26	.987	52	.734
27	.974	53	.726
28	.961	54	.718
29	.948	55	.710
30	.935	56	.704
31	.922	57	.698
32	.909	58	.692
33	.896	59	.686
34	.883	60	.680
35	.870	61	.674
36	.862	62	.668
37	.854	63	.662
38	.846	64	.656
39	.838	65	.650

Adapted from Astrand, I. *Acta Physiologica Scandinavica* 49 (1960). Supplementum 169:45-60.

INTERPRETING YOUR MAXIMAL OXYGEN UPTAKE RESULTS

After obtaining your maximal oxygen uptake by taking any of the three cardiovascular endurance tests, you can determine your current level of cardiovascular fitness in Table 2.6. Locate the maximal oxygen uptake in your respective age category, and on the top row you will find your present level of cardiovascular fitness. For example, a nineteen-year-old male with a maximal oxygen uptake of 41 ml/kg/min would be classified in the average cardiovascular fitness category. Once you have established your maximal oxygen uptake and cardiovascular fitness category, record this information in Figure 2.7 in this chapter and Figure A.1 in Appendix A. After you initiate your personal exercise program, you may wish to retake the test periodically to evaluate your progress.

BASIC PRINCIPLES OF CARDIOVASCULAR EXERCISE PRESCRIPTION

All too often there are individuals who are exercising, but when they take a cardiovascular endurance test, they are surprised to find that they may not be as conditioned as they thought they

Table 2.6.
Cardiovascular Fitness Classification according to Maximal Oxygen Uptake in ml/kg/min

		Fitness Classification				
Sex	Age	Poor	Fair	Average	Good	Excellent
Men	<29	<25	25-33	34-42	43-52	53+
	30-39	<23	23-30	31-38	39-48	49+
	40-49	<20	20-26	27-35	36-44	45+
	50-59	<18	18-24	25-33	34-42	43+
	60-69	<16	16-22	23-30	31-40	41+
Women	<29	<24	24-30	31-37	38-48	49+
	30-39	<20	20-27	28-33	34-44	45+
	40-49	<17	17-23	24-30	31-41	42+
	50-59	<15	15-20	21-27	28-37	38+
	60-69	<13	13-17	18-23	24-34	35+

Reproduced with permission. *Exercise Testing and Training of Apparently Healthy Individuals: A Handbook for Physicians.* American Heart Association.

Figure 2.7. *Cardiovascular Endurance Report*

Name: ______________________ Age: __________ Sex: __________

Date	Test Used	Max VO_2	Fitness Classification

were. Although these individuals may be exercising regularly, they most likely are not following the basic principles for cardiovascular exercise prescription; therefore, they do not reap significant benefits.

For a person to develop the cardiovascular system, the heart muscle has to be overloaded like any other muscle in the human body. Just as the biceps muscle in the upper arm is developed by doing weight-lifting exercises, the heart muscle also has to be exercised to increase in size, strength, and efficiency. In order to better understand how the cardiovascular system can be developed, four basic principles that govern this development must be discussed. These principles are intensity, mode, duration, and frequency of exercise.

Intensity of Exercise

The intensity of exercise is perhaps the most commonly ignored factor when trying to develop the cardiovascular system. This principle refers to how hard a person has to exercise to improve cardiovascular fitness. Muscles have to be overloaded to a given point for them to develop. While the training stimuli to develop the biceps muscle can be accomplished with simple curl-up exercises, the stimuli for the cardiovascular system is provided by making the heart pump at a higher rate for a certain period of time. Research has shown that cardiovascular development occurs when working at about 60 to 90 percent of the heart's reserve capacity. Many experts, however, prefer to prescribe exercise between 70 and 85 percent of this capacity. This is done to insure better and faster development (70 percent) and for safety reasons (85 percent), so that unconditioned individuals will not work too close to maximum capacity. The 70 and 85 percentages can be easily calculated and training can be monitored by checking your pulse. To determine your own intensity for exercise, follow the next few steps.

1. Check your resting heart rate (RHR) sometime after you have been sitting quietly for fifteen to twenty minutes. You can take your pulse for thirty seconds and multiply by two or take it for a full minute.

   Write down your own RHR:

   ____ beats per minute (bpm)

2. Estimate your maximal heart rate (MHR). This heart rate is almost entirely dependent on your age. The formula to estimate MHR for women is 220 minus age (220-age) and for men, 205 minus one half the age (205-½ age).

   Your estimated MHR: ____ - ____ = ____ bpm

3. Determine your heart rate reserve (HRR). This is done by taking your maximal heart rate and subtracting the resting heart rate from it (HRR = MHR - RHR). Your heart rate reserve indicates the amount of beats that your heart has available to go from resting conditions to an all-out maximal effort.

   Your HRR: ____ - ____ = ____ beats

4. Compute your own work intensity (WI) by multiplying your heart rate reserve by 70 percent and 85 percent (HBR x .70 and HRR x .85). Using both percentages will allow you to stay within the optimal range during exercise.

   70% WI: ____ x .70 = ____ beats

   85% WI: ____ x .85 = ____ beats

5. Determine your cardiovascular training zone (CTZ). Your training zone is computed by adding your resting heart rate to the 70 and 85 percent work intensities (RHR + .70WI and RHR + .85WI). This will give you your target heart rates (THR) at 70 and 85 percent of maximum. Your CTZ is then found between these two target heart rates.

   70% THR: ____ (.70WI) + ____ (RHR) = ____ bpm

   85% THR: ____ (.85WI) + ____ (RHR) = ____ bpm

   Cardiovascular training zone: ____to____bpm

6. Example. The cardiovascular training zone for a twenty-four-year-old male with a resting heart rate of seventy-two bpm would be:

   MHR: 205 – 24/2 = 193 bpm
   HRR: 193 – 72 = 121 beats
   70% WI: 121 x .70 = 85 beats
   85% WI: 121 x .85 = 103 beats
   70% THR: 85 + 72 = 157 bpm
   85% THR: 103 + 72 = 175 bpm

   Cardiovascular training zone: 157 to 175 bpm

The target training zone indicates that whenever you exercise to improve the cardiovascular system, you have to maintain your heart rate between those two target rates to obtain adequate development. After a few weeks of training, you may experience a significant reduction in resting heart rate; therefore, you should recompute your target zone periodically. Once you have reached an ideal level of cardiovascular endurance, training in that same zone will allow you to maintain your fitness level.

Exercise heart rate should be monitored regularly during exercise to make sure that you are training in the respective zone. Wait until you are about five minutes into your exercise session before taking your first rate. When you check the heart rate, count your pulse for ten seconds and then multiply by six to get the per-minute pulse rate. Exercise heart rate will remain at the same level for about fifteen seconds following exercise. After fifteen seconds, heart rate will drop rapidly. Do not hesitate to stop during your exercise bout to check your pulse. If the rate is too low, increase the intensity of the exercise. If the rate is too high, slow down. To develop the cardiovascular system, you do not have to exercise above the 85 percent rate. From a health standpoint, training above this number will not add any extra benefits, but may actually be unsafe for some individuals. For unconditioned adults, it is recommended that cardiovascular training be conducted around the 70 percent rate. This lower rate is recommended to reduce potential problems associated with high-intensity exercise.

Rate of Perceived Exertion

Since many people do not check their heart rate during exercise, an alternate method of prescribing intensity of exercise has become more popular in recent years. This method uses a rate of perceived exertion (RPE) scale developed by Gunnar Borg. Using the scale shown in Figure 2.8, a person subjectively rates the perceived exertion or difficulty of exercise when training in the appropriate target zone. The exercise heart rate is then associated with the corresponding RPE value. For example, if the training intensity requires a heart rate zone between 150 and 170 bpm, the person would associate this with training between hard and very hard. However, some individuals may perceive less exertion than others when training in the correct zone. Therefore, associate your own inner perception of the task with the phrases given on the scale. You may then proceed to exercise at that rate of perceived exertion. It is important that you cross-check your target zone with your perceived exertion in the initial weeks of your exercise program. To help you develop this association, keep a regular record of your activities using the form provided in Figure 2.10. After several weeks of training, you should be able to predict your exercise heart rate just by your own perceived exertion of the exercise session.

Whether you monitor the intensity of exercise by checking your pulse or through rate of perceived exertion, be aware that changes in normal exercise conditions will affect the training zone. For example, exercising on a hot and/or humid day, or at altitude, increases the heart rate response to a given task. Consequently, make the necessary adjustments in the intensity of your exercise.

Figure 2.8. *Rate of Perceived Exertion Scale.*

6			
7	Very, very light	14	
8		15	Hard
9	Very light	16	
10		17	Very hard
11	Fairly light	18	
12		19	Very, very hard
13	Somewhat hard	20	

From Borg, G. "Perceived Exertion: A Note on History and Methods." Medicine and Science in Sports and Exercise 5:90-93, 1973.

Mode of Exercise

Earlier in the chapter, it was mentioned that the type of exercise that develops the cardiovascular system has to be aerobic in nature. Once you have established your target training zone, any activity or combination of activities that will get your heart rate up to that training zone and keep it there for as long as you exercise will yield adequate development. Examples of such activities are walking, jogging, aerobic dancing, swimming, cross-country skiing, rope skipping, cycling, racquetball, stair climbing, and stationary running or cycling.

The activity that you choose should be based on your personal preferences, what you enjoy doing best, and your physical limitations. There may be a difference in the amount of strength or flexibility developed through the use of different activities, but as far as the cardiovascular system is concerned, the heart doesn't know whether you are walking, swimming, or cycling. All the heart knows is that it has to pump at a certain rate, and as long as that rate is in the desired range, cardiovascular development will occur.

Duration of Exercise

According to the existing evidence regarding the duration of exercise, it is recommended that a person train between fifteen and sixty minutes per session. The duration is based on how intensely a person trains. If the training is done around 85 to 90 percent, fifteen to twenty minutes are sufficient. At the 60 to 70 percent intensity, the person should train for at least thirty minutes. As mentioned earlier, under intensity of training, unconditioned adults should train at the lower percentage; therefore, a minimum of thirty minutes of exercise is required.

As a part of the training session, always include a five-minute warm-up and a five-minute cool-down period. Your warm-up should consist of general calisthenics, stretching exercises, or exercising at a lower intensity level than the actual target zone. To cool down, gradually decrease the intensity of exercise. Do not stop abruptly. This will cause blood to pool in the exercised body parts, thereby diminishing the return of blood to the heart. A decreased blood return can cause dizziness, faintness, or even induce cardiac abnormalities.

Frequency of Exercise

Ideally, a person should engage in aerobic exercise four to five times per week. Research has indicated that to maintain cardiovascular fitness, a training session should be conducted about every forty-eight hours. As little as three training sessions per week, done on nonconsecutive days, will maintain cardiovascular endurance. For faster development in the initial stages, four to six times per week is recommended.

TIPS FOR GETTING STARTED AND ADHERING TO AN EXERCISE PROGRAM

Having learned the basic principles of cardiovasular exercise prescription, you can proceed to Figure 2.9 and fill out your own prescription. In this figure, a gradual program is used to improve your fitness level. While you could go ahead and attempt to train five or six times per week for thirty minutes at a time, if you have not been exercising regularly, you may find this discouraging and may drop out before getting too far. The reason for this is that as you initiate the program, you will probably develop some muscle soreness and stiffness, and possibly minor injuries. According to one report, more than 65 percent of those who begin an exercise program drop out in the initial six weeks due to injuries. Muscle soreness, stiffness, and the risk for injuries can be reduced or eliminated by progressively increasing the intensity, duration, and frequency of exercise as outlined in Figure 2.9.

Now that you have completed your exercise prescription, the difficult part begins: starting and sticking to a lifetime exercise program. Although you are probably motivated after reading the benefits derived through physical activity, it takes a lifetime of dedication and perseverance to reap and maintain good fitness. The first few weeks are probably the most difficult. However, "if there is a will, there is a way." Once you begin to see positive changes, it won't be as difficult. Very soon you will develop a habit for exercise that will bring about a deep satisfaction and sense of self-accomplishment. The following suggestions have been used successfully by others.

1. Select aerobic activities that you enjoy doing. Picking an activity that you don't enjoy decreases your chances for exercise adherence. Don't be afraid of trying out a new activity, even if that means learning new skills.
2. Use a combination of different activities. You can train by using two or three different activities the same week. For some people this decreases the monotony of repeating the same activity every day. Try lifetime sports. Many endurance sports such as racquetball, basketball, soccer, badminton, rollerskating, cross-country skiing, and surfing (paddling the board) provide a nice break from regular workouts.
3. Set aside a regular time for exercise. If you don't plan ahead, it is a lot easier to skip. Holding your exercise hour "sacred" helps you adhere to the program.
4. Obtain adequate equipment for exercise. A poor pair of shoes, for example, can increase the risk for injury, leading to discouragement right from the beginning.
5. Find a friend or group of friends to exercise with. The social interaction will make exercise more fulfilling. Besides, it's harder to skip if someone else is waiting for you.
6. Set goals and share them with others. It is tougher to quit when someone else knows what you are trying to accomplish. When you reach a particular goal, reward yourself with a new pair of shoes or a jogging suit.
7. Don't become a chronic exerciser. Learn to listen to your body. Overexercising can lead to chronic fatigue and injuries. Exercise should be enjoyable, and in the process you need to "stop and smell the roses."
8. Exercise in different places and facilities. This practice will add variety to your workouts.
9. Keep a regular record of your activities. In this manner, you will be able to monitor your progress and compare with previous months and years.
10. Conduct periodic assessments. Improving to a higher fitness category is a reward by itself.
11. See a physician when health problems arise. When in doubt, "it is better to be safe than sorry."

Remember that the benefits of fitness can only be maintained through a regular lifetime program. Exercise is not like putting money in the bank. It does not help to exercise four or five hours on Saturday, and not do anything else the rest of the week. If anything, exercising only once a week is unsafe for unconditioned adults. Even the greatest athlete on earth, if he stops exercising, after only a few years would be at a similar risk for disease as someone else who has never done any physical activity. Staying with a physical fitness program long enough will cause positive physiological and psychological changes, and once you are there, you will not want to have it any other way.

References

1. Allsen, P. E., J. M. Harrison, and B. Vance. *Fitness for Life: An Individualized Approach.* Dubuque, IA: Wm. C. Brown, 1984.
2. American Heart Association Committee on Exercise. *Exercise Testing and Training of Apparently Healthy Individuals: A Handbook for Physicians.* New York: American Heart Association, 1972.
3. Astrand, I. *Acta Physiologica Scandinavica* 49, 1960. Supplementum 169:45-60, 1960.
4. Astrand, P. O., and K. Rodahl. *Textbook of Work Physiology.* New York: McGraw-Hill, 1977.
5. Borg, G. Perceived Exertion: "A Note on History and Methods." *Medicine and Science in Sports and Exercise* 5:90-93, 1973.
6. Cooper, K. H. "A Means of Assessing Maximal Oxygen Intake." *JAMA* 203:201-204, 1968.
7. Cooper, K. H. *The Aerobics Program for Total Well Being.* New York: Mount Evans and Co., 1982.
8. Getchell, B. *Physical Fitness: A Way of Life.* New York: John Wiley & Sons, Inc., 1983.
9. Hoeger, W. W. K. *Ejercicio, Salud y Vida [Exercise, Health and Life].* Caracas, Venezuela: Editorial Arte, 1980.
10. Karvonen, M. J., E. Kentala, and O. Mustala. "The Effects of Training on the Heart Rate, a Longitudinal Study." *Annales Medicinae Experimentalis et Biologiae Fenniae* 35: 307-315, 1957.
11. McArdle, W. D., F. I. Katch, and V. L. Katch. *Exercise Physiology: Energy, Nutrition and Human Performance.* Philadelphia: Lea and Febiger, 1981.
12. Mirkin, G., and M. Shangold. "Getting Back in Shape." *Nation's Business* 71:36, 1983.
13. Pollock, M. L., J. H. Wilmore, and S. M. Fox III. *Health and Fitness Through Physical Activity.* New York: John Wiley & Sons, 1978.
14. Wilmore, J. H. *Training for Sport and Activity.* Boston: Allyn and Bacon, Inc., 1982.

Figure 2.9. *Personalized Cardiovascular Exercise Prescription*

1. Name: ______________________ 2. Age: ____ 3. Date: ________

4. Maximal Heart Rate: _____ bpm 5. Resting Heart Rate: _____ bpm

6. Current Fitness Classification: ______________________

7. Cardiovascular Training Zone: ____________ (70%) to ____________ (85%) bpm

8. Ten-Second Pulse Count (divide both rates under #7 by six):

____________ (70%) to ____________ (85%) beats

9. Rate of Perceived Exertion: ______________________

10. Mode of Exercise: ______________________

____

The following is your weekly program for cardiovascular fitness development. If you are in the average, good, or excellent category, you may start at week five. After completing this program, in order for you to maintain your fitness level, you should exercise in the desired training zone for about thirty minutes, a minimum of three times per week, on nonconsecutive days.

Week	Duration (min.)	Frequency	Training Intensity	10-Sec. Pulse Count[a]
1	15	3	Approximately 60%[b]	
2	15	4	Approximately 60%	
3	20	4	Approximately 60%	_____ beats
4	20	5	Approximately 60%	
5	20	4	About 70%	
6	20	5	About 70%	
7	30	4	About 70%	_____ beats
8	30	5	About 70%	
9	30	4	Between 70% and 85%	
10	30	5	Between 70% and 85%	
11	30-40	5	Between 70% and 85%	_____ to _____ beats
12	30-40	5-6	Between 70% and 85%	

[a] Fill out your own 10-sec. pulse count under this column.
[b] To obtain the approximate 60 percent rate, subtract twelve beats from your 70% target heart rate in bpm (#7) or two beats from your 70% 10-sec. pulse count (#8).

Figure 2.10. *Cardiovascular Exercise Record Sheet*

Month ______

Date	Body Weight	Exercise Heart Rate	Type of Exercise	Distance in Miles	Time Hrs/Min	RPE
1						
2						
3						
4						
5						
6						
7						
8						
9						
10						
11						
12						
13						
14						
15						
16						
17						
18						
19						
20						
21						
22						
23						
24						
25						
26						
27						
28						
29						
30						
31						
			Total			

Month ______

Date	Body Weight	Exercise Heart Rate	Type of Exercise	Distance in Miles	Time Hrs/Min	RPE
1						
2						
3						
4						
5						
6						
7						
8						
9						
10						
11						
12						
13						
14						
15						
16						
17						
18						
19						
20						
21						
22						
23						
24						
25						
26						
27						
28						
29						
30						
31						
			Total			

Figure 2.10. *Cardiovascular Exercise Record Sheet* (continued)

Month ______

Date	Body Weight	Exercise Heart Rate	Type of Exercise	Distance in Miles	Time Hrs/Min	RPE
1						
2						
3						
4						
5						
6						
7						
8						
9						
10						
11						
12						
13						
14						
15						
16						
17						
18						
19						
20						
21						
22						
23						
24						
25						
26						
27						
28						
29						
30						
31						
			Total			

Month ______

Date	Body Weight	Exercise Heart Rate	Type of Exercise	Distance in Miles	Time Hrs/Min	RPE
1						
2						
3						
4						
5						
6						
7						
8						
9						
10						
11						
12						
13						
14						
15						
16						
17						
18						
19						
20						
21						
22						
23						
24						
25						
26						
27						
28						
29						
30						
31						
			Total			

CHAPTER THREE

Muscular Strength Assessment and Prescription

Many people are still under the impression that muscular strength and endurance are only necessary for athletes and other individuals who hold jobs that require heavy muscular work. However, strength and endurance are important components of total physical fitness and have become an integral part of everyone's life.

Adequate levels of strength significantly enhance a person's health and well-being throughout life. Strength is important in daily activities such as sitting, walking, running, lifting and carrying objects, and doing housework. Strength is also of great value in improving posture, personal appearance, and self-image in developing sports skills, and in meeting certain emergencies in life where strength is necessary to cope effectively. From a health standpoint, strength helps maintain muscle tissue and a higher resting metabolism, decreases the risk for injury, helps prevent and eliminate chronic low back pain, and is an important factor in childbearing.

RELATIONSHIP BETWEEN STRENGTH AND METABOLISM

Perhaps one of the most significant benefits of maintaining a good strength level is its relationship to human metabolism. Metabolism is defined as all energy and material transformations that occur within living cells. A primary result of a strength-training program is an increase in muscle size (lean body mass), known as muscle hypertrophy. Several studies have shown that there is a direct relationship between oxygen consumption as a result of metabolic activity and amount of lean body mass. Muscle tissue uses energy even at rest, while fatty tissue uses very little energy and may be considered metabolically inert from the point of view of caloric use. As muscle size increases, so does the resting metabolism or the amount of energy (expressed in calories) required by an individual during resting conditions to sustain proper cell function. Even small increases in muscle mass increase resting metabolism. All other factors being equal, if one takes two individuals at 150 pounds with different amounts of muscle mass, the one with the greater muscle size will have a higher resting metabolic rate, allowing this person to eat more calories in order to maintain the muscle tissue.

Lack of physical activity is also a reason for the decrease in metabolism as people grow older. Contrary to some beliefs, metabolism does not slow down with aging. It is not so much that metabolism slows down as is the fact that *we* slow down. Lean body mass decreases with sedentary living, which in turn slows down the resting metabolic rate. If people continue eating at the same rate, body fat increases. Hence, participating in a strength-training program is an important factor in the prevention and reduction of obesity.

WOMEN AND STRENGTH TRAINING

Due to the increase in muscle mass, many women feel that strength-training programs are counterproductive because they will make them too muscular and less feminine-looking. The thought that strength training will make women less feminine is as false as to think that playing basketball will turn them into giants. Masculinity and femininity are established by genetic inheritance and not by the amount of physical activity. Variations in the degree of masculinity and femininity are determined by individual differences in hormonal secretions of androgen, estrogen, progesterone, and testosterone. Women with a bigger-than-average build are often inclined to participate in sports because of their natural physical advantage. As a result, many women have associated sports and strength participation with increased masculinity.

As the number of women that participate in sports has steadily increased in the last few years, the myth that strength training masculinizes women has gradually been disappearing. For example, per pound of body weight, women gymnasts are considered to be among the strongest athletes in the world. These athletes engage in very serious strength-training programs and for their body size are most likely twice as strong as the average male. Yet, lady gymnasts are among the most graceful and feminine of all women. In recent years, increased femininity has become the rule rather than the exception for women who participate in strength-training programs.

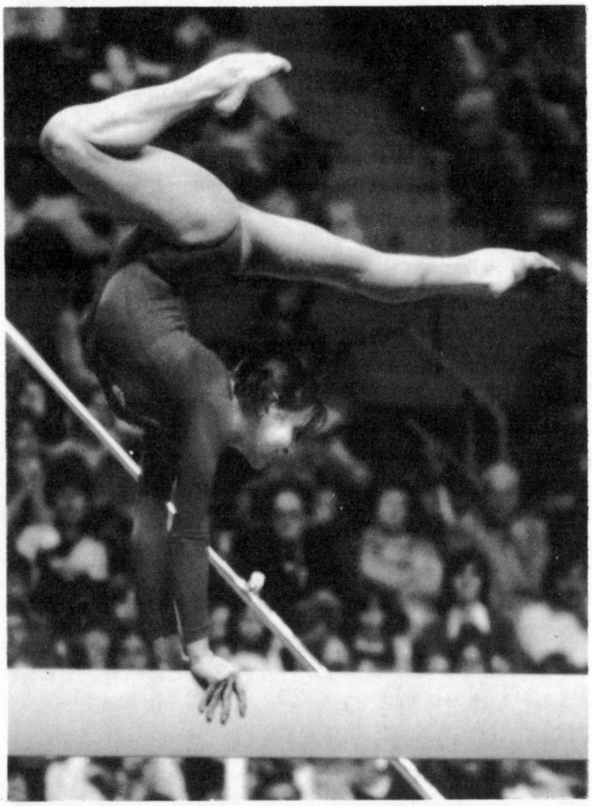

Figure 3.1. *Female gymnast performing a strength part on the balance beam. Contrary to some beliefs, high levels of strength do not masculinize women. (Courtesy of Universal Gym Equipment, Inc., 930 27th Ave., S.W. Cedar Rapids, Iowa).*

Another benefit of strength training, which is accentuated even more when combined with aerobic exercise, is a decrease in adipose or fatty tissue around the muscle fibers themselves. Research has shown that in women the decrease in fatty tissue is greater than the amount of muscle hypertrophy. Therefore, it is not at all uncommon to lose inches and yet not lose body weight. Figure 3.2 represents a graphical illustration of the reduction in fatty tissue and the increase in muscle size as a result of a conditioning program. However, since muscle tissue is more dense than fatty tissue, and in spite of the fact that inches are being lost, women often become discouraged because the results cannot be readily seen on the scale. This discouragement can be easily offset by regularly determining the amount of body fat loss (as will be explained in Chapter 5).

MUSCULAR STRENGTH VERSUS MUSCULAR ENDURANCE

Although muscular strength and endurance are interrelated, a basic difference exists between the two. Strength is the capacity of a muscle to exert maximal force against a resistance. Endurance is the capacity of a muscle to exert submaximal force repeatedly over a period of time. Keeping these two principles in mind, strength tests and training programs have been developed to measure and develop absolute muscular strength, muscular endurance, or a combination of both. Absolute strength is usually determined by the maximal amount of resistance (one repetition maximum or 1 RM) that an individual can lift in a single effort. Muscular endurance is commonly determined by the number of repetitions that an individual can perform against a submaximal resistance or by the length of time that a given contraction can be sustained.

MUSCULAR STRENGTH AND ENDURANCE ASSESSMENT

As with the cardiovascular fitness assessment, you will be given a choice of three tests to

Figure 3.2. *Changes in Body Composition as a Result of a Combined Aerobic and Strength-Training Program.*

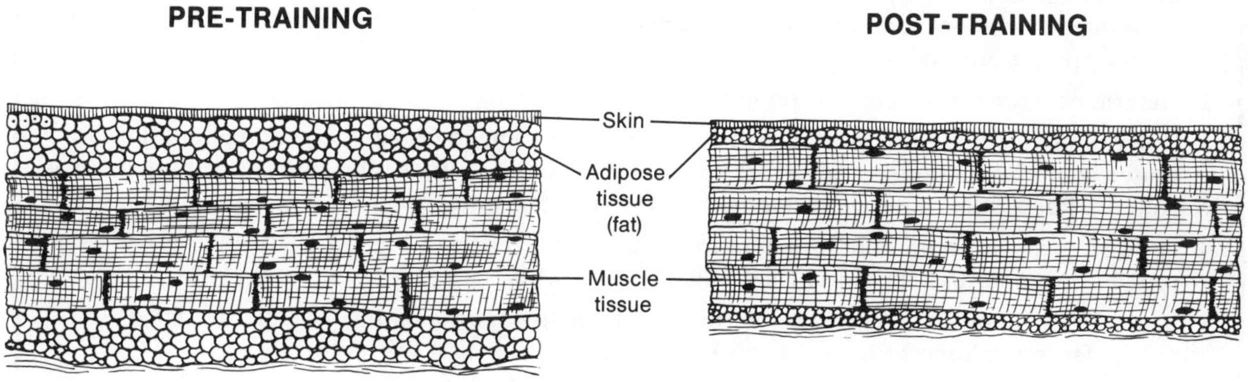

determine your strength and/or endurance level. Your selection of test should be based primarily on the facilities available to you, and secondly, whether you have been on a strength-training program recently. Since there is a small increased risk of injury for individuals attempting a maximal contraction if they have not been lifting regularly, it is perhaps best for these individuals to avoid an absolute-strength test. After you have selected your test, go directly to the procedures that explain the respective test. For safety reasons, always take a friend or group of friends with you whenever you train with weights or conduct any type of strength assessment. Also, remember that since these are three different tests, to make valid comparisons, use the same test for pre- and post-assessments. The following are your three strength-testing options:

1. **Muscular strength and endurance test.** Using submaximal resistance based on body weight, a strength-endurance rating is determined according to six selected lifts. To conduct the assessment, you will need a gym machine that will allow you to do each lift. If you are not familiar with the different lifts, Appendix B provides a graphic illustration of each lift.

2. **Muscular endurance test.** This test has been developed to measure muscular endurance rather than absolute strength. Five different exercises are used to determine the endurance of specific muscle groups. The advantage of this test is that the only equipment needed is a chinning bar and a sixteen-inch-high bench.

3. **Strength-to-body weight ratio test.** This is an absolute strength test that will require you to determine your 1 RM on six different lifts. Since 1 RM is determined through trial and error, individual assessments require about fifteen to twenty minutes or longer to conduct. As with the first test, a gym machine is needed to gather the data.

After you have established your strength fitness category, record this information in Figure 3.9 and in your fitness and wellness profile in Appendix A. If you wish to conduct periodic strength assessments, additional blanks have been provided in Figure 3.9 for you to monitor your improvements.

Figure 3.3. *Procedures for the Muscular Strength and Endurance Test.*

1. Familiarize yourself with the six lifts used for this test: bench press, arm curl, lateral pull-down, quadriceps lift, leg curl, and sit-up. (A graphic illustration for each lift is given in Appendix B. For the leg curl exercise, the knees should be flexed to ninety degrees. For the sit-up exercise, use a horizontal plane, hold the weight behind the neck, have someone hold your feet, and keep the knees flexed at a 100-degree angle. For the lateral pull-down exercise, use a sitting position and have someone hold you down by the waist or shoulders. On the quadriceps lift, maintain the trunk in an upright position).
2. Determine your body weight in pounds.
3. Determine the amount of resistance to be used on each lift. To obtain this number, multiply your body weight by the percent given for each lift in Figure 3.4, under the percent of body weight column. Record this number in the next column under resistance.
4. Perform the maximum continuous number of repetitions possible on each lift. Record your repetitions under the appropriate column in Figure 3.4.
5. Based on the number of repetitions performed, look up your percentile ranking for each exercise on the far left column of Table 3.1. Also record this information in Figure 3.4.
6. Total the percentile scores obtained for each exercise, and divide by six to obtain an average score. Determine your overall strength fitness category according to the following ratings:

Average Score	Strength Category
80+	Excellent
60-79	Good
40-59	Average
20-39	Fair
<19	Poor

From Hoeger, W. W. K. and D. R. Hopkins. "A Six-Item Muscular Strength Test Based on Selected Percentages of Body Weight." Data collected at The University of Texas of the Permian Basin, Odessa, Texas, 1985.

Figure 3.4. *Data Form for the Muscular Strength and Endurance Test.*

Name: ______________________ Sex: __________ Date: ______________

Body Weight: ______________ lbs.

Lift	% Body Weight		Resistance	Repetitions	% Rank
	Men	Women			
Lat. Pull-Down	.70	.45			
Quad. Lift	.65	.50			
Bench Press	.75	.45			
Sit-Up	.16	.10			
Leg Curl	.32	.25			
Arm Curl	.35	.18			

Total:

Average Percentile Rank (divide total by 6): ______________

Overall Strength Category: ______________

Table 3.1.
Muscular Strength and Endurance Scoring Table

MEN*

Percentile Rank	LPD**	QL	BP	SU	LC	AC
99	30	25	26	30	24	25
95	25	20	21	26	20	21
90	19	19	19	23	19	19
80	16	15	16	17	15	15
70	13	14	13	14	13	12
60	11	13	11	12	11	10
50	10	12	10	10	10	9
40	9	10	7	8	8	8
30	7	9	5	5	6	7
20	6	7	3	3	4	5
10	4	5	1	2	3	3
5	3	3	0	1	1	2

WOMEN*

Percentile Rank	LPD**	QL	BP	SU	LC	AC
99	30	25	27	32	20	25
95	25	20	21	27	17	21
90	21	18	20	22	12	20
80	16	13	16	14	10	16
70	13	11	13	11	9	14
60	11	10	11	6	7	12
50	10	9	10	5	6	10
40	9	8	5	4	5	8
30	7	7	3	2	4	7
20	6	5	1	1	3	6
10	3	3	0	0	1	3
5	2	1	0	0	0	2

*Men: n = 101, Women: n = 113.
**LPD = Lateral Pull Down, QL = Quadriceps Lift, BP = Bench Press, SU = Sit-Up, LC = Leg Curl, AC = Arm Curl.

Figure 3.5. *Procedures for the Muscular Endurance Test*

This muscular endurance test is adapted from work conducted by Robert V. Hockey[5], and the procedures are as follows:

1. Five different exercises (see Figure 3.6) are conducted on this test, and depending on the description of each one you will be asked to:
   (a) perform a maximum number of continuous repetitions
   (b) perform a maximum number of repetitions in a given period of time
   (c) hold a particular contraction as long as possible

2. Perform each exercise as described and record your results in Figure 3.6.
   (a) Bent-leg sit-up. Bend both legs at the knees at approximately ninety degrees. Having someone hold your feet flat on the floor, attempt to do as many repetitions as possible in a one-minute period. At the start of each sit-up, the back of the head has to come in contact with the floor. At the top, at least one elbow must touch one knee.
   (b) Push-up. The men perform as many continuous push-ups as possible. The body must be kept straight, the chest must touch the floor each time, and arms must be fully extended at the end of each repetition. Men and women alike perform a static push-up for as long as possible. This is done by lowering the body until the arms are flexed to ninety degrees or less (two or three inches above the floor). The entire body must be kept straight and off the floor with the exception of hands and feet.
   (c) Pull-up. Men perform as many continuous pull-ups as possible. Grasp the bar with the palms forward. On each repetition, the chin has to raise above the bar. The knees cannot be raised, nor are you allowed to kick with the legs when attempting the pull-ups. Women perform a modified pull-up by using a bar chest high, grasping the bar with palms forward, and sliding the feet under until the arms form a right angle with the body. Conduct as many continuous repetitions as possible, touching the bar with the chin or forehead on each repetition.
   (d) Flexed-arm hang. Women perform a flexed-arm hang by raising the chin to the level of the bar and holding this position as long as possible. Time stops once the chin cannot be kept level with the bar.
   (e) Bench jumps. Using a sixteen-inch bench, attempt to jump up and down the bench as many times as possible in a one-minute period. If you cannot jump the full minute, you may step up and down. A repetition is counted each time both feet return to the floor.

3. Based on your results, look up your percentile ranking for each exercise on the far left column of Table 3.2. Record this information in Figure 3.6.

4. Total the percentile scores obtained for each exercise, and divide by five to obtain an average score. Determine your own overall endurance fitness category according to the following ratings:

Average Score	Endurance Category
80+	Excellent
60-79	Good
40-59	Average
20-39	Fair
<19	Poor

Figure 3.6. *Data Form for the Muscular Endurance Test.*

Name: ______________________ Sex: ________ Date: ______________

Men			Women		
Exercise	Score	% Rank	Exercise	Score	% Rank
Sit-up			Sit-up		
Push-ups			Static Push-ups		
Static Push-ups			Flx.-Arm Hang		
Pull-ups			Mod. Pull-ups		
Bench Jumps			Bench Jumps		
	Total:			Total:	

Average Percentile Rank (divide total by 5): ______________________

Overall Endurance Category: ______________________

Table 3.2.
Muscular Endurance Scoring Table

MEN

Percentile Rank	Bent-leg Sit-ups (1 Minute Maximum)	Push-ups	Static Push-ups	Pull-ups	Bench Jumps
95	50	53	97	14	38
90	47	49	72	12	36
80	44	44	67	10	34
70	41	41	63	9	33
60	39	38	60	8	31
50	37	35	57	7	30
40	35	32	54	6	29
30	33	29	51	5	27
20	30	26	47	4	26
10	27	21	42	2	24
5	24	17	37	0	22

WOMEN

Percentile Rank	Bent-leg Sit-ups (1 Minute Maximum)	Static Push-ups	Flexed Arm Hang	Modified Pull-ups	Bench Jumps
95	36	38	34	43	28
90	33	35	28	40	26
80	30	32	19	36	24
70	28	30	14	33	22
60	26	28	10	30	21
50	24	26	8	28	20
40	22	24	6	26	19
30	20	22	4	23	18
20	18	20	2	20	16
10	15	17	1	16	14
5	12	14	0	13	12

Reproduced with permission from Hockey, R. V. *Physical Fitness: The Pathway to Healthful Living.* St. Louis: Times Mirror/Mosby College Publishing, 1985.

Figure 3.7. *Procedures for the Strength-to-Body Weight Ratio Test.*[4]

1. Familiarize yourself with the six lifts used for this test: bench press, leg press, arm curl, lateral pull-down, leg extension, and leg curl (a graphic illustration of each lift is given in Appendix B).

2. Determine your body weight in pounds.

3. Determine your one repetition maximum (1 RM) for each lift. This is done through trial and error. Estimate the amount of resistance (weight) that you think you will be able to lift. If the load is too light, increase the resistance by five to ten pounds; if it is too heavy, decrease by the same amount. Allow two to three minutes between trials. Continue the process until you have determined the maximal amount of resistance that you can lift in one single effort. Record this information under the 1 RM column in Figure 3.8.

4. Express each 1 RM as a percentage of your body weight. To obtain this number, divide the 1 RM for each lift by your weight. Enter this number under the ratio column in Figure 3.8. For example, the strength-to-body weight ratio for a 150-pound male who bench pressed 180 pounds would be 1.20 (180 divided by 150).

5. Using Table 3.3, look up on the far right column the number of points scored for the ratio obtained on each lift. In the case of the previous example, a ratio of 1.2 on the bench press for a male would score seven points. Record this information on the appropriate points column in Figure 3.8.

6. Total the number of points obtained on each lift, and determine your overall strength fitness category according to the following ratings:

Total Points	Strength Category
48+	Excellent
37-47	Good
25-36	Average
13-24	Fair
<12	Poor

Figure 3.8. *Data Form for the Strength-to-Body Weight Ratio Test.*

Name: ______________________ Sex: __________ Date: ______________

Body Weight: ______________ lbs.

Lift	1 RM	Ratio	Points
Bench Press			
Leg Press			
Arm Curl			
Lateral Pull-Down			
Leg Curl			
Leg Extension			

Overall Strength Category

____

Total Points:

____

Table 3.3.
Strength-to-Body Weight Ratio Scoring Table

BENCH PRESS	ARM CURL	LATERAL PULL-DOWN	LEG PRESS	LEG EXTENSION[a]	LEG CURL	POINTS
			MEN			
1.50	0.70	1.20	3.00	0.80	1.40	10
1.40	0.65	1.15	2.80	0.75	1.30	9
1.30	0.60	1.10	2.60	0.70	1.20	8
1.20	0.55	1.05	2.40	0.65	1.15	7
1.10	0.50	1.00	2.20	0.60	1.00	6
1.00	0.45	0.95	2.00	0.55	0.90	5
0.90	0.40	0.90	1.80	0.50	0.80	4
0.80	0.35	0.85	1.60	0.45	0.70	3
0.70	0.30	0.80	1.40	0.40	0.60	2
0.60	0.25	0.75	1.20	0.35	0.50	1
			WOMEN			
0.90	0.50	0.85	2.70	0.70	1.05	10
0.85	0.45	0.80	2.50	0.65	1.00	9
0.80	0.42	0.75	2.30	0.60	0.95	8
0.70	0.38	0.73	2.10	0.55	0.90	7
0.65	0.35	0.70	2.00	0.52	0.85	6
0.60	0.32	0.65	1.80	0.50	0.80	5
0.55	0.28	0.63	1.60	0.45	0.75	4
0.50	0.25	0.60	1.40	0.40	0.70	3
0.45	0.21	0.55	1.20	0.35	0.65	2
0.35	0.18	0.50	1.00	0.30	0.60	1

From Heyward, V. H. *Designs for Fitness.* Minneapolis, MN, 1984.

[a]Leg extension ratios adapted with permission by the author. (This exercise is also referred to as Quadriceps Left)

Figure 3.9. *Muscular Strength Report.*

Name: ______________________ Age: __________ Sex: __________

Date	Test Used	Score	Fitness Classification

PHYSIOLOGICAL FACTORS INVOLVED IN MUSCULAR CONTRACTION

There are several important physiological factors related to muscle contraction and subsequent strength gains. These factors are neural stimulation, muscle fiber type, overload principle, and specificity of training. Basic knowledge of these factors is important in order to understand the principles involved in strength training.

Neural Stimulation

Within the neuromuscular system, single motor neurons (nerves traveling from the central nervous system to the muscle) branch and attach to multiple muscle fibers. The combination of the motor neuron and the fibers that it innervates is called a motor neuron. The number of fibers that a motor neuron can innervate varies from just a few to as many as 200. Stimulation of a motor neuron causes the muscle fibers to contract maximally or not at all. Variations in the number of fibers innervated and the frequency of their stimulation determine the strength of the muscle contraction. As the number of fibers innervated and frequency of stimulation increase, so does the strength of the muscular contraction.

Fiber Types

There are primarily two types of muscle fibers that determine muscle response: type I or slow twitch and type II or fast twitch. Type I fibers have a greater capacity for aerobic work. Type II fibers have a greater capacity for anaerobic work and produce a greater overall force. The latter are important for quick and powerful movements commonly used in strength-training activities.

During muscular contraction, type I fibers are always recruited first. As the force and speed of muscle contraction increase, the relative importance of the type II fibers also increases. An activity must be intense and powerful in order for activation of the type II fibers to occur.

Overload Principle

Strength gains are achieved in two ways: first, through an increased ability of individual muscle fibers to elicit a stronger contraction, and second, by recruiting a greater proportion of the total available fibers for each contraction. The development of these two factors can be accomplished by the use of the overload principle. This principle states that in order for strength improvements to occur, the demands placed on the muscle must be systematically and progressively increased over a period of time, and the resistance must be of a magnitude significant enough to cause physiologic adaptation. In simpler terms, just like all other organs and systems of the human body, muscles have to be taxed beyond their regular accustomed loads to increase in physical capacity.

Specificity of Training

Another important aspect of training is the concept of specificity of training. This principle indicates that for a muscle to increase in strength or endurance, the training program must be specific in order to obtain the desired effects. In like manner, in order to increase static (isometric) versus dynamic (isotonic) strength, an individual must use static against dynamic training procedures to achieve the appropriate results.

PRINCIPLES OF STRENGTH-TRAINING PRESCRIPTION

Similar to the prescription of cardiovascular exercise, several principles need to be observed to improve muscular strength and endurance. These principles are mode, resistance and quantity, and frequency of training.

Mode of Training

There are three basic types of training methods used to improve strength: isometric, isotonic, and isokinetic. Isometric training refers to a muscle contraction producing little or no movement, such as pushing or pulling against immovable objects. Isotonic training refers to a muscle contraction with movement, such as lifting an object over your head. During isotonic training, the resistance is kept constant as the limb moves through the full range of motion at the particular joint. Isokinetic training is a form of isotonic training but uses a special apparatus that provides maximum resistance through the full range of motion.

The mode of training used by different individuals depends largely on the type of equipment available and the specific objective that the training program is attempting to accomplish.

Isometric training does not require much equipment and was commonly used several years ago, but its popularity has significantly decreased in recent years. Since strength gains with isometric training are specific to the angle at which the contraction is being performed, this type of training is quite beneficial in a sport like gymnastics where static contractions are regularly used during routines.

Isotonic training is the most popular mode used in weight training. The primary advantage is that strength gains occur through the full range of motion. Most of our daily activities are isotonic in nature. We are constantly lifting, pushing, and pulling objects, where strength is needed through a complete range of motion. Another advantage is that improvements are easily measured by the amount lifted.

The benefits of isokinetic training are similar to isotonic training. Theoretically, strength gains should be better because maximum resistance is constantly applied. However, research has not shown this type of training to be more effective than an isotonic program. Many people enjoy isokinetic training because of the impressive equipment used in the program. A real disadvantage is that the equipment is very expensive and not readily available to most people.

Resistance and Quantity

Resistance and quantity in strength training are the equivalent of intensity and duration in cardiovascular exercise prescription. The amount of resistance (or weight) used will depend on whether the individual is trying to develop muscular strength or muscular endurance.

To stimulate strength development, it is recommended that you use a resistance of approximately 80 percent of the maximum capacity (1 RM). For example, if you can bench press 150 pounds, you should work with at least 120 pounds (150 x .80). Using less than 80 percent will help you increase muscular endurance rather than strength. Because of the time factor involved in constantly determining your 1 RM on each lift to insure that you are indeed working above 80 percent, a rule of thumb widely accepted by many authors and coaches is that individuals should perform between six and ten repetitions maximum for adequate strength gains. In other words, if you are training with a resistance of 100 pounds, and you cannot lift it more than ten times, your training stimulus is adequate for strength development. Once you can lift this weight more than ten times, you should increase the resistance by five to ten pounds and again build up to ten repetitions. If you work with more than ten repetitions, you will improve muscular endurance to a greater extent instead of muscular strength.

The quantity or amount of strength training is given in number of sets rather than length of time involved. A set has been defined as a number of repetitions performed for a given exercise. For example, if you can lift 100 pounds eight times, you have done one set of eight repetitions. The number of sets recommended for optimum development is anywhere from three to five sets with about ninety seconds recovery time between each set. Due to the physiology of muscle fiber, there is a limit to the number of sets that can be done. As the number of sets increases, so does the amount of muscle fatigue and subsequent recovery time; therefore, strength gains may be lessened if too many sets are performed. A recommended program for beginners in their first year of training is three heavy sets (up to the maximum number of repetitions) preceded by one or two light warm-up sets.

To make your exercise program more time-effective, alternate two or three exercises that require different muscle groups at the time (also referred to as circuit training). In this manner, you would not have to wait the full ninety seconds before proceeding to the next set. For example, you may combine bench press, leg extensions, and sit-ups. This way you can go almost directly from one set of exercises to the next.

Additionally, to avoid muscle soreness and stiffness at the beginning stages of the program, build up gradually to your three sets of maximal repetitions. This can be accomplished by only doing one set of each exercise with a lighter resistance on the first day. On your second session, do two sets of each exercise, one light, and the second with the regular resistance. On the third day you may proceed to three sets, one light and two heavy ones. By your fourth training session, you should be able to do three heavy sets.

Frequency of Training

Strength training should be done either with a total body workout three times per week, or more frequently if a split routine (upper body one day and lower body the next) is used. Following a maximum workout, it is necessary to rest the muscle at least forty-eight hours to allow adequate recovery. If you have not recovered in two or three days, you are most likely overtraining and therefore slowing down your progress. In such a case, a decrease in the total number of sets performed on the previous workout is recommended.

In order to achieve significant strength gains, a minimum of eight weeks of consecutive training is needed. Of course, if you continue training, you will reap greater benefits. Once you have achieved an ideal level of strength, you will only need to conduct one training session per week to maintain your new strength level.

STRENGTH-TRAINING PROGRAMS

Two strength-training programs have been outlined in Appendix B. These programs have been developed to provide a complete body workout. Only a minimum of equipment is required for the first program, "Strength Training Exercises Without Weights" (Exercises 1 through 9). This program can be conducted within the walls of your own home. Your body weight is used as the primary resistance for most exercises. In a few instances, a friend's help or some basic implements from around your home are used to provide a greater stimulus. The second program, "Strength Training Exercises With Weights" (Exercises 10 through 24), requires the use of a gym machine or free weights. On this second program, the first eight exercises are recommended to get a complete workout — the rest are optional. However, if one of the optional exercises involves the same body parts, you may substitute the latter for one of the basic eight.

With either of the two programs that you choose, you will have to decide on the resistance and the number of repetitions based on whether you wish to increase muscular strength or muscular endurance. Remember — up to ten repetitions maximum are used for strength gains, and more than ten for muscular endurance. Since both strength and endurance are required in daily activities, it is recommended that you conduct your training around ten repetitions. In this manner you will obtain good strength gains and yet be close to the endurance threshold as well. Perhaps the only exercise where more than ten repetitions are recommended is the abdominal curl-up exercise. The abdominal muscles are considered primarily antigravity or postural muscles, hence, a little more endurance is required. Usually twenty to thirty repetitions are done on this exercise. As noted earlier, three sets are recommended for each exercise. You may also use the form provided in Figure 3.10 to keep a record of your training sessions.

References

1. Berger, R. A. *Introduction to Weight Training*. Englewood Cliffs, NJ: Prentice-Hall, Inc., 1984.
2. Fox, E. L. *Sports Physiology*. Philadelphia: Saunders College Publishing, 1979.
3. Fox, E. L., and D. K. Mathews. *The Physiological Basis of Physical Education and Athletics*. Philadelphia: Saunders College Publishing, 1981.
4. Heyward, V. H. *Designs for Fitness*. Minneapolis, MN: Burgess Publishing Co., 1984.
5. Hockey, R. V. *Physical Fitness: The Pathway to Healthful Living*. St. Louis: Times Mirror/Mosby College Publishing, 1985.
6. Hoeger, W. W. K. *Ejercicio, Salud y Vida* [Exercise, Health and Life]. Caracas, Venezuela: Editorial Arte, 1980.
7. Lamb, D. R. *Physiology of Exercise: Responses and Adaptations*. New York: McMillan Publishing Co., 1984.
8. McArdle, W. D., F. I. Katch, and V. L. Katch. *Exercise Physiology: Energy, Nutrition and Human Performance*. Philadelphia: Lea and Febiger, 1981.
9. O'Shea, J. P. *Scientific Principles and Methods of Strength Fitness*. Reading, MA: Addison-Wesley Publishing Co., 1976.

Figure 3.10. *Muscular Strength Record Sheet.*

			Resistance																	
		Date:																		
Exercise	Sets	Reps.																		
1.																				
2.																				
3.																				
4.																				
5.																				
6.																				
7.																				
8.																				
9.																				
10.																				
11.																				
12.																				

Figure 3.10. *Muscular Strength Record Sheet.*

			Resistance																	
		Date:																		
Exercise	Sets	Reps.																		
1.																				
2.																				
3.																				
4.																				
5.																				
6.																				
7.																				
8.																				
9.																				
10.																				
11.																				
12.																				

CHAPTER FOUR

Muscular Flexibility Assessment and Prescription

Flexibility has been defined as the ability of a joint to move freely through its full range of motion. The contribution of muscular flexibility to overall fitness and preventive health care has been generally underestimated and overlooked by health care professionals, practitioners, and even coaches and athletes.

Total range of motion about a joint is highly specific and varies significantly from one joint to the other (hip, trunk, shoulder), as well as from one individual to the next. The amount of flexibility possessed by individuals seems to be related to genetic factors and physical activity. Because of the specificity of flexibility, it is difficult to precisely indicate how much is ideal. However, the development and maintenance of some level of flexibility are important parts of everyone's health enhancement program, and even more so during the aging process.

THE VALUE OF MUSCULAR FLEXIBILITY

Sports medicine specialists have indicated that many muscular skeletal problems and injuries, especially among adults, are related to a lack of flexibility. Approximately 80 percent of all low back problems in the United States are due to improper alignment of the vertebral column and pelvic girdle — a direct result of inflexible and weak muscles. As noted in Chapter 1, this backache syndrome cost American industry in excess of $1 billion each year in lost productivity and services alone, and an extra $225 million in Workmen's Compensation. Additionally, in daily life we are often required to make rapid or strenuous movements that we are not accustomed to make, leading to potential injury. Physical therapists have also indicated that improper body mechanics are often the result of inadequate flexibility levels.

Most experts agree that participating in a regular flexibility program will help a person maintain good joint mobility, increase resistance to muscle injury and soreness, prevent low back and other spinal column problems, improve and maintain good postural alignment, enhance proper and graceful body movement, improve personal appearance and self-image, and facilitate the development and maintenane of motor skills throughout life. Flexibility exercises have also been used successfully in the treatment of patients suffering from dysmenorrhea and general neuromuscular tension. Furthermore, stretching exercises in conjunction with calisthenics are helpful in warm-up routines to prepare the human body for more vigorous aerobic or strength-training exercises, as well as subsequent cool-down routines to help the organism return to the normal resting state.

FACTORS AFFECTING FLEXIBILITY

Flexibility seems to be determined by heredity and exercise. Joint range of motion is limited by such factors as joint structure, ligaments, tendons, muscles, skin, tissue injury, adipose tissue, body temperature, age, sex, and index of physical activity.

The range of motion about a given joint depends largely on the structure of that particular joint. Fortunately, greater range of motion is attainable and can be accomplished through "plastic" and/or "elastic" elongation. Plastic elongation refers to a permanent lengthening of soft tissue. Even though joint capsules, ligaments, and tendons are primarily nonelastic in nature, they can undergo plastic elongation. This permanent lengthening leads to increases in joint range of motion and is best attained using slow-sustained stretching exercises. Muscle tissue, on the other hand, has elastic properties and will respond to stretching exercises by undergoing elastic or temporary lengthening. This form of elongation increases the extensibility of the muscles.

Changes in muscle temperature can increase or decrease flexibility by as much as 20 percent. Properly warmed-up individuals exhibit better flexibility levels as compared to non-warmed-up subjects. Cool temperatures have the opposite effect, decreasing joint range of motion. Because of the effects of temperature on muscular flexibility, many people prefer to conduct their stretching exercises following the aerobic phase of their workout. Aerobic activities raise the temperature of connective tissue facilitating plastic elongation.

Another factor that influences flexibility is the amount of adipose tissue in and around joints and muscle tissue. Large amounts of adipose tissue not only increase resistance to movement, but the additional bulk restricts joint mobility because of the premature contact between contiguous body surfaces.

On the average, women enjoy higher flexibility levels than men and seem to retain this advantage throughout life. Aging decreases the extensibility of soft tissue, resulting in decreased flexibility. However, the most significant contributors to decrements in flexibility are sedentary living and lack of physical activity. As physical activity decreases, muscles lose elasticity, and tendons and ligaments tighten and shorten. In addition, inactivity frequently leads to an increase in adipose tissue, which further decreases joint range of motion.

Finally, injury to muscle tissue and/or tight skin resulting in excessive scar tissue has a negative effect on joint range of motion.

FLEXIBILITY ASSESSMENT TECHNIQUES

There are many flexibility tests available in the literature, but most of them are specific to certain sports and are not practical for use with the general population. For example, the bridge-up test and the front-to-rear splits test (see Figures 4.1 and 4.2) were developed to determine flexibility of the spine (hyperextension) and front-to-rear leg extension, respectively. Both tests have applications in sports like gymnastics and several track and field events, but they are not indicative of actions encountered by most people in daily life. Because of the lack of pratical flexibility tests, many health and fitness programs have been limited in the choice of tests available and have relied strictly on the sit-and-reach test (see Figure 4.3), which only measures flexibility of the lower back and the hamstring muscles (back of the thigh).

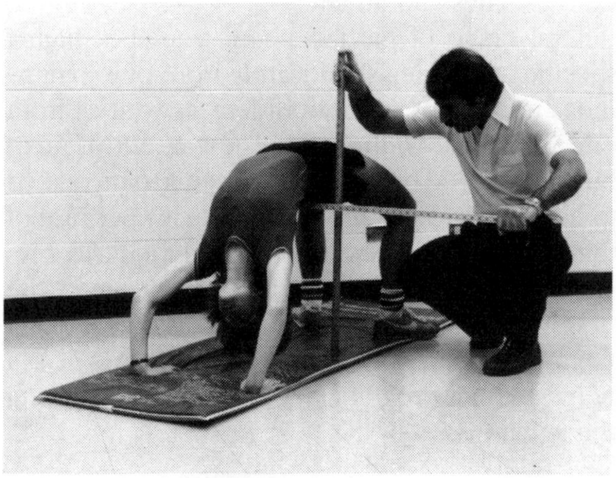

Figure 4.1. *The bridge-up test.*

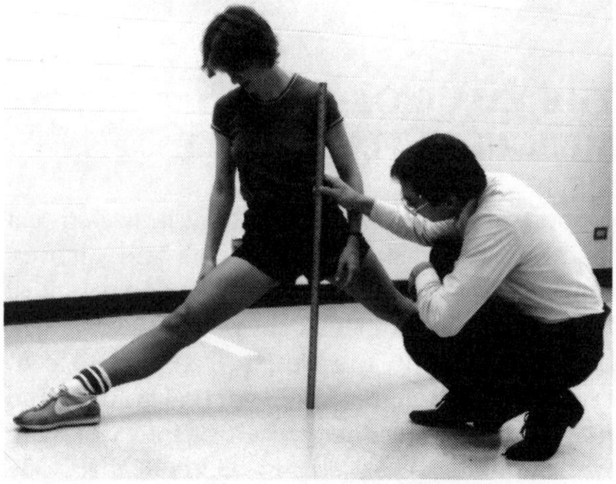

Figure 4.2. *Front-to-rear splits test.*

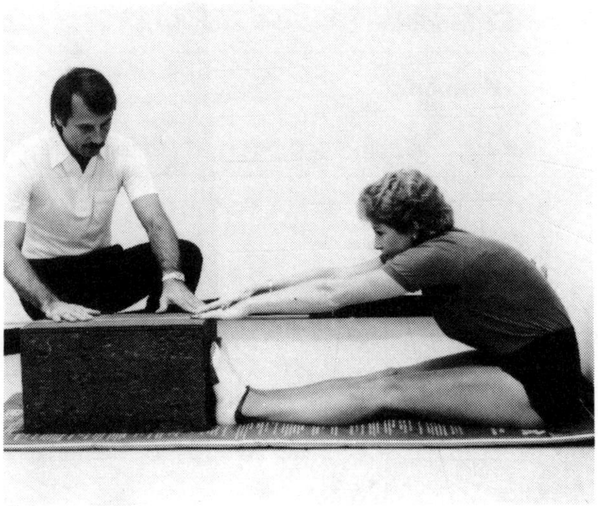

Figure 4.3. *The sit-and-reach test.*

Since flexibility is joint specific and a high degree in one joint does not necessarily indicate a high degree in other joints, two recently developed tests that are indicative of everyday movements, such as reaching, bending, and turning, have been included to determine your flexibility profile. These tests were adapted from previous work done by other researchers[5,9,10] and have a practical application in a health and fitness setting. These two tests are the trunk rotation test[5,10] and the shoulder rotation test[9].

For the flexibility profile, instead of a choice of tests, you will need to take all three tests. The tests are quite simple to administer and require very little equipment. You may now go directly to the procedures of each test outlined in Figures 4.4 through 4.6 and make the necessary arrangements to take each test. Make sure that you warmup properly by doing some gentle stretching exercises prior to taking the tests.

Figure 4.4. *Procedures for the Modified Sit-and-Reach Test*[a]

1. Place a yardstick on top of a box approximately twelve inches high.
2. Sit on the floor with your back and head against the wall and legs fully extended, with the bottom of the feet against the box (remove your shoes for this test).
3. As illustrated in Figure 4.4a, place the hands one on top of the other, and reach forward as far as possible without letting your head and back come off the wall (you may round your shoulders as much as possible, but neither head nor back should come off the wall). Have someone else slide the yardstick along the top of the box until the end touches your fingers. The yardstick must then be held firmly in place throughout the rest of the test.
4. Allow your back and head to come off the wall. Bob forward three times, the third time stretching forward as far as possible on the yardstick, and hold the final position for at least two seconds (see Figure 4.3). Record the final number of inches reached to the nearest one-half inch.
5. Repeat the procedure three times and use the average of the three trials as the test score. Using Table 4.1, determine your percentile rank and flexibility classification for this test. Record this information in Figure 4.7.

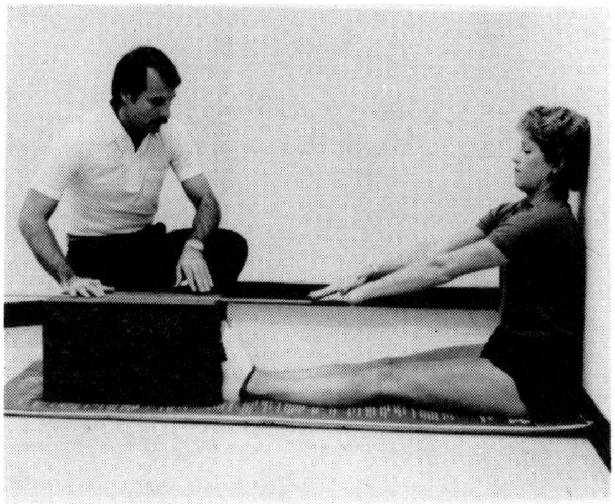

Figure 4.4a. *Determining the starting position for the sit-and-reach test.*

From Hopkins, D. R., and W. W. K. Hoeger. "The Modified Sit-and-Reach Test." Data collected at The University of Texas of The Permian Basin, Odessa, Texas, 1985.

[a] Unlike the traditional sit-and-reach test, the modified protocol used for this test varies in that the arm and leg lengths are taken into consideration to determine your score. In the original test procedures, the fifteen-inch mark of the yardstick is always set at the edge of the box where the feet are placed. This procedure does not differentiate between an individual with long arms and/or short legs and someone with short arms and/or long legs. All other factors being equal, the individual with the longer arms and/or shorter legs would receive a better rating because of the structural advantage.

Table 4.1.
Percentile Scores and Flexibility Classification for the Modified Sit-and-Reach Test

Percentile Rank	AGE	Men < 35[a]	Men 35+[b]	Women < 35[c]	Women 35+[b]	Fitness Classification
99		23.0	19.5	19.0	20.5	Excellent
95		19.0	16.5	18.0	17.5	
90		18.5	16.0	17.5	16.5	
80		17.0	14.5	16.5	15.0	
70		16.0	13.5	16.0	14.0	Good
60		15.0	12.5	15.5	13.5	
50		14.0	11.5	15.0	12.5	Average
40		13.0	10.5	14.5	11.5	
30		12.0	10.0	13.5	10.5	Fair
20		11.0	9.0	12.0	9.5	
10		9.5	8.0	10.0	8.0	Poor
5		8.0	7.5	9.0	7.0	

[a]n = 107 [b]n = 113 [c]n = 117 [d]n = 110

Figure 4.5. *Procedures for the Trunk Rotation Test.*

1. A measuring scale with a sliding panel is placed on the wall at shoulder height. The scale should be adjustable to accommodate individual differences in height. Two measuring tapes are glued in place above and below the sliding panel and centered at the fifteen-inch mark. Each tape should be at least thirty inches long. If no sliding panel is available, simply tape the measuring tapes onto the wall. A line is then drawn on the floor which must also be centered with the fifteen-inch mark (see Figures 4.5a, 4.5b, 4.5c, and 4.5d).
2. Stand sideways two to three feet away from the wall (depending on arm length), with your feet straight ahead and slightly separated. The arm opposite to the wall is held out horizontally from the body, making a fist with the hand. The measuring scale or tapes should be shoulder height at this time.
3. Rotate the trunk, the extended arm going backward (always maintaining a horizontal plane) and making contact with the panel, sliding it forward as far as possible. If you do not have a panel, slide your fist alongside the tapes (see Figures 4.5b and 4.5c). The final position should be held for at least two seconds. The hand should be positioned with the little finger side forward during the entire sliding movement, as illustrated in Figure 4.5e. During the test, the knees can be slightly bent, feet should not be moved, and the body must be kept as straight (vertical) as possible.
4. The test is conducted for both the right and left sides of the body. Each participant is allowed three trials on each side. The furthest point reached, measured to the nearest one-half inch, and held for at least two seconds, is recorded. The average of the three trials on each side is used as the final test score. Using Table 4.2, determine your percentile rank and flexibility classification for the right and left sides of the body. Record this information in Figure 4.7.

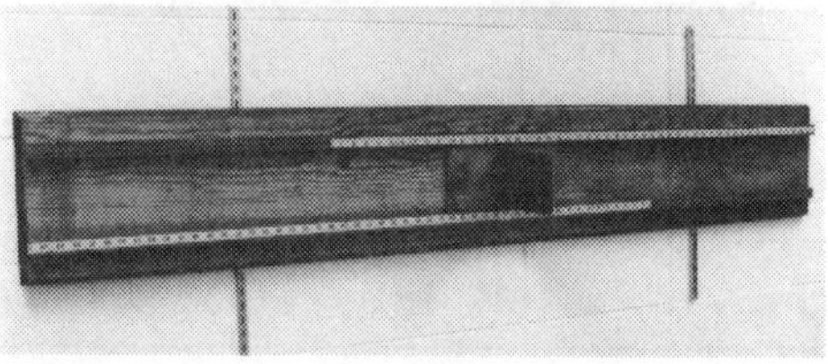

Figure 4.5a. *Measuring device for the trunk rotation test.*

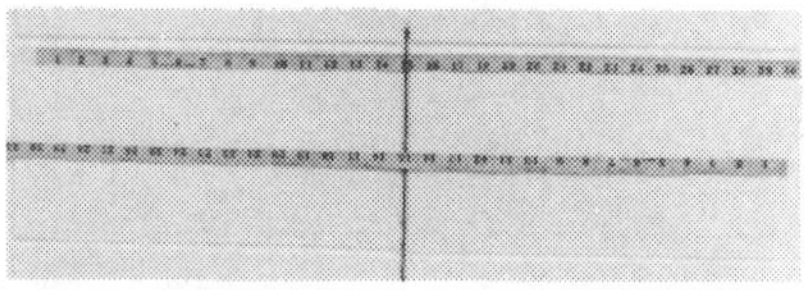

Figure 4.5b. *Measuring tapes used for trunk rotation test.*

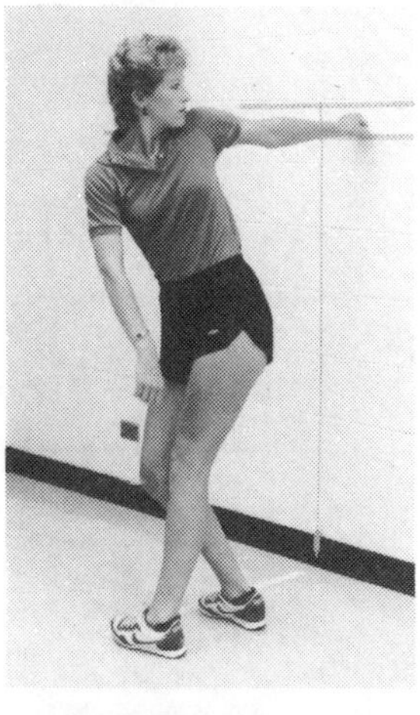

Figure 4.5c. *Trunk rotation test using simple measuring tapes.*

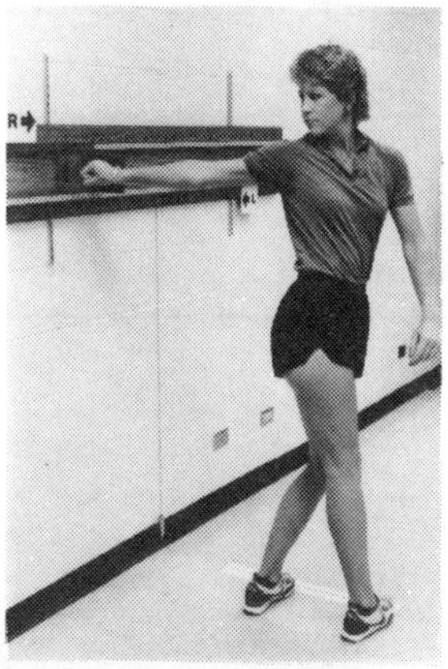

Figure 4.5d. *Trunk rotation test using a sliding panel device.*

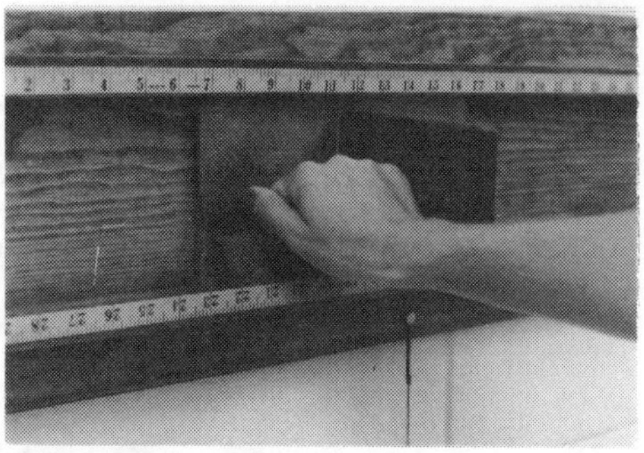

Figure 4.5e. *Proper hand position during trunk rotation test.*

From Hoeger, W. W. K., and D. R. Hopkins. "Trunk Rotation and Shoulder Rotation Flexibility Tests." Data collected at The University of Texas of the Permian Basin, Odessa, Texas, 1985.

Table 4.2.
Percentile Scores and Flexibility Classification for the Trunk Rotation Test

MEN

Percentile Rank	AGE < 35[a] Right	AGE < 35[a] Left	AGE 35+[b] Right	AGE 35+[b] Left	Fitness Classification
99	28.0	28.0	26.0	28.5	Excellent
95	26.0	25.0	23.5	23.0	
90	24.5	23.5	21.5	22.0	
80	22.5	22.0	18.5	18.5	
70	21.0	20.5	16.5	16.5	Good
60	19.0	19.5	15.5	15.5	
50	17.5	18.0	14.5	14.5	Average
40	16.5	17.0	13.5	13.5	
30	15.5	15.0	11.5	12.0	Fair
20	13.5	13.5	10.5	10.5	
10	12.0	11.0	4.2	5.5	Poor
5	10.5	9.0	2.0	2.5	

WOMEN

Percentile Rank	AGE < 35[c] Right	AGE < 35[c] Left	AGE 35+[d] Right	AGE 35+[d] Left	Fitness Classification
99	28.5	26.5	27.0	28.5	Excellent
95	23.5	23.0	22.0	23.5	
90	22.0	22.0	20.0	21.5	
80	20.0	20.5	18.5	19.0	
70	19.0	19.5	17.0	18.0	Good
60	17.5	18.5	16.0	17.0	
50	17.0	17.5	14.0	15.5	Average
40	16.0	16.5	13.0	14.0	
30	15.5	15.5	11.5	12.0	Fair
20	14.0	14.5	7.5	9.5	
10	10.5	13.0	3.5	4.5	Poor
5	8.5	6.5	2.0	3.0	

[a]n = 105 [b]n = 105 [c]n = 114 [d]n = 110

Figure 4.6. *Procedures for the Shoulder Rotation Test.*

1. With the aid of a large caliper, measure the biacromial width to the nearest one-fourth inch (biacromial width is measured between the lateral edges of the acromion processes of the shoulders, as shown in Figure 4.6a). If a caliper is not available, you may construct your own by using three regular yardsticks. Nail and glue two of the yardsticks at one end at a ninety-degree angle. Use the third one as the sliding end of the caliper.
2. Place a sixty-inch measuring tape on an aluminum or wood stick, starting at about six or seven inches from the end to allow the subject gripping space with the hand.
3. Using a reverse grip, hold on to the stick behind your back, as shown in Figure 4.6b. Place the right hand against the start of the tape and grasp firmly. Hold on to the other end of the stick with the left hand.
4. Standing straight up and extending both arms to full length, with elbows locked, bring the stick over the head, until you can see it in front of you (see Figure 4.6c). Depending on the resistance encountered when rotating the shoulders, move the left grip in one-half to one inch at a time, and repeat the task (always keep the right-hand grip against the beginning of the tape). The trials are repeated until the subject can no longer rotate the shoulders, or starts bending the elbows to do so. Measure the last successful trial to the nearest one-half of an inch.
5. The final score for this test is determined by subtracting the biacromial width from the best score (shortest distance) between both hands on the rotation test. For example, if the best score is thirty-five inches and the biacromial width is fifteen inches, the final score would be twenty inches (35 – 15 = 20). Using Table 4.3, determine your percentile rank and flexibility classification for this test. Record this information in Figure 4.7.

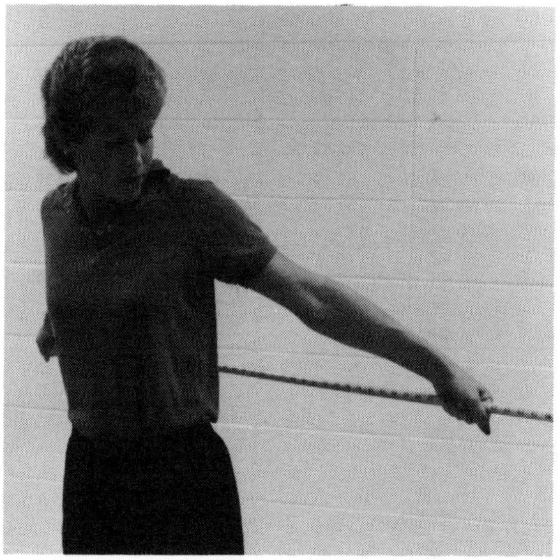

Figure 4.6b. *Reverse grip used during shoulder rotation test.*

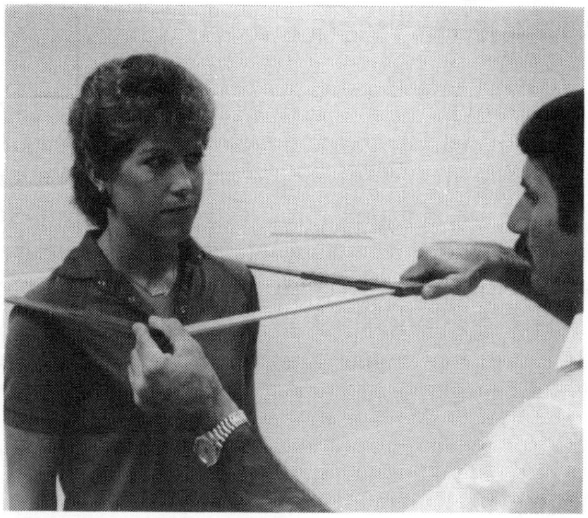

Figure 4.6a. *Measuring biacromial width.*

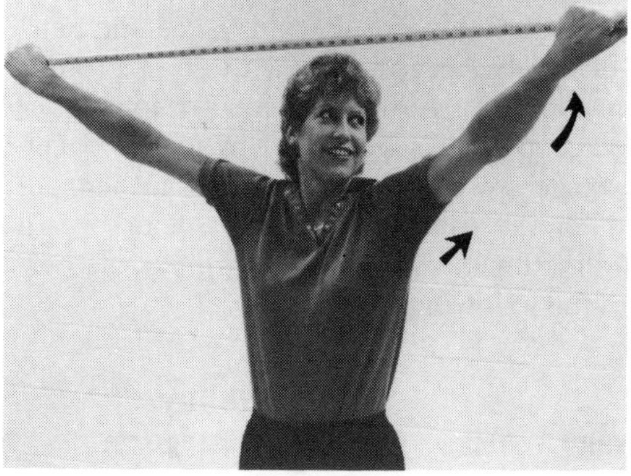

Figure 4.6c. *Shoulder rotation test.*

From Hoeger, W. W. K., and D. R. Hopkins, "Trunk Rotation and Shoulder Rotation Flexibility Tests." Data collected at The University of Texas of the Permian Basin, Odessa, Texas, 1985.

Table 4.3.
Percentile Scores and Flexibility Classification for the Shoulder Rotation Test

Percentile Rank	AGE	Men < 35[a]	Men 35+[b]	Women < 35[c]	Women 35+[b]	Fitness Classification
99		6.0	20.0	4.0	10.5	Excellent
95		14.5	20.5	9.5	15.5	
90		16.0	21.5	12.5	17.5	
80		18.5	24.5	15.0	21.0	
70		20.5	27.5	17.5	23.0	Good
60		23.0	28.5	19.0	24.0	
50		24.5	30.0	19.5	24.5	Average
40		25.5	30.5	21.5	25.5	
30		27.0	31.0	24.0	28.0	Fair
20		28.5	32.0	25.0	30.5	
10		31.5	34.0	29.0	32.0	Poor
5		33.0	36.5	30.0	33.5	

[a]n = 106 [b]n = 99 [c]n = 105 [d]n = 106

INTERPRETATION OF THE FLEXIBILITY TESTS

After determining your score, percentile rank, and flexibility category for each test, record this information in Figure 4.7. Thereafter, total all of the percentile ranks and divide by four to obtain an average score (two scores, right and left, are given for the trunk rotation test). Your overall flexibility fitness category is determined according to the following ratings:

Average Score	Flexibility Fitness Category
80+	Excellent
60-79	Good
40-59	Average
20-39	Fair
<19	Poor

PRINCIPLES OF MUSCULAR FLEXIBILITY PRESCRIPTION

The overload and specificity of training principles also apply to the development of muscular flexibility. In order to increase the total range of motion of a given joint, the specific muscles around that particular joint have to be progressively stretched beyond their normal accustomed length. The principles of mode, intensity, duration, and frequency of exercise are also used for the prescription of flexibility programs.

Mode of Exercise

There are three modes of stretching exercises commonly used to increase flexibility. These are: (a) ballistic stretching, (b) slow-sustained stretching, and (c) propioceptive neuromuscular

Figure 4.7. *Muscular Flexibility Report*

Name: ______________________ Age: ________ Sex: ________

Date: ______________

Test	Score	% Rank	Fitness Classification
Sit-and-Reach			
Right Trunk Rotation			
Left Trunk Rotation			
Shoulder Rotation			

Total:

Average Percentile Rank (divide total by 4): ______________

Overall Flexibility Category: ______________

Date: ______________

Test	Score	% Rank	Fitness Classification
Sit-and-Reach			
Right Trunk Rotation			
Left Trunk Rotation			
Shoulder Rotation			

Total:

Average Percentile Rank (divide total by 4): ______________

Overall Flexibility Category: ______________

Date: ______________

Test	Score	% Rank	Fitness Classification
Sit-and-Reach			
Right Trunk Rotation			
Left Trunk Rotation			
Shoulder Rotation			

Total:

Average Percentile Rank (divide total by 4): ______________

Overall Flexibility Category: ______________

facilitation stretching. Although research has indicated that all three types of stretching are effective in developing better flexibility, there are certain advantages and disadvantages to each technique.

Ballistic or dynamic stretching exercises are performed using jerky, rapid, and bouncy movements that provide the necessary force to lengthen the muscles. In spite of the fact that studies have indicated that this type of stretching helps to develop flexibility, the ballistic actions may lead to increased muscle soreness and injury due to small tears to the soft tissue. In addition, proper precautions must be taken not to overstretch ligaments, since they undergo plastic or permanent elongation. If the magnitude of the stretching force cannot be adequately controlled, as in fast, jerky movements, ligaments can be easily overstretched. This, in turn, leads to excessively loose joints, increasing the risk for injuries, including joint dislocation and sublaxation (partial dislocation). Consequently, most authorities do not recommend ballistic exercises for flexibility development.

With the slow-sustained stretching technique, muscles are gradually lengthened through a joint's complete range of motion, and the final position is held for a few seconds. Using a slow-sustained stretch causes the muscles to relax; hence, greater length can be achieved. This type of stretch causes relatively little pain and has a very low risk of injury. Slow-sustained stretching exercises are the most frequently used and recommended for flexibility development programs.

Proprioceptive neuromuscular facilitation (PNF) stretching has become more popular in the last few years. This technique is based on a "contract and relax" method and requires the assistance of another person. The procedure used is as follows:

1. The person assisting with the exercise provides an initial force by slowly pushing you in the direction of the desired stretch. The initial stretch does not cover the entire range of motion.
2. You (the person being stretched) then apply force in the opposite direction of the stretch, against the assistant, who will try to hold you as close as possible at the initial degree of stretch achieved. In other words, an isometric contraction is being performed at that angle.
3. After four or five seconds of isometric contraction, completely relax the muscle(s) being stretched. The assistant will slowly increase the degree of stretch to a greater angle.
4. Now repeat the isometric contraction for another four or five seconds and relax again. Your friend can then slowly increase the degree of stretch one more time. This procedure can be repeated anywhere from two to five times until mild discomfort occurs. On the last trial, the final stretched position should be held for several seconds.

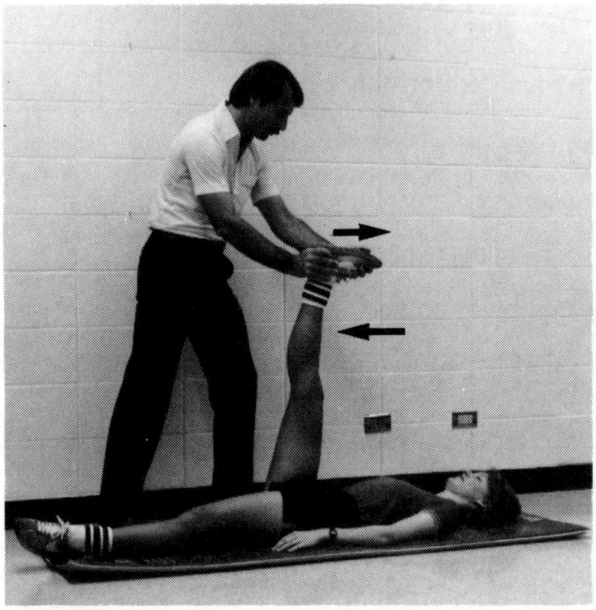

Figure 4.8. *Proprioceptive neuromuscular facilitation stretching technique.*

Theoretically, with the PNF technique, the isometric contraction aids in the relaxation of the muscle(s) being stretched, which results in greater muscle length. While some researchers have indicated that PNF is more effective than slow-sustained stretching, the disadvantages are that the degree of pain incurred with PNF is greater, a second person is required to perform the exercises, and a greater period of time is needed to conduct each session.

Intensity of Exercise

Before starting any flexibility exercises, always warm up the muscles adequately with some calisthenic exercises. A good time to do flexibility exercises is following your aerobic workout. Increased body temperature can significantly increase joint range of motion. Failing to conduct a proper warmup increases the risk for muscle pulls and tears.

The intensity or degree of stretch when doing flexibility exercises should only be to a point of mild discomfort. Pain does not have to be a part of the stretching routine. Excessive pain is an indication that the load is too high and may lead to injury. Stretching should only be done to slightly below the pain threshold. As you reach this point, try to relax the muscle being stretched as much as possible. After completing the stretch, bring the body part gradually back to the original starting point.

Duration of Exercise

The duration of exercise refers to the number of repetitions for each exercise and the length of time that each repetition (final stretched position) must be held. The general recommendations are that each exercise be done four or five times, and each time the final position should be held for five to ten seconds. As the flexibility levels increase, you can progressively increase the time that each repetition is held, up to a maximum of one minute at a time.

At least one stretching exercise should be used for each major muscle group. A complete set of exercises for the development of muscular flexibility is given in Appendix C. Depending on the number and the length of the repetitions performed, a complete workout will last between ten and twenty minutes.

Frequency of Exercise

Flexibility exercises should be conducted five to six times per week in the initial stages of the program. After a minimum of six to eight weeks of almost daily stretching, flexibility levels can be maintained with only two or three sessions per week, using about three repetitions of ten to fifteen seconds each.

PREVENTION AND REHABILITATION OF LOW BACK PAIN

Very few people make it through life without suffering from low back pain at some point in their lifetime. Current estimates indicate that 75 million Americans suffer from chronic low back pain each year. Unfortunately, approximately 80 percent of the time, backache syndrome is preventable and is caused by: (a) physical inactivity, (b) poor postural habits and body mechanics, and (c) excessive body weight.

Lack of physical activity is the most common cause contributing to chronic low back pain. The deterioration or weakening of the abdominal and gluteal muscles, along with a tightening of the lower back (erector spine) muscles, bring about an unnatural forward tilt of the pelvis. This tilt puts extra pressure on the spinal vertebrae, causing pain in the lower back (*see* Figure 4.9). In addition, excessive accumulation of fat around the midsection of the body contributes to the forward tilt of the pelvis, which further aggravates the condition.

Low back pain is also frequently associated with faulty posture and improper body mechanics. This refers to the use of correct body positions in all of daily life's activities, including sleeping, sitting, standing, walking, driving, working, and exercising. Incorrect posture and poor mechanics, as explained in Figure 4.10, lead to increased strain placed not only on the lower back, but on many other bones, joints, muscles, and ligaments.

The incidence and frequency of low back pain can be greatly reduced by including some specific stretching and strengthening exercises in your regular fitness program. When suffering from backache, in most cases pain is only present with movement and physical activity. If the pain is severe and persists even at rest, the initial step is to consult a physician. Your doctor will initially rule out any disc damage and most likely prescribe correct bed rest using several pillows under your knees for adequate leg support (*see* Figure 4.10). This position helps release muscle spasms by stretching the muscles involved. Additionally, he may prescribe a muscle relaxant, and/or anti-inflammatory medication, and/or some type of physical therapy. Once you are pain-free in the resting state, you need to start correcting the muscular imbalance by stretching the tight muscles and strengthening weak ones (stretching exercises are always performed first). Because of the significance of these exercises in the prevention and rehabilitation of the backache syndrome, the exercises have been included separately in Appendix D. You should conduct these exercises twice or more daily when suffering from backache. Under normal conditions, three to four times per week is sufficient to prevent the syndrome.

Figure 4.9. *A comparison of incorrect (left) and correct (right) pelvic alignment.*

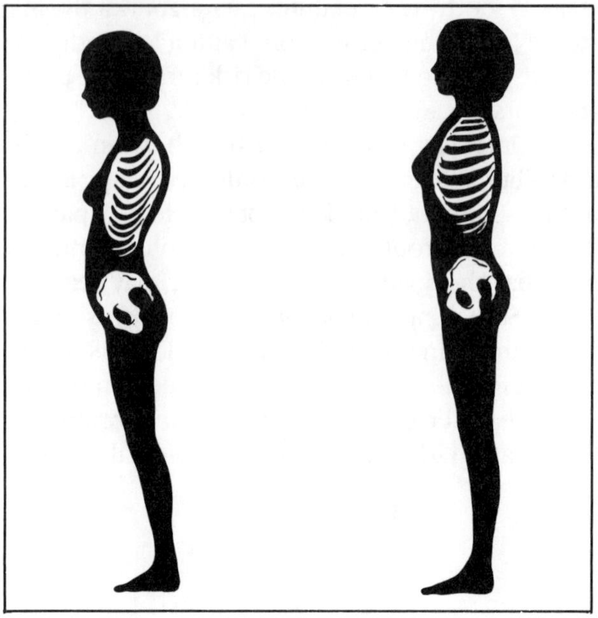

References

1. Billing, H., and E. Loewendahl. *Mobilization of the Human Body.* Palo Alto, CA: Stanford University Press, 1949.
2. Chapman, E. A., H. A. deVries, and R. Swezey. "Joint Stiffness: Effects of Exercise on Young and Old Men." *Journal of Gerontology* 27:218-221, 1972.
3. deVries, H. A. "Evaluation of Static Stretching Procedures for Improvements of Flexibility." *Research Quarterly* 33:222-229, 1962.
4. Dickerson, R. V. "The Specificity of Flexibility." *Research Quarterly* 39: 792-794, 1968.
5. Fleishman, E. A. *Examiners Manual for Basic Fitness Tests.* Englewood Cliffs, NJ: Prentice-Hall, Inc., 1964.
6. Fox, E. L., and D. K. Mathews. *The Physiological Basis of Physical Education and Athletics.* Philadelphia: Saunders College Publishing, 1981.
7. Holt, L. E., T. M. Travis, and T. Okita. "Comparative Study of Three Stretching Techniques." *Perceptual and Motor Skills* 31:611-616, 1970.
8. Johns, R. J., and V. Wright. "Relative Importance of Various Tissues in Joint Stiffness." *Journal of Applied Physiology* 17:824-828, 1962.
9. Johnson, B. L., and J. K. Nelson. *Practical Measurements for Evaluation in Physical Education.* Minneapolis, MN: Burgess Publishing Co., 1979.
10. Johnson, L. C. "Trunk Rotation Flexibility Test." Unpublished test protocol. Lake Geneva, WI: Fitness Monitoring Preventive Medicine Clinic, 1979.
11. Kraus, H., and W. Raab. *Hypokinetic Disease.* Springfield, IL: Charles C. Thomas, 1961.
12. McCue, B. F. "Flexibility of College Women." *Research Quarterly* 24: 316-324, 1953.
13. Sapega, A. A., T. C. Quedenfeld, R. A. Moyer, and R. A. Butler, "Biophysical Factors in Range-of-Motion Exercise." *Physician and Sportsmedicine* 9:57-65, 1981.
14. Wright, V., and R. J. Johns. "Physical Factors Concerned with Stiffness of Normal and Diseased Joints." *Bulletin of Johns Hopkins Hospital* 106: 215-231, 1960.

Figure 4.10.

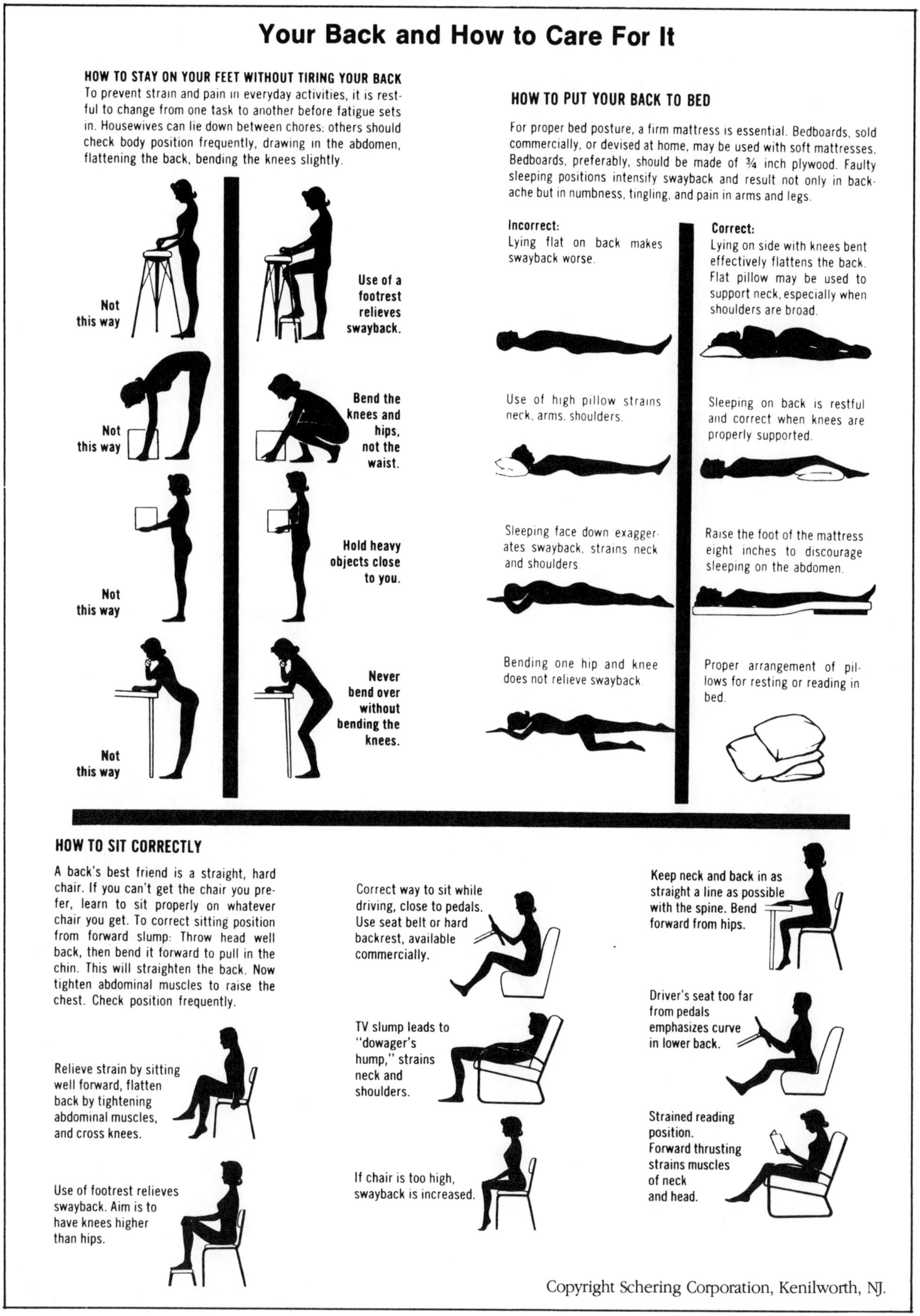
Your Back and How to Care For It
HOW TO STAY ON YOUR FEET WITHOUT TIRING YOUR BACK
To prevent strain and pain in everyday activities, it is restful to change from one task to another before fatigue sets in. Housewives can lie down between chores; others should check body position frequently, drawing in the abdomen, flattening the back, bending the knees slightly.
Not this way
Use of a footrest relieves swayback.
Not this way
Bend the knees and hips, not the waist.
Not this way
Hold heavy objects close to you.
Not this way
Never bend over without bending the knees.
HOW TO PUT YOUR BACK TO BED
For proper bed posture, a firm mattress is essential. Bedboards, sold commercially, or devised at home, may be used with soft mattresses. Bedboards, preferably, should be made of ¾ inch plywood. Faulty sleeping positions intensify swayback and result not only in backache but in numbness, tingling, and pain in arms and legs.
Incorrect:
Lying flat on back makes swayback worse.
Use of high pillow strains neck, arms, shoulders.
Sleeping face down exaggerates swayback, strains neck and shoulders.
Bending one hip and knee does not relieve swayback.
Correct:
Lying on side with knees bent effectively flattens the back. Flat pillow may be used to support neck, especially when shoulders are broad.
Sleeping on back is restful and correct when knees are properly supported.
Raise the foot of the mattress eight inches to discourage sleeping on the abdomen.
Proper arrangement of pillows for resting or reading in bed.
HOW TO SIT CORRECTLY
A back's best friend is a straight, hard chair. If you can't get the chair you prefer, learn to sit properly on whatever chair you get. To correct sitting position from forward slump: Throw head well back, then bend it forward to pull in the chin. This will straighten the back. Now tighten abdominal muscles to raise the chest. Check position frequently.
Relieve strain by sitting well forward, flatten back by tightening abdominal muscles, and cross knees.
Use of footrest relieves swayback. Aim is to have knees higher than hips.
Correct way to sit while driving, close to pedals. Use seat belt or hard backrest, available commercially.
TV slump leads to "dowager's hump," strains neck and shoulders.
If chair is too high, swayback is increased.
Keep neck and back in as straight a line as possible with the spine. Bend forward from hips.
Driver's seat too far from pedals emphasizes curve in lower back.
Strained reading position. Forward thrusting strains muscles of neck and head.
Copyright Schering Corporation, Kenilworth, NJ.

Figure 4.10

Your Back and How to Care For It

CHAPTER FIVE

Body Composition Assessment

Obesity has become a health hazard of epidemic proportions in most developed countries around the world. Statistical estimates indicate that 35 percent of the adult population in developed countries is obese. Current U.S. estimates indicate that approximately 50 percent of all adults have a weight problem. The evidence further shows that the prevalence is still increasing. Consider the following two facts. The average weight of American adults increased by about fifteen pounds in just the last decade. When Yankee Stadium in New York was renovated in 1976, total seating capacity had to be reduced in order to accommodate the wider bodies of our adult population!

Obesity by itself has been associated with several serious health problems and accounts for 15 to 20 percent of the annual U.S. Mortality rate. Obesity has long been recognized as a major risk factor for diseases of the cardiovascular system, including coronary heart disease, hypertension, congestive heart failure, elevated blood lipids, atherosclerosis, strokes, thromboembolitic disease, varicose veins, and intermittent claudication.

New evidence now points toward a possible link between obesity and cancer of the colon, rectum, prostate, gallbladder, breast, uterus, and ovaries. It is interesting to note that if all deaths from cancer could be eliminated, the average life span would increase by approximately two years. If obesity was eliminated, life span could increase by as many as seven years. In addition, obesity has been associated with diabetes, osteoarthritis, ruptured intervertebral discs, gallstones, gout, respiratory insufficiency, and complications during pregnancy and delivery. Furthermore, it can lead to psychological maladjustment and increased accidental death rate. Life insurance companies are also quick to point out that there is a 150 percent greater mortality rate among overweight males as compared to the average mortality rate.

THE ROLE OF BODY COMPOSITION

The term "body composition" is used in reference to the fat and nonfat components of the human body. The fat component is usually referred to as fat mass or percent body fat. The nonfat component is referred to as lean body mass. Although for many years people have relied on height/weight charts to determine ideal body weight, we now know that these tables can be highly inaccurate for many people. The proper way of determining ideal weight is through body composition, that is, by finding out what percent of total body weight is fat, and what amount is lean tissue. Once the fat percentage is known, ideal body weight can be calculated from ideal body fat, or the recommended amount of fat where there is no detriment to human health.

In spite of the fact that different techniques used to determine percent body fat were developed several years ago, many people are still unaware of these procedures and continue to depend on height/weight charts to find out what their "ideal" body weight should be. These standard height/weight tables were first published in 1912 and were based on average weights (including shoes and clothing) for men and women who obtained life insurance policies between 1888 and 1905. The ideal weight on the tables is obtained according to sex, height, and frame size. Since no scientific guidelines to determine frame size are given, most people choose their size based on the column where their body weight is found.

To determine whether people are truly obese or "falsely" at ideal body weight, body composition must be established. Obesity is related to excessive body fat accumulation. If body weight is used as the only criteria, an individual can easily be overweight according to height/weight charts, and yet not be obese. This is commonly seen among football players, body builders, weight lifters, and other athletes with large muscle size. Some of these athletes in reality have very little body fat and appear to be twenty or thirty pounds overweight.

The inaccuracy of the height/weight charts in predicting ideal weight for many people was clearly illustrated when a young man that weighed about 225 pounds applied to join a city police force, but was turned down without having been granted an interview. The reason: he was "too fat" according to the height/weight charts. When this young man's body composition was later assessed at a preventive medicine clinic, he was shocked to find out that only 5 percent of his total body weight was in the form of fat (considerably below the ideal standard). In the words of the technical director of the clinic, "The only way that this fellow could come down to the chart's target weight would have been through surgical removal of a large amount of his muscle tissue."

On the other end of the spectrum, some people who weigh very little and are viewed by many as "skinny" or underweight can actually be classified as obese because of their high body fat content. Not at all uncommon are cases of people weighing as little as 100 pounds who are over 30 percent fat (about one-third of their total body weight). Such cases are more readily observed among sedentary people and those who are constantly dieting. Both physical inactivity and constant negative caloric balance lead to a loss in lean body mass. It is clear from these examples that plain body weight does not always tell the true story.

ESSENTIAL AND STORAGE FAT

Total fat in the human body is classified into two types, essential fat and storage fat. The essential fat is needed for normal physiological functions, and without it, human health begins to deteriorate. This essential fat constitutes about 3 percent of the total fat in men and 10 to 12 percent in women. The percentage is higher in women because it includes sex-specific fat, such as found in the breast tissue, the uterus, and other sex-related fat deposits. The amount varies from 10 to 12 percent in women because of morphological (body build) differences from one woman to another.

Storage fat constitutes the fat that is stored in adipose tissue, mostly beneath the skin (subcutaneous fat) and around major organs in the body. This fat serves three basic functions: (a) as an insulator to retain body heat, (b) as energy substrate for metabolism, and (c) as padding against physical trauma to the body. The amount of storage fat does not differ between men and women, except that men tend to store fat around the waist, and women more so around the hips and thighs.

TECHNIQUES FOR ASSESSING BODY COMPOSITION

There are several different procedures whereby body composition can be determined. The most

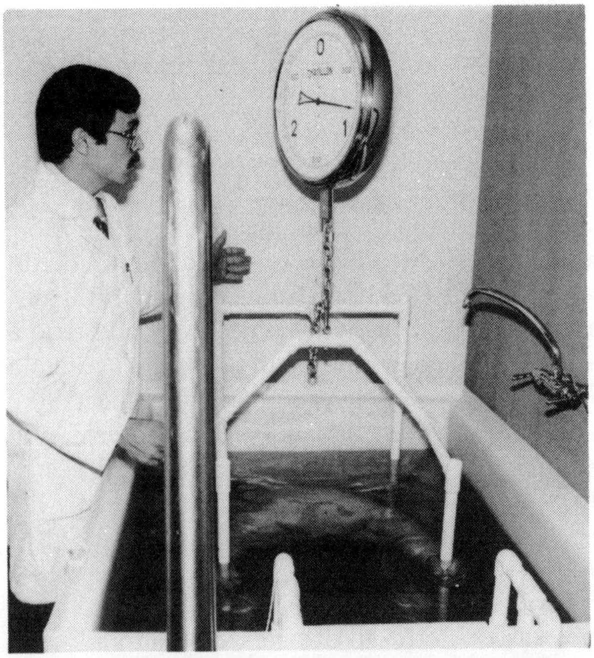

Figure 5.1. *Hydrostatic weighing technique for body composition assessment. (Courtesy of Fitness Monitoring Preventive Medicine Clinic, Lake Geneva, Wisconsin.)*

common techniques are: (a) hydrostatic or underwater weighing, (b) measurement of body volume, (c) skinfold thickness, and (d) circumference measurements.

Hydrostatic weighing and measurement of body volume are the most accurate techniques available to assess body composition, but they also require a considerable amount of time, skill, space, equipment, and complex procedures. The current circumference measurements techniques available, although quite easy to administer, have questionable validity. As a result, most health and fitness programs prefer the use of the skinfold thickness technique, which correlates quite well with hydrostatic weighing and provides a quick, simple, and inexpensive estimate of body composition.

The Skinfold Thickness Technique

The assessment of body composition using skinfold thickness is based on the principle that approximately 50 percent of the fatty tissue in the body is deposited directly beneath the skin. If this tissue is estimated validly and reliably, a good indication of percent body fat can be obtained. This procedure is regularly performed with the aid of pressure calipers (*see* Figure 5.2), and several sites must be measured to reflect the total percentage of fat.

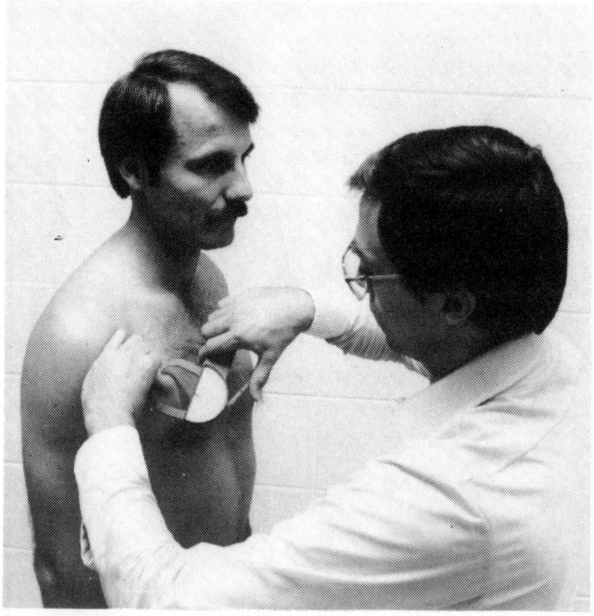

Figure 5.2. *Skinfold thickness technique for body composition assessment.*

Nevertheless, even with the skinfold technique, a minimum amount of training is necessary to achieve accurate measurements. Also, variations in measurements on the same subject may be found when these are taken by different observers. Therefore, it is recommended that pre- and post-measurements be conducted by the same technician. Furthermore, measurements should be taken at the same time of the day, preferably in the morning, since water hydration changes due to activity and exercise can increase skinfold girth up to 15 percent. The procedures for assessing percent body fat using skinfold thickness are outlined in Figure 5.3. If skinfold calipers are available to you, you may proceed to assess your percent body fat with the help of your instructor or an experienced technician (this instrument should be available at most colleges and universities around the country).

DETERMINING LEAN BODY MASS AND IDEAL BODY WEIGHT

After finding out your percent body fat, you can determine your current body composition classification according to Table 5.4. In this same table you can find the healthy or ideal amount of fat that you should have under the ideal column on the left side of the table. For example, the ideal fat percentage for a twenty-year-old female is 18 percent. As noted earlier, optimal percent body fat is established at the point where there is no detriment to your health. This ideal percentage does not mean that you cannot be somewhat below this number. Many highly trained male athletes are as low as 3 percent, and some female distance runners have been found around 6 percent body fat.

Although there is little disagreement regarding a greater mortality rate among obese people, some evidence seems to indicate that the same is true for underweight people. Being underweight and thin does not necessarily mean the same thing, though. A healthy thin person is someone with total body fat around the ideal percentage, yet an underweight person is an individual with extremely low body fat, even to the point of compromising the essential fat. The 3 percent essential fat for men and 10 to 12 percent for women are the lower limits for most people to maintain good health. Below these percentages,

Figure 5.3. *Procedures for Body Fat Assessment According to Skinfold Thickness Technique.*

1. Select the proper anatomical sites. For men, chest, abdomen, and thigh skinfolds are used. For women, use triceps, suprailium, and thigh skinfolds (see Figure 5.3a). All measurements should be taken on the right side of the body with the subject standing. The correct anatomical landmarks for skinfolds are:

   Chest: a diagonal fold halfway between the shoulder crease and the nipple.

   Abdomen: a vertical fold taken about one inch to the right of the umbilicus.

   Triceps: a vertical fold on the back of the upper arm, halfway between the shoulder and the elbow.

   Thigh: a vertical fold on the front of the thigh, midway between the knee and hip.

   Suprailium: a diagonal fold above the crest of the ilium (on the side of the hip).

2. Measure each site by grasping a double thickness of skin firmly with the thumb and forefinger, pulling the fold slightly away from the muscular tissue. The calipers are held perpendicular to the fold, and the measurement is taken one-half inch below the finger hold. Each site is measured three times and the values are read to the nearest .1 to .5 mm. The average of the two closest readings is recorded as the final value. The readings should be taken without delay to avoid excessive compression of the skinfold. Releasing and refolding the skinfold is required between readings.

3. When doing pre-and post-assessments, the measurement should be conducted at the same time of day. The best time is early in the morning to avoid water hydration changes resulting from activity or exercise.

4. Percent fat is obtained by adding together all three skinfold measurements and looking up the respective values on Tables 5.1 for women, 5.2 for men under forty, and 5.3 for men over forty.

5. For example, if the skinfold measurements for an eighteen-year-old female are: (a) triceps = 16, (b) suprailium = 14, and (c) thigh = 20 (total = 50), the percent body fat would be 20.6 percent.

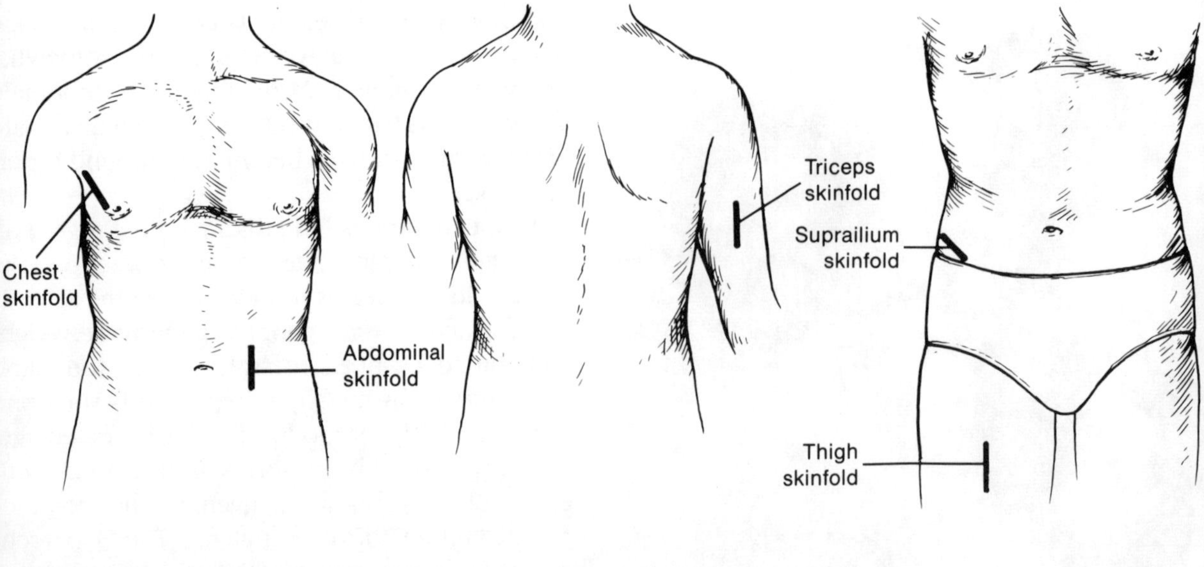

Figure 5.3a. *Anatomical landmarks for skinfolds*

Table 5.1.
Percent Fat Estimates for Women

	Age to the Last Year								
Sum of 3 Skinfolds	**Under 22**	**23 to 27**	**28 to 32**	**33 to 37**	**38 to 42**	**43 to 47**	**48 to 52**	**53 to 57**	**Over 58**
23- 25	9.7	9.9	10.2	10.4	10.7	10.9	11.2	11.4	11.7
26- 28	11.0	11.2	11.5	11.7	12.0	12.3	12.5	12.7	13.0
29- 31	12.3	12.5	12.8	13.0	13.3	13.5	13.8	14.0	14.3
32- 34	13.6	13.8	14.0	14.3	14.5	14.8	15.0	15.3	15.5
35- 37	14.8	15.0	15.3	15.5	15.8	16.0	16.3	16.5	16.8
38- 40	16.0	16.3	16.5	16.7	17.0	17.2	17.5	17.7	18.0
41- 43	17.2	17.4	17.7	17.9	18.2	18.4	18.7	18.9	19.2
44- 46	18.3	18.6	18.8	19.1	19.3	19.6	19.8	20.1	20.3
47- 49	19.5	19.7	20.0	20.2	20.5	20.7	21.0	21.2	21.5
50- 52	20.6	20.8	21.1	21.3	21.6	21.8	22.1	22.3	22.6
53- 55	21.7	21.9	22.1	22.4	22.6	22.9	23.1	23.4	23.6
56- 58	22.7	23.0	23.2	23.4	23.7	23.9	24.2	24.4	24.7
59- 61	23.7	24.0	24.2	24.5	24.7	25.0	25.2	25.5	25.7
62- 64	24.7	25.0	25.2	25.5	25.7	26.0	26.2	26.4	26.7
65- 67	25.7	25.9	26.2	26.4	26.7	26.9	27.2	27.4	27.7
68- 70	26.6	26.9	27.1	27.4	27.6	27.9	28.1	28.4	28.6
71- 73	27.5	27.8	28.0	28.3	28.5	28.8	29.0	29.3	29.5
74- 76	28.4	28.7	28.9	29.2	29.4	29.7	29.9	30.2	30.4
77- 79	29.3	29.5	29.8	30.0	30.3	30.5	30.8	31.0	31.3
80- 82	30.1	30.4	30.6	30.9	31.1	31.4	31.6	31.9	32.1
83- 85	30.9	31.2	31.4	31.7	31.9	32.2	32.4	32.7	32.9
86- 88	31.7	32.0	32.2	32.5	32.7	32.9	33.2	33.4	33.7
89- 91	32.5	32.7	33.0	33.2	33.5	33.7	33.9	34.2	34.4
92- 94	33.2	33.4	33.7	33.9	34.2	34.4	34.7	34.9	35.2
95- 97	33.9	34.1	34.4	34.6	34.9	35.1	35.4	35.6	35.9
98-100	34.6	34.8	35.1	35.3	35.5	35.8	36.0	36.3	36.5
101-103	35.2	35.4	35.7	35.9	36.2	36.4	36.7	36.9	37.2
104-106	35.8	36.1	36.3	36.6	36.8	37.1	37.3	37.5	37.8
107-109	36.4	36.7	36.9	37.1	37.4	37.6	37.9	38.1	38.4
110-112	37.0	37.2	37.5	37.7	38.0	38.2	38.5	38.7	38.9
113-115	37.5	37.8	38.0	38.2	38.5	38.7	39.0	39.2	39.5
116-118	38.0	38.3	38.5	38.8	39.0	39.3	39.5	39.7	40.0
119-121	38.5	38.7	39.0	39.2	39.5	39.7	40.0	40.2	40.5
122-124	39.0	39.2	39.4	39.7	39.9	40.2	40.4	40.7	40.9
125-127	39.4	39.6	39.9	40.1	40.4	40.6	40.9	41.1	41.4
128-130	39.8	40.0	40.3	40.5	40.8	41.0	41.3	41.5	41.8

Body density calculated based on the generalized equation for predicting body density of women developed by A. S. Jackson, M. L. Pollock, and A. Ward. *Medicine and Science in Sports and Exercise* 12:175-182, 1980. Percent body fat determined from the calculated body density using the Siri formula.[13]

Table 5.2.
Percent Fat Estimates for Men Under 40

		Age to the Last Year						
Sum of 3 Skinfolds	**Under 19**	**20 to 22**	**23 to 25**	**26 to 28**	**29 to 31**	**32 to 34**	**35 to 37**	**38 to 40**
8- 10	.9	1.3	1.6	2.0	2.3	2.7	3.0	3.3
11- 13	1.9	2.3	2.6	3.0	3.3	3.7	4.0	4.3
14- 16	2.9	3.3	3.6	3.9	4.3	4.6	5.0	5.3
17- 19	3.9	4.2	4.6	4.9	5.3	5.6	6.0	6.3
20- 22	4.8	5.2	5.5	5.9	6.2	6.6	6.9	7.3
23- 25	5.8	6.2	6.5	6.8	7.2	7.5	7.9	8.2
26- 28	6.8	7.1	7.5	7.8	8.1	8.5	8.8	9.2
29- 31	7.7	8.0	8.4	8.7	9.1	9.4	9.8	10.1
32- 34	8.6	9.0	9.3	9.7	10.0	10.4	10.7	11.1
35- 37	9.5	9.9	10.2	10.6	10.9	11.3	11.6	12.0
38- 40	10.5	10.8	11.2	11.5	11.8	12.2	12.5	12.9
41- 43	11.4	11.7	12.1	12.4	12.7	13.1	13.4	13.8
44- 46	12.2	12.6	12.9	13.3	13.6	14.0	14.3	14.7
47- 49	13.1	13.5	13.8	14.2	14.5	14.9	15.2	15.5
50- 52	14.0	14.3	14.7	15.0	15.4	15.7	16.1	16.4
53- 55	14.8	15.2	15.5	15.9	16.2	16.6	16.9	17.3
56- 58	15.7	16.0	16.4	16.7	17.1	17.4	17.8	18.1
59- 61	16.5	16.9	17.2	17.6	17.9	18.3	18.6	19.0
62- 64	17.4	17.7	18.1	18.4	18.8	19.1	19.4	19.8
65- 67	18.2	18.5	18.9	19.2	19.6	19.9	20.3	20.6
68- 70	19.0	19.3	19.7	20.0	20.4	20.7	21.1	21.4
71- 73	19.8	20.1	20.5	20.8	21.2	21.5	21.9	22.2
74- 76	20.6	20.9	21.3	21.6	22.0	22.2	22.7	23.0
77- 79	21.4	21.7	22.1	22.4	22.8	23.1	23.4	23.8
80- 82	22.1	22.5	22.8	23.2	23.5	23.9	24.2	24.6
83- 85	22.9	23.2	23.6	23.9	24.3	24.6	25.0	25.3
86- 88	23.6	24.0	24.3	24.7	25.0	25.4	25.7	26.1
89- 91	24.4	24.7	25.1	25.4	25.8	26.1	26.5	26.8
92- 94	25.1	25.5	25.8	26.2	26.5	26.9	27.2	27.5
95- 97	25.8	26.2	26.5	26.9	27.2	27.6	27.9	28.3
98-100	26.6	26.9	27.3	27.6	27.9	28.3	28.6	29.0
101-103	27.3	27.6	28.0	28.3	28.6	29.0	29.3	29.7
104-106	27.9	28.3	28.6	29.0	29.3	29.7	30.0	30.4
107-109	28.6	29.0	29.3	29.7	30.0	30.4	30.7	31.1
110-112	29.3	29.6	30.0	30.3	30.7	31.0	31.4	31.7
113-115	30.0	30.3	30.7	31.0	31.3	31.7	32.0	32.4
116-118	30.6	31.0	31.3	31.6	32.0	32.3	32.7	33.0
119-121	31.3	31.6	32.0	32.3	32.6	33.0	33.3	33.7
122-124	31.9	32.2	32.6	32.9	33.3	33.6	34.0	34.3
125-127	32.5	32.9	33.2	33.5	33.9	34.2	34.6	34.9
128-130	33.1	33.5	33.8	34.2	34.5	34.9	35.2	35.5

Body density calculated based on the generalized equation for predicting body density of men developed by A. S. Jackson and M. L. Pollock. *British Journal of Nutrition* 40:497-504, 1978. Percent body fat determined from the calculated body density using the Siri formula.[13]

Table 5.3.
Percent Fat Estimates for Men Over 40

	Age to the Last Year							
Sum of 3 Skinfolds	**41 to 43**	**44 to 46**	**47 to 49**	**50 to 52**	**53 to 55**	**56 to 58**	**59 to 61**	**Over 62**
8- 10	3.7	4.0	4.4	4.7	5.1	5.4	5.8	6.1
11- 13	4.7	5.0	5.4	5.7	6.1	6.4	6.8	7.1
14- 16	5.7	6.0	6.4	6.7	7.1	7.4	7.8	8.1
17- 19	6.7	7.0	7.4	7.7	8.1	8.4	8.7	9.1
20- 22	7.6	8.0	8.3	8.7	9.0	9.4	9.7	10.1
23- 25	8.6	8.9	9.3	9.6	10.0	10.3	10.7	11.0
26- 28	9.5	9.9	10.2	10.6	10.9	11.3	11.6	12.0
29- 31	10.5	10.8	11.2	11.5	11.9	12.2	12.6	12.9
32- 34	11.4	11.8	12.1	12.4	12.8	13.1	13.5	13.8
35- 37	12.3	12.7	13.0	13.4	13.7	14.1	14.4	14.8
38- 40	13.2	13.6	13.9	14.3	14.6	15.0	15.3	15.7
41- 43	14.1	14.5	14.8	15.2	15.5	15.9	16.2	16.6
44- 46	15.0	15.4	15.7	16.1	16.4	16.8	17.1	17.5
47- 49	15.9	16.2	16.6	16.9	17.3	17.6	18.0	18.3
50- 52	16.8	17.1	17.5	17.8	18.2	18.5	18.8	19.2
53- 55	17.6	18.0	18.3	18.7	19.0	19.4	19.7	20.1
56- 58	18.5	18.8	19.2	19.5	19.9	20.2	20.6	20.9
59- 61	19.3	19.7	20.0	20.4	20.7	21.0	21.4	21.7
62- 64	20.1	20.5	20.8	21.2	21.5	21.9	22.2	22.6
65- 67	21.0	21.3	21.7	22.0	22.4	22.7	23.0	23.4
68- 70	21.8	22.1	22.5	22.8	23.2	23.5	23.9	24.2
71- 73	22.6	22.9	23.3	23.6	24.0	24.3	24.7	25.0
74- 76	23.4	23.7	24.1	24.4	24.8	25.1	25.4	25.8
77- 79	24.1	24.5	24.8	25.2	25.5	25.9	26.2	26.6
80- 82	24.9	25.3	25.6	26.0	26.3	26.6	27.0	27.3
83- 85	25.7	26.0	26.4	26.7	27.1	27.4	27.8	28.1
86- 88	26.4	26.8	27.1	27.5	27.8	28.2	28.5	28.9
89- 91	27.2	27.5	27.9	38.2	28.6	28.9	29.2	29.6
92- 94	27.9	28.2	28.6	28.9	29.3	29.6	30.0	30.3
95- 97	28.6	29.0	29.3	29.7	30.0	30.4	30.7	31.1
98-100	29.3	29.7	30.0	30.4	30.7	31.1	31.4	31.8
101-103	30.0	30.4	30.7	31.1	31.4	31.8	32.1	32.5
104-106	30.7	31.1	31.4	31.8	32.1	32.5	32.8	33.2
107-109	31.4	31.8	32.1	32.4	32.8	33.1	33.5	33.8
110-112	32.1	32.4	32.8	33.1	33.5	33.8	34.2	34.5
113-115	32.7	33.1	33.4	33.8	34.1	34.5	34.8	35.2
116-118	33.4	33.7	34.1	34.4	34.8	35.1	35.5	35.8
119-121	34.0	34.4	34.7	35.1	35.4	35.8	36.1	36.5
122-124	34.7	35.0	35.4	35.7	36.1	36.4	36.7	37.1
125-127	35.3	35.6	36.0	36.3	36.7	37.0	37.4	37.7
128-130	35.9	36.2	36.6	36.9	37.3	37.6	38.0	38.5

Body density calculated based on the generalized equation for predicting body density of men developed by A. S. Jackson and M. L. Pollock. *British Journal of Nutrition* 40:497-504, 1978. Percent body fat determined from the calculated body density using the Siri formula.[13]

normal physiologic functions can be seriously impaired. In addition, some experts point out that a little storage fat (over the essential fat) is better than none at all. As a result, the standards for ideal percent fat in Table 5.4 are set higher than the minimum essential fat requirements, at a point that is conducive to good health. Additionally, because lean tissue decreases with age, one extra percentage point is allowed for every additional decade of life.

The previous discussion on ideal percent body fat is important, because ideal body weight is computed based on the ideal fat percentage for your respective age and gender. To compute ideal body weight, the following steps are taken (use Figure 5.4 for your computations):

1. Determine the pounds of body weight in fat (FW). This is done by multiplying your body weight (BW) by the percent fat (%F) expressed in decimal form (FW=BW x %F).
2. Determine lean body mass (LBM) by subtracting your weight in fat from your total body weight (LBM=BW–FW). Remember that anything which is not fat must be part of the lean component.
3. Look up on Table 5.4 what your ideal percent fat (IPF) should be.
4. To compute ideal body weight (IBW), use the following formula: IBW = LBM/(1.0–IFP)

An example of these computations may be helpful. A nineteen-year-old male that weighs 186 pounds and is 25 percent fat would like to know what his ideal body weight should be.

Sex: male

Age: 19

BW=186 pounds

%F=25% (.25 in decimal form)

1. FW=BW x %F FW=186 x .25=46.5 lbs.
2. LBM=BW–FW LBM=186–46.5=139.5 lbs.
3. IPF: 12% (.12 in decimal form)
4. IBW=LBM/(1.0–IFP) IBW=139.5/(1.0–.12)
   IBW=139.5/.88=158.5 lbs.

Now it is your turn. Calculate your own ideal body weight using the form provided in Figure 5.4. Extra spaces are provided for you to repeat your computations at regular intervals. If you initiate a diet/exercise program, it is recommended that you repeat the computations about once a month to monitor changes in body composition. This is important, because lean body mass is affected by weight reduction programs as well

Table 5.4.
Body Composition Classification According to Percent Body Fat

Age	Ideal	Good	Moderate	Fat	Obese
MEN					
<19	12	12.5-17.0	17.5-22.0	22.5-27.0	27.5+
20-29	13	13.5-18.0	18.5-23.0	23.5-28.0	28.5+
30-39	14	14.5-19.0	19.5-24.0	24.5-29.0	29.5+
40-49	15	15.5-20.0	20.5-25.0	25.5-30.0	30.5+
50+	16	16.5-21.5	21.5-26.0	26.5-31.0	31.5+
WOMEN					
Age	**Ideal**	**Good**	**Moderate**	**Fat**	**Obese**
<19	17	17.5-22.0	22.5-27.0	27.5-32.0	32.5+
20-29	18	18.5-23.0	23.5-28.0	28.5-33.0	33.5+
30-39	19	19.5-24.0	24.5-29.0	29.5-34.0	34.5+
40-49	20	20.5-25.0	25.5-30.0	30.5-35.0	35.5+
50+	21	21.5-26.5	26.5-31.0	31.5-36.0	36.5+

as by physical activity. As lean body mass changes, so will your ideal body weight. The initial data on percent body fat, ideal body weight, and body composition classification should also be recorded in Appendix A, as has been done with the other fitness components.

An example of the changes in body composition resulting from a weight control/exercise program was seen in a coed aerobic dance course taught at The University of Texas of the Permian Basin. The class was taught during a six-week summer term, and students participated in aerobic dance routines four times per week for sixty minutes each time. The first and last day of classes were used to assess several physiological parameters, including body composition. Students were also given information on diet and nutrition and basically followed their own weight control program. At the end of the six weeks, the average weight loss for the entire class was only three pounds. However, since body composition was assessed, members of the class were surprised to find out that in reality the average fat loss was six pounds, accompanied by a three-pound increase in lean body mass.

When dieting, body composition should be reassessed periodically due to the effects of negative caloric intake on lean body mass. These effects will be explained in more detail in Chapter 6, but dieting does decrease lean body mass. This lean body mass loss can be reduced or eliminated if a sensible diet is combined with physical exercise.

Figure 5.4. *Computation Form for Ideal Body Weight*

Name: ______________________ Age: ________ Sex: ________

Date				
Body Weight (BW)				
Percent Fat (% F)*				
Fat Weight (FW) FW = BW x % F				
Lean Body Mass (LBM) LBM = BW - FW				
Ideal Percent Fat (IPF)*				
Ideal Body Weight (IBW) IBW = LBM/(1-IPF)				
Body Composition Category				

*Express percentages in decimal form (e.g., 25% = .25)

References

1. Angel, A., and D. A. K. Roncari. "Medical Complications of Obesity." *Canada Medical Association Journal* 119:1408-1411, 1978.
2. Cooper, K. H. *The Aerobics Program for Total Well-Being.* New York: Mount Evans and Co., 1982.
3. Craddock, D. *Obesity and its Management.* New York: Churchill Livingston, 1978.
4. Hubert, H. B., M. Feinleib, R. M. McNamara, and W. P. Castelli. "Obesity As An Independent Risk Factor for Cardiovascular Disease: A 26-Year Follow-Up of Participants in the Framingham Heart Study." *Circulation* 67:968-977, 1983.
5. Jackson, A. S., and M. L. Pollock. "Generalized Equations for Predicting Body Density of Men." *British Journal of Nutrition* 40:497-504, 1978.
6. Jackson, A. S., M. L. Pollock, and A. Ward. "Generalized Equations for Predicting Body Density of Women." *Medicine and Science in Sports and Exercise* 3:175-182, 1980.
7. Jensen, C. R., and A. G. Fisher. *Scientific Basis of Athletic Conditioning.* Philadelphia: Lea and Febiger, 1979.
8. Lamb, D. R. *Physiology of Exercise: Responses and Adaptations.* New York: McMillan Publishing Co., 1984.
9. McArdle, W. D., F. I. Katch, and V. L. Katch. *Exercise Physiology: Energy, Nutrition, and Human Performance.* Philadelphia: Lea and Febiger, 1981.
10. Petit, D. W. "The Psychological Consequences of Obesity." In Bray, G. A., and J. E. Bethune, editors, *Treatment and Management of Obesity.* New York: Harper and Row, 1974.
11. Pollock, M. L., J. H. Wilmore, and S. M. Fox III. *Exercise in Health and Disease.* Philadelphia: W. B. Saunders Co., 1984.
12. Powers, P. S. *Obesity: The Regulation of Weight.* Baltimore: Williams and Williams, 1980.
13. Siri, W. E. *Body Composition from Fluid Spaces and Density.* Berkeley, CA: Donner Laboratory of Medical Physics, University of California, 19 March 1956.
14. Wilmore, J. H., C. H. Brown, and J. A. Davis. "Body Physique and Composition of the Female Distance Runner." *Annals of the New York Academy of Sciences* 301:764-776, 1980.

CHAPTER SIX

Nutrition for Weight Control and Wellness

The science of nutrition studies the relationship of foods to optimal health and performance. Ample scientific evidence has long linked good nutrition to overall health and well-being. Proper nutrition signifies that a person's diet is supplying all of the essential nutrients to carry out normal tissue growth, repair, and maintenance. It also implies that the diet will provide sufficient substrates to obtain the energy necessary for work, physical activity, and relaxation. Unfortunately, the typical American diet is too high in calories, sugars, fats, and sodium, and not high enough in fiber; none of which is conducive to good health.

NUTRIENTS

The essential nutrients required by the human body are carbohydrates, fats, protein, vitamins, minerals, and water. The first three have been referred to as fuel nutrients because they are the only substances used to supply the energy necessary for work and normal body functions. Vitamins, minerals, and water have no caloric value but are still essential for normal body functions and maintenance of good health. In addition, many nutritionists like to add a seventh nutrient to this list that has received a great deal of attention recently — dietary fiber.

Carbohydrates

Carbohydrates are the major source of calories used by the body to provide energy for work, cell maintenance, and heat. They also play a crucial role in the digestion and regulation of fat and protein metabolism. Each gram of carbohydrates provides the human body with approximately four calories. Carbohydrates are found primarily in breads, cereals, fruits, and vegetables.

Carbohydrates are classified into two types. Simple carbohydrates (frequently denoted as sugar) are formed by simple or double sugar units with little nutritive value (e.g., candy, ice cream, pop, cakes, etc.). Eating too many simple carbohydrates can take up the place of more nutritive foods in the diet. Complex carbohydrates are formed by complex sugar chains and not only provide many valuable nutrients to the body, but can also be an excellent source of fiber or roughage.

Fats

Fats or lipids are also used as a source of energy in the human body. They are the most concentrated source of energy. Each gram of fat supplies nine calories to the body. Fats are also a part of the cell structure. They are used as stored energy and, as an insulator for body heat preservation. They provide shock absorption, supply essential fatty acids, and carry the fat-soluble vitamins A, D, E, and K. The basic sources of fat are milk, dairy products, and meats and alternates.

Depending on the source, fats can be classified into saturated and polyunsaturated (or unsaturated) fats. The saturated fats are those that do not melt at room temperature (e.g., meats, cheese, butter). Polyunsaturated fats are in liquid form at room temperature. In general, saturated fats increase the blood cholesterol level, while polyunsaturated fats decrease the cholesterol content (the role of cholesterol in health and disease will be discussed in Chapter 7).

Proteins

Proteins are the main substances used to build and repair tissues such as muscles, blood, internal organs, skin, hair, nails, and bones. They are a part of hormones, enzymes, and antibodies and help maintain normal body fluid balance. Proteins can also be used as a source of energy, but only if there are not enough carbohydrates and fats available. Each gram of protein yields about four calories of energy, and the primary sources are meats and alternates, milk, dairy products, and some breads and cereals.

Vitamins

Vitamins are organic substances essential for normal metabolism, growth, and development of the body. They are classified into two types based on their solubility: fat-soluble vitamins (A, D, E, and K), and water-soluble vitamins (B complex and C). Vitamins cannot be manufactured by the body; hence, they can only be obtained through a well-balanced diet. A description of the functions of each vitamin is presented in Figure 6.1.

Minerals

Minerals are inorganic elements found in the body and in food. They serve several important functions. Minerals are constituents of all cells, especially those found in hard parts of the body (bones, nails, teeth). They are crucial in the maintenance of water balance and the acid-base balance. They are essential components of respiratory pigments, enzymes, and enzyme systems, and they regulate muscular and nervous tissue excitability. The specific functions of some of the most important minerals are contained in Figure 6.2.

Water

Approximately 70 percent of total body weight is water. It is the most important nutrient and is involved in almost every vital body process. Water is used in digestion and absorption of food, in the circulatory process, in removing waste products, in building and rebuilding cells, and in the transport of other nutrients. Water is contained in almost all foods, but primarily in liquid foods, fruits, and vegetables. Besides the natural content in foods, it is recommended that every person drink at least eight to ten glasses of fluids a day.

Dietary Fiber

Dietary fiber is basically a type of complex carbohydrate made up of plant material that cannot be digested by the human body. It is mainly present in leaves, skins, roots, and seeds. Processing and refining foods removes almost all of the natural fiber. In our daily diets, the main sources of dietary fiber are whole grain cereals and breads, fruits, and vegetables.

Fiber is important in the diet because it binds water, yielding a softer stool that decreases transit time of food residues in the intestinal tract. Many researchers feel that speeding up the passage of food residues through the intestines decreases the risk for colon cancer, primarily because of the decreased time that cancer-causing agents remain in contact with the intestinal wall. The increased water content of the stool may also dilute the cancer-causing agents, decreasing the potency of these substances.

The risk for coronary disease also decreases with increased fiber intake. This decreased risk can be attributed to two factors. First, all too often saturated fats take the place of dietary fiber in the diet, therefore increasing cholesterol absorption and/or formation. Second, some specific water-soluble fibers such as pectin and guar gum found in beans, oats, corn, and fruits seem to bind cholesterol in the intestines, thereby preventing its absorption. In addition, several other health disorders have been linked to low fiber intake, including constipation, diverticulitis, hemorrhoids, ulcerative colitis, gallbladder disease, appendicitis, and obesity.

Determining the amount of fiber in your diet can be confusing at times, because it is often measured as crude fiber rather than dietary fiber. Crude fiber is the smaller portion of the dietary fiber that actually remains after chemical extraction in the digestive tract. The recommended amount of dietary fiber is about twenty-five grams per day, or the equivalent of seven grams of crude fiber.

Figure 6.1. *Major Functions of Vitamins*

NUTRIENT	GOOD SOURCES	MAJOR FUNCTIONS	DEFICIENCY SYMPTOMS
Vitamin A	Milk, cheese, butter, fortified margarine, eggs, liver orange/ yellow/dark green fruits and vegetables	Required for healthy bones, teeth, skin, gums, and hair. Maintenance of inner mucous membranes, thus increasing resistance to infection. Adequate vision in dim light	Night blindness, decreased growth, decreased resistance to infection, rough-dry skin
Vitamin D	Fortified milk, cod liver oil, salmon, tuna, egg yolk	Necessary for bones and teeth. Needed for calcium and phosphorus absorption	Rickets (bone softening), fractures and muscle spasms
Vitamin E	Vegetable oils, yellow and green leafy vegetables, margarine, wheat germ, whole grain breads and cereals	Related to oxydation and normal muscle and red blood cell chemistry	Leg cramps, red blood cell breakdown
Vitamin K	Green leafy vegetables, cauliflower, cabbage, eggs, peas, and potatoes	Essential for normal blood clotting	Hemorrhaging
Vitamin B_1 (Thiamine)	Enriched bread, lean meat, fish, liver, pork, poultry, organ meats, legumes, nuts, dried yeast, and milk	Assists in proper use of carbohydrates. Normal functioning of nervous system. Maintenance of good appetite	Loss of appetite, nausea, confusion, cardiac abnormalities, muscle spasms
Vitamin B_2 (Riboflavine)	Eggs, milk, leafy green vegetables, whole grains, lean meats, dried beans and peas	Contributes to energy release from carbohydrates, fats, and proteins. Needed for normal growth and development, good vision and healthy skin	Cracking of the corners of the mouth, inflammation of the skin, impaired vision
Vitamin B_6 (Pyridoxine)	Vegetables, meats, whole grain cereals, soybeans, peanuts, and potatoes	Necessary for protein and fatty acids metabolism, and normal red blood cell formation	Depression, irritability, muscle spasms, nausea
Vitamin B_{12}	Meat, poultry, fish, liver, organ meats, eggs, shellfish, milk, and cheese	Required for normal growth, red blood cell formation, nervous system and digestive tract functioning	Impaired balance, weakness, drop in red blood cell count
Niacin	Liver and organ meats, meat, fish, poultry, whole grains, enriched breads, nuts, green leafy vegetables, and dried beans and peas	Contribute to energy release from carbohydrates, fats, and proteins. Normal growth and development, and formation of hormones and nerve-regulating substances	Confusion, depression, weakness, weight loss
Biotin	Liver, kidney, eggs, yeast, legumes, milk, nuts, dark green vegetables	Essential for carbohydrate metabolism and fatty acid synthesis	Inflamed skin, muscle pain, depression, weight loss
Folic Acid	Leafy green vegetables, organ meats, whole grains and cereals, and dried beans	Needed for cell growth and reproduction and red blood cell formation	Decreased resistance to infection
Pantothenic Acid	All natural foods, especially liver, kidney, eggs, nuts, yeast milk, dried peas and beans, and green leafy vegetables	Related to carbohydrate and fat metabolism	Depression, low blood sugar, leg cramps, nausea, headaches
Vitamin C (Ascorbic Acid)	Fruits and vegetables	Helps protect against infection. Formation of collagenous tissue. Normal blood vessels, teeth and bones	Slow healing wounds, loose teeth, hemorrhaging, rough-scaly skin, irritability

Figure 6.2. *Major Functions of Minerals*

NUTRIENT	GOOD SOURCES	MAJOR FUNCTIONS	DEFICIENCY SYMPTOMS
Calcium	Milk, cheese, green leafy vegetables, dried beans, sardines, salmon, and citrus fruits	Required for strong teeth and bone formation. Maintenance of good muscle tone, heart beat, and nerve function	Bone pain and fractures, periodontal disease, muscle cramps
Iron	Organ meats, lean meats, seafoods, eggs, dried peas and beans, nuts, whole and enriched grains, and green leafy vegetables	Major component of hemoglobin. Aids in energy utilization	Nutritional anemia, and overall weakness
Phosphorus	Meats, fish, milk, eggs, dried beans and peas, whole grains, and processed foods	Required for bone and teeth formation. Energy release regulation	Bone pain and fracture, weight loss, and weakness
Zinc	Milk, meat, seafood, whole grains, nuts, eggs, and dried beans	Essential component of hormones, insulin, and enzymes. Used in normal growth and development	Loss of appetite, slow healing wounds, and skin problems
Magnesium	Green leafy vegetables, whole grains, nuts, soybeans, seafood, and legumes	Needed for bone growth and maintenance. Carbohydrate and protein utilization. Nerve function. Temperature regulation	Irregular heartbeat, weakness, muscle spasms, and sleeplessness
Sodium	Table salt, processed foods, and meat	Body fluid regulation. Transmission of nerve impulse. Heart action	Rarely seen
Potassium	Legumes, whole grains, bananas, orange juice, dried fruits, and potatoes	Heart action. Bone formation and maintenance. Regulation of energy release. Acid-base regulation	Irregular heartbeat, nausea, weakness

Since most nutrition labels list the fiber content in terms of crude fiber, you should be careful to use the seven-gram guideline (*see* Table 6.1). Also, pay particular attention not to consume too much fiber, since excessive amounts can lead to increased loss of calcium, phosphorus, and iron, not to mention increased gastrointestinal discomfort. It is also important to increase fluid intake when dietary fiber is increased, since too little fluid can lead to dehydration and/or constipation.

THE BALANCED DIET

Most people would like to live life to its fullest, maintain good health, and lead a productive life. One of the fundamental ways to accomplish this goal is eating a well-balanced diet.

Generally, the daily caloric intake should be distributed in such a way that 50 to 60 percent of the calories come from complex carbohydrates, 25 to 30 percent from fat, and 15 to 20 percent

Table 6.1.
Crude Fiber Content of Selected Foods

Food	Serving Size	Crude Fiber (gr)
Almonds	½ cup	1.9
Apple	1 medium	1.5
Banana	1 medium	0.3
Beans (cooked)		
Kidney	½ cup	1.4
Lima	½ cup	1.3
White	½ cup	1.4
Blackberries	½ cup	3.0
Beets (cooked)	½ cup	0.7
Bran	2 tbsp.	0.9
Brazil nuts	½ cup	2.1
Broccoli (cooked)	½ cup	1.2
Brown rice (cooked)	½ cup	0.3
Carrots (cooked)	½ cup	0.8
Cashew nuts	½ cup	1.0
Cauliflower (cooked)	½ cup	0.6
Corn (cooked)	½ cup	0.6
Eggplant (cooked)	½ cup	0.9
Graham Crackers	2	0.4
Lettuce	3 leafs	0.3
Orange	1 medium	0.9
Parsnips (cooked)	½ cup	1.5
Peanuts (roasted)	½ cup	1.7
Pear	1 medium	2.2
Peas (cooked)	½ cup	1.5
Popcorn	3 cups	0.4
Potato (cooked)	1 medium	0.9
Rye Wafers	2	0.3
Strawberries	½ cup	0.9
Stringbeans (cooked)	½ cup	0.8
Summer squash (cooked)	½ cup	0.6
Watermelon	1 cup	0.4
Zucchini (cooked)	½ cup	0.7

Source: Calculated from Composition of Foods, Agriculture Handbook No. 8 and Nutritive Value of American Foods in Common Units, Agriculture Handbook No. 456. U.S. Dept. of Agriculture.

from protein. Less than half of your fat calories should come from saturated fats. In addition, all of the vitamins, minerals, and water must be provided. Achieving and maintaining a balanced diet is not as difficult as most people think. The difficult part is retraining yourself to eat the right type of foods and avoid those that have little or no nutritive value. Yet, most people are not willing to change their eating patterns. Even when faced with such conditions as obesity, elevated blood lipids, hypertension, etc., people still do not change. The motivating factor seems to be when a major health breakdown actually occurs (e.g., a heart attack, a stroke, cancer). By this time the damage has already been done. In many cases it is irreversible and for some, fatal.

Dietary Analysis

The initial step to rate your present diet can be done by conducting a nutritional analysis. This analysis can be quite an educational experience, because most people do not realize how detrimental and non-nutritious many common foods are. To analyze your own diet in terms of total nutrition, keep a three-day record of everything that you eat. Record this information in Figure E.1, found in Appendix E. At the end of each day, look up the nutrient content for everything that you ate in "The Nutritive Value of Selected Foods" chart, also contained in Appendix E. This information should be recorded in the respective spaces provided in your three-day listing of foods in Figure E.1. If you do not find a particular food in the list given in Appendix E, the information is often provided on the food container itself, or you may refer to the references given at the end of the Appendix. After recording the nutritive values for each day, add up each column and record the totals at the bottom of the chart. Following the third day, use Figure E.2 and compute an average for the three days. You may now compare your results against the Recommended Dietary Allowance (RDA) given at the end of Figure E.2. The results of your analysis will give you a good indication of areas of strength and deficiency in your current diet. The only question that still remains to be answered is whether your total caloric intake is adequate. This question will be answered later in this chapter.

Achieving a Balanced Diet

If you have read in detail Figures 6.1 and 6.2 (Vitamins and Minerals) and have done a careful analysis of your diet, you have probably found out that in order to have a good/balanced diet you must eat a variety of foods as well as decrease the daily intake of fats and sweets.

Although balancing a diet may seem very complex, simple guidelines to achieve an optimal diet are given in Figure 6.3. The basic rules of this "New American Eating Guide" are (a) to eat the minimum number of servings required for each one of the four basic food groups, and (b) obtain a final positive ("+") score at the end of each day. If these two simple principles are met, your diet will most likely have all of the required nutrients for proper body functions.

Figure 6.3. *The New American Eating Guide*

NEW AMERICAN EATING GUIDE

Instructions

Eating can be a real joy, especially when you know that your diet is keeping you healthy. Eat foods from each of the four groups every day. Each food group contains different nutrients that your body needs. But each group has some foods that are better than others. This figure will help you pick the foods that best contribute to good health. A good diet consists of vegetalbes, fruits, whole wheat bread and grains, potatoes, beans, lean meat, fish, poultry, and low-fat dairy products. This diet is high in nutrients and low in fat, sugar, salt and cholesterol. Pick plenty of ANYTIME foods— they should be the backbone of your diet. They are low in fat whole grains, and therefore high in fiber and trace minerals. Next best are the IN MODERATION foods. They contain moderate amounts of either saturated fats[1] or unsaturated fats[2]. Some items contain large amounts of fat, but mostly mono-unsaturated or polyunsaturated[3]. (The small numbers listed after items in the chart denote a food's drawbacks.) Eat small portions of NOW & THEN foods and eat them less often than the other foods. They are usually high in fat, with large amounts of saturated fats[4], or they are very high in added sugar[5], salt[6], or cholesterol[7]. Foods that are sometimes high in salt, depending on the manufacturer or recipe, are designated[(6)]. Try to eat only two NOW & THEN foods a day. Foods that contain low to moderate amounts of fat but are high in sugar, salt, cholesterol, or refined grains[8], are usually moved one or sometimes two categories to the right. You can make a game out of rating your diet by keeping track of the foods you eat for one or several days. ANYTIME foods get one point; IN MODERATION foods do not get any points; and NOW & THEN foods lose one point. If you have a "+" score, congratulations! If you have a "-" score, shape up! BON APPETIT!

1—moderate fat, saturated 2—moderate fat, unsaturated 3—high fat, unsaturated 4—high fat, saturated 5—high in added sugar
6—high in salt or sodium (6)—may be high in salt or sodium 7—high in cholesteral 8—refined grains

	Anytime	In Moderation	Now & Then
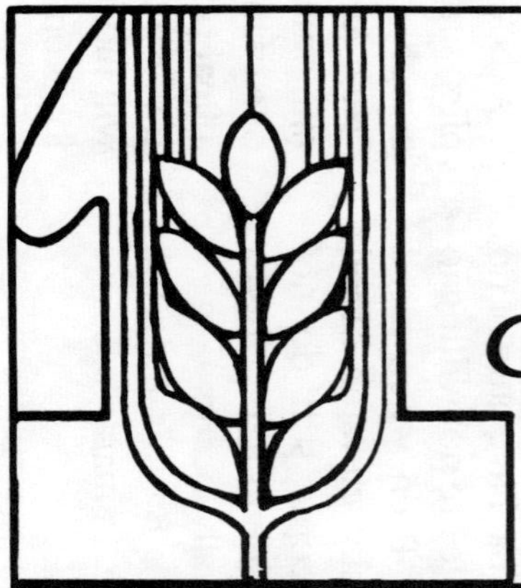 *group 1* **Beans, Grains & Nuts** FOUR OR MORE SERVINGS/DAY	bread & rolls (whole grain) bulghur dried beans & peas (legumes) lentils oatmeal pasta, whole wheat rice, brown rye bread sprouts whole grain hot & cold cereals whole wheat matzoh	cornbread - 8 flour tortilla - 8 granola cereals - 1 or 2 hominy grits - 8 macaroni and cheese - 1, (6), 8 matzoh - 8 nuts - 3 pasta, except whole wheat - 8 peanut butter - 3 pizza - 6, 8 refined, unsweetened cereals - 8 refried beans, commercial - 1, or homemade in oil - 2 seeds - 3 soybeans - 2 tofu - 2 waffles or pancakes with syrup - 5, (6), 8 white bread and rolls - 8 white rice - 8	croissant - 4, 8 doughnut (yeast-leavened) - 3 or 4, 5, 8 presweetened breakfast cereals - 5, 8 sticky buns - 1 or 2, 5, 8 stuffing (made with butter) - 4, (6), 8
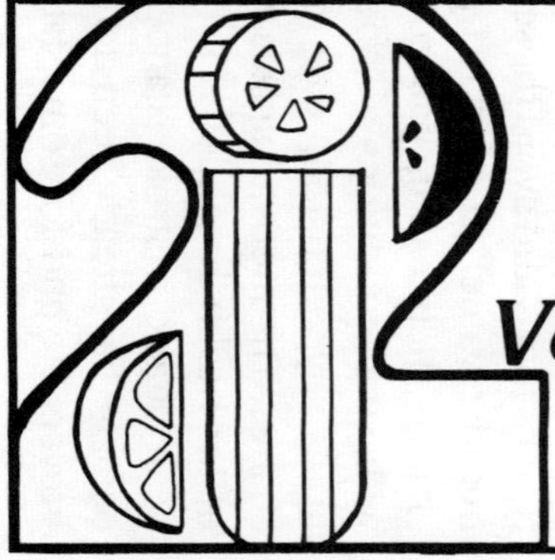 *group 2* **Fruits & Vegetables** FOUR OR MORE SERVINGS/DAY	all fruits and vegetables except those listed at right applesauce (unsweetened) unsweetened fruit juices unsalted vegetable juices potatoes, white or sweet	avocado - 3 cole slaw - 3 cranberry sauce (canned) - 5 dried fruit french fries, homemade in vegetable oil - 2, commercial - 1 fried eggplant (vegetable oil) - 2 fruits canned in syrup - 5 gazpacho - 2, (6) glazed carrots - 5, (6) guacamole - 3 potatoes au gratin - 1, (6) salted vegetable juices - 6 sweetened fruit juices - 5 vegetables canned with salt - 6	coconut - 4 pickles - 6

 group 3 **Milk Products** **CHILDREN: 3 TO 4 SERVINGS/DAY** **ADULTS: 2 SERVINGS/DAY**	buttermilk made from skim milk lassi (low-fat yogurt & fruit juice drink) low-fat cottage cheese low-fat milk, 1% milkfat low-fat yogurt non-fat dry milk skim milk cheeses - (6) skim milk skim milk & banana shake	cocoa made with skim milk - 5 cottage cheese, regular, 4% milkfat - 1 frozen lowfat yogurt - 5 ice milk - 5 low-fat milk, 2% milkfat - 1 low-fat yogurt, sweetened - 5 mozzarella cheese, part-skim type only - 1, (6)	cheesecake - 4, 5 cheese fondue - 4, (6) cheese souffle - 4, (6), 7 egg nog - 1, 5, 7 hard cheeses: bleu, brick, camembert, cheddar, muenster, swiss - 4, (6) ice cream - 4, 5 processed cheeses - 4, 6 whole milk - 4 whole milk yogurt - 4
 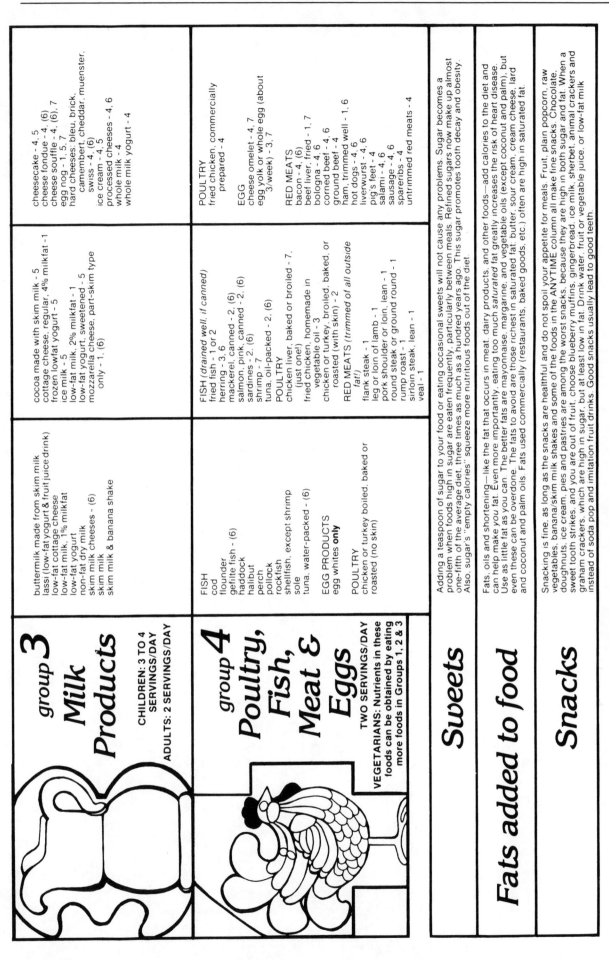 group 4 **Poultry, Fish, Meat & Eggs** **TWO SERVINGS/DAY** **VEGETARIANS: Nutrients in these foods can be obtained by eating more foods in Groups 1, 2 & 3**	FISH cod flounder gefilte fish - (6) haddock halibut perch pollock rockfish shellfish, except shrimp sole tuna, water-packed - (6) EGG PRODUCTS egg whites **only** POULTRY chicken or turkey boiled, baked or roasted (no skin)	FISH *(drained well, if canned)* fried fish - 1 or 2 herring - 3, 6 mackerel, canned - 2, (6) salmon, pink, canned - 2, (6) sardines - 2, (6) shrimp - 7 tuna, oil-packed - 2, (6) POULTRY chicken liver, baked or broiled - 7, (just one!) fried chicken, homemade in vegetable oil - 3 chicken or turkey, broiled, baked, or roasted (with skin) - 2 RED MEATS *(trimmed of all outside fat!)* flank steak - 1 leg or loin of lamb - 1 pork shoulder or loin, lean - 1 round steak or ground round - 1 rump roast - 1 sirloin steak, lean - 1 veal - 1	POULTRY fried chicken, commercially prepared - 4 EGG cheese omelet - 4, 7 egg yolk or whole egg (about 3/week) - 3, 7 RED MEATS bacon - 4, (6) beef liver, fried - 1, 7 bologna - 4, 6 corned beef - 4, 6 ground beef - 4 ham, trimmed well - 1, 6 hot dogs - 4, 6 liverwurst - 4, 6 pig's feet - 4 salami - 4, 6 sausage - 4, 6 spareribs - 4 untrimmed red meats - 4

Sweets

Adding a teaspoon of sugar to your food or eating occasional sweets will not cause any problems. Sugar becomes a problem when foods high in sugar are eaten frequently, particularly between meals. Refined sugars now make up almost one-fifth of the average diet, three times as much as a hundred years ago. This sugar promotes tooth decay and obesity. Also, sugar's "empty calories" squeeze more nutritious foods out of the diet.

Fats added to food

Fats, oils and shortening—like the fat that occurs in meat, dairy products, and other foods—add calories to the diet and can help make *you* fat. Even more importantly, eating too much *saturated* fat greatly increases the risk of heart disease. Use as little fat as you can. The better fats are mayonnaise, margarine, and vegetable oils (except coconut and palm), but even these can be overdone. The fats to avoid are those richest in saturated fat: butter, sour cream, cream cheese, lard and coconut and palm oils. Fats used commercially (restaurants, baked goods, etc.) often are high in saturated fat.

Snacks

Snacking is fine, as long as the snacks are healthful and do not spoil your appetite for meals. Fruit, plain popcorn, raw vegetables, banana/skim milk shakes and some of the foods in the ANYTIME column all make fine snacks. Chocolate, doughnuts, ice cream, pies and pastries are among the worst snacks, because they are high in both sugar and fat. When a sweet tooth strikes, and you are out of fruit, choose blueberry muffins, gingerbread, ice milk, sherbet, animal crackers and graham crackers, which are high in sugar, but at least low in fat. Drink water, fruit or vegetable juice, or low-fat milk instead of soda pop and imitation fruit drinks. Good snacks usually lead to good teeth.

One serving equals: Group 1 = 1 slice of bread, 1 cup ready-to-eat cereal, ½ cup cooked cereal/pasta/grits, or equivalent; Group 2 = ½ cup cooked or juice, 1 cup raw, or 1 medium size fruit; Group 3 = 1 cup milk/yogurt, 1½ oz. cheese, 1 cup pudding/ice cream, 2 cups cottage cheese, or equivalent; Group 4 = 2 oz. cooked lean meat/fish/poultry, 2 eggs, or equivalent.

Figure 6.4. *Daily Diet Record Form*

Name: ____________________ **Dates:** ________ **to** ________

Daily Caloric Intake: ____________ **calories**[1]

Day of Month

Food Group	Code[2]	Scr.[3]	Cal.[4]	Code	Scr.	Cal.	Code	Scr.	Cal.	Code	Scr.	Cal.	Code	Scr.	Cal.	Code	Scr.	Cal.	Code	Scr.	Cal.	Code	Scr.	Cal.
Group 1 **Beans, Grains** **& Nuts** **4 Servings**																								
Meet Req. Serv.																								
Group 2 **Fruits &** **Vegetables** **4 Servings**																								
Meet Req. Serv.																								
Group 3 **Milk Products** **2 Servings** (children 3-4 Serv.)																								
Meet Req. Serv.																								
Group 4 **Poultry, Meat** **Fish & Eggs** **2 Servings**																								
Meet Req. Serv.																								
Totals																								

[1]Refer to Figure 6.5. [2]Code, use Appendix E. [3]Scr. = Score ("+", "NP", "-"), use Figure 6.3. [4]Cal. = Calories, refer to Appendix E.

Figure 6.4. *Daily Diet Record Form*

Name: ______________________ **Dates:** ________ **to** ________

Daily Caloric Intake: ____________ **calories**[1]

Day of Month

Food Group	Code[2]	Scr.[3]	Cal.[4]	Code	Scr.	Cal.	Code	Scr.	Cal.	Code	Scr.	Cal.	Code	Scr.	Cal.	Code	Scr.	Cal.	Code	Scr.	Cal.	Code	Scr.	Cal.
Group 1 **Beans, Grains** **& Nuts** **4 Servings**																								
Meet Req. Serv.																								
Group 2 **Fruits &** **Vegetables** **4 Servings**																								
Meet Req. Serv.																								
Group 3 **Milk Products** **2 Servings** (children 3-4 Serv.)																								
Meet Req. Serv.																								
Group 4 **Poultry, Meat** **Fish & Eggs** **2 Servings**																								
Meet Req. Serv.																								
Totals																								

[1]Refer to Figure 6.5. [2]Code, use Appendix E. [3]Scr. = Score ("+", "NP", "-"), use Figure 6.3. [4]Cal. = Calories, refer to Appendix E.

Figure 6.4. *Daily Diet Record Form*

Name: ______________________ **Dates:** ________ **to** ________

Daily Caloric Intake: ____________ **calories**[1]

Day of Month

Food Group	Code[2]	Scr.[3]	Cal.[4]	Code	Scr.	Cal.	Code	Scr.	Cal.	Code	Scr.	Cal.	Code	Scr.	Cal.	Code	Scr.	Cal.	Code	Scr.	Cal.	Code	Scr.	Cal.
Group 1 **Beans, Grains** **& Nuts** **4 Servings**																								
Meet Req. Serv.																								
Group 2 **Fruits &** **Vegetables** **4 Servings**																								
Meet Req. Serv.																								
Group 3 **Milk Products** **2 Servings** (children 3-4 Serv.)																								
Meet Req. Serv.																								
Group 4 **Poultry, Meat** **Fish & Eggs** **2 Servings**																								
Meet Req. Serv.																								
Totals																								

[1]Refer to Figure 6.5. [2]Code, use Appendix E. [3]Scr. = Score ("+", "NP", "-"), use Figure 6.3. [4]Cal. = Calories, refer to Appendix E.

To aid you in the achievement of this goal the log contained in Figure 6.4 can be used to record your data. This record sheet will be much easier to keep than the complete dietary analysis. First, make a copy of Figure 6.3 and post it somewhere visible in the kitchen or keep it with you at all times. Now use Figure 6.4, and whenever you have something to eat, record the code of the food and the "+", "NP" (no points), or "–" characters in the corresponding spaces provided for each day. If you are on a weight reduction program, you should also record the caloric content of each food. This information can be obtained from Appendix E, the food container itself, or some of the references given at the end of the Appendix. Try to record all the information immediately after each meal, since it will be easier to keep track of foods and the amount eaten. If you eat twice the amount of a particular serving, make sure that you double the calories and also record the two "+", "–" or "NP" characters. At the end of the day, evaluate your diet by checking whether you have eaten the minimum required servings for each group, and by adding up the "+" and "–" points accumulated. If you have met the required servings and ended up with a positive score, you are "well" on your way toward a well-balanced diet. Additional tips on nutrition as related to cardiovascular disease, cancer prevention, and weight control will be outlined in Chapters 7, 8, and 11.

NUTRITION AND WEIGHT CONTROL

Achieving and maintaining ideal body weight (ideal body fat percentage) is a major objective of a good physical fitness and wellness program. Next to poor cardiovascular fitness, obesity is the most common problem encountered in fitness and wellness assessments. Estimates indicate that only 5 percent of all the people that ever initiate a traditional weight loss program are able to lose the desired weight, and worse yet, only one in 200 is able to keep the weight off for a significant period of time. You may ask why the traditional diets have failed. The answer, as you will learn in this chapter, is that very few diets teach the importance of lifetime changes in food selection and the role of exercise as the keys to successful weight loss. Although only a few years ago the principles that govern a weight loss and maintenance program seemed to be pretty clear, we now know that the final answers are not yet in.

The basic concepts related to weight control have been centered around three assumptions: (1) that balancing food intake against output allows a person to achieve ideal weight, (2) that fat people just eat too much, and (3) that it really does not matter to the human body how much (or little) fat is stored. While there may be a lot of truth to these statements, they are still open to much debate and research.

The Energy-Balancing Equation

The energy-balancing equation basically states that as long as caloric input equals caloric output, the person will not gain or lose weight. If caloric intake exceeds the output, the individual will gain weight. When output exceeds input, weight is lost. This principle is quite simple, and if daily energy requirements could be accurately determined, it seems reasonable that the conscious mind could be used to balance caloric intake versus output. Unfortunately, this is not always the case. There are individual differences, genetic- and lifestyle-related, that will affect different people in different ways.

Perhaps some examples may help explain this. It is well known that one pound of fat equals 3,500 calories. Assuming that the basic daily caloric expenditure for a given person is 2,500 calories, if this person decreased the daily intake by 500 calories per day, one pound of fat should be lost in seven days (500 x 7 = 3,500). Research has shown, however, and many dieters have probably experienced, that even when caloric input is carefully balanced against caloric ouptut, weight loss does not always come as predicted. Furthermore, two people with similar measured caloric intake and output will not necessarily lose weight at the same rate.

The most common explanation given by many in the past regarding individual differences in weight loss or weight gain was variations in human metabolism from one person to the other. We have all seen people that can eat all day long and yet not gain an ounce of weight, while others cannot even "dream" about food without gaining weight. Since many experts did not believe that such extreme differences could be accounted to human metabolism alone, several theories have been developed that may better explain these individual variations.

Setpoint Theory

Recent scientific research has indicated that there is a weight-regulating mechanism (WRM) located in the hypothalamus of the brain that regulates how much the body should weigh. This mechanism has a setpoint that controls both appetite and the amount of fat stored. It is hypothesized that the setpoint works like a thermostat for body fat, maintaining body weight fairly constant because it knows at all times the exact amount of adipose tissue stored in the fat cells. Some people have high settings, and others are quite low. If body weight decreases (as in dieting), this change is sensed by the setpoint, which in turn triggers the WRM to increase the person's appetite or make the body conserve energy to maintain the "set" weight. The opposite may also be true. Some people who consciously try to gain weight have an extremely difficult time in doing so. In this case, the WRM decreases appetite or causes the body to waste energy to maintain the lower weight.

Dieting Can Make You Fat!

Every person has his or her own certain body fat percentage (as established by the setpoint) that the body attempts to maintain. The genetic instinct to survive tells the body that fat storage is vital, and therefore it sets an inherently acceptable fat level. This level of fat remains pretty constant or may gradually climb due to poor lifestyle habits. For instance, under strict caloric reductions, the body may make extreme metabolic adjustments in an effort to maintain its setpoint for fat. The basal metabolic rate may drop dramatically against a consistent negative caloric balance, and a person may be on a plateau for days or even weeks without losing much weight. Dietary restriction alone will not lower the setpoint even though weight and fat may be lost. When the dieter goes back to a normal or even below normal caloric intake, at which the weight may have been stable for a long period of time, the fat loss is quickly regained as the body strives to regain a comfortable fat store.

Let us use a practical illustration. You would like to lose some body fat and assume that you have presently reached a stable weight at an average daily caloric intake of 1,800 calories (you do not gain or lose weight at this daily intake). You now start a strict low-calorie diet, or even worse, a near-fasting diet in an attempt to achieve rapid weight loss. Immediately the body activates its survival mechanism and readjusts its metabolism to a lower caloric balance. After a few weeks of dieting at less than 400 to 600 calories per day, the body can now maintain its normal functions at 1,000 calories per day. Having lost the desired weight, you terminate your diet, but know that if you go back to your original caloric intake of 1,800 calories per day, the weight may be gained back. Therefore, to adjust to the new lower body weight, you restrict your intake to 1,500 calories per day and may be surprised that even at this lower intake (300 fewer calories), you are gaining weight back at a rate of one pound every one to two weeks. This new lowered metabolic rate, as pointed out in a recent Swedish study, may take a year or more after terminating the diet to kick back up to its normal level.

From this explanation, it is clear that individuals should never go on very low-calorie diets. Not only will this practice decrease your resting metabolic rate, but it will also deprive the body of the basic daily nutrients required for normal physiological functions. Under no circumstances should a person ever engage in diets below 1,200 and 1,500 calories for women and men, respectively. Remember that weight (fat) is gained over a period of months and years and not overnight. Equally, weight loss should be accomplished gradually and not abruptly. Daily caloric intakes of 1,200 to 1,500 calories will still provide the necessary nutrients if properly distributed over the four basic food groups (meeting the daily required servings from each group). Of course, the individual will have to learn which foods meet the requirements, and yet are low in calories. This can be easily learned after only a few days of dieting using the "New American Eating Guide," as well as keeping track of the total number of calories consumed.

Setpoint and Nutrition

Other researchers feel that a second way in which the setpoint may work is by keeping track of the nutrients and calories that you consume on a daily basis. Your body, like a cash register, records the daily food intake, and the brain will not feel satisfied until the calories and nutrients have been "registered."

For some people this setpoint for calories and nutrients seems to work regardless of the amount of physical activity that they do, as long as it is not too exhausting. Numerous studies have shown that appetite does not increase with moderate physical activity. Hence, you can choose to lose weight by either going hungry, or by only reducing somewhat your caloric intake (not to offset the setpoint), along with an increase in daily physical (aerobic) activity. The increased number of calories burned through exercise will help decrease body fat.

The most common question that individuals seem to have regarding the setpoint is how can it be lowered so that the body will feel comfortable at a lower fat percentage. Several factors seem to have a direct effect on the setpoint. Aerobic exercise and a diet high in complex carbohydrates, nicotine, and amphetamines all have been shown to decrease this fat thermostat. The last two, however, are more destructive than the overfatness, thereby eliminating themselves as reasonable alternatives (it has been said that as far as the extra strain on the heart is concerned, smoking one pack of cigarettes per day is the equivalent of carrying fifty to seventy-five pounds of excess body fat). On the other hand, a diet high in fats and refined carbohydrates, near-fasting diets, and even artificial sweeteners seem to increase the setpoint. Therefore, it looks as though the only practical and effective way to lower the setpoint and lose fat weight is through a combination of aerobic exercise and a diet high in complex carbohydrates.

Yellow Fat Versus Brown Fat

For years it has been known that there are two different types of fat, yellow and brown. The proportion of yellow to brown could be another factor that influences weight regulation. The average ratio is about 99 percent yellow fat to 1 percent brown fat. The difference between the two is that yellow fat simply stores energy in the form of fat, while brown fat has a high amount of the iron-containing hemoglobin pigment found in red blood cells. The brown cells do not store fat, but rather have the capacity to produce body heat by burning the fat. Under resting conditions, brown fat produces an estimated 25 percent of the total body heat, and according to Dr. George A. Bray of the Los Angeles Medical Center at Harbour University of California, the brown fat can actually produce as much heat as the entire rest of the body.

The fact that brown fat converts food energy to heat may also explain why some individuals simply do not gain weight. Even though the amount of brown fat is genetically determined and cannot be changed throughout life, people with only slightly higher levels may have an advantage when it comes to weight control. It is also possible that even if the percentage is the same, some indivduals may have active brown cells that generate more heat. Perhaps you have come across thin people who are warm even when everyone else seems quite comfortable. On the contrary, since one of the basic functions of fat is body heat preservation, obese people who are successful in losing weight but have a lower proportion or less active brown fat may feel cold when it is actually pleasantly warm.

Diet and Metabolism

Fat can be lost with dietary restrictions and/or aerobic exercise. However, when weight loss is pursued by means of dietary restrictions alone, there will always be a decrease in lean body mass (muscle protein, along with vital organ protein). The amount of lean body mass lost depends exclusively on the caloric restriction of your diet. In near-fasting diets, up to 50 percent of the weight loss can be lean body mass, and the other 50 percent will be actual fat loss. When diet is combined with exercise, 98 percent of the weight loss will be in the form of fat, and there may actually be an increase in lean tissue. Lean body mass loss is never desirable because it weakens the organs and muscles and slows down the metabolism.

Contrary to some beliefs, metabolism does not decrease with age. It has been shown that basal metabolism is directly related to lean body weight. The greater the lean tissue, the higher the metabolic rate. What happens is that as a result of sedentary living and less physical activity, the lean component decreases and fat tissue increases. The organism, though, continues to use the same amount of oxygen per pound of lean body mass. Since fat is considered metabolically inert from the point of view of caloric use, the lean tissue uses most of the oxygen even at rest.

Consequently, as muscle and organ mass decreases, the energy requirements at rest also decrease.

Decreases in lean body mass are commonly seen with aging (due to physical inactivity) and severely restricted diets. The loss of lean body mass may also account for the lower metabolic rate described under "dieting makes you fat" and the lengthy period of time that it takes to kick back up. There are no diets with caloric intakes below 1,200 to 1,500 calories that can insure no loss of lean body mass. Even at this intake, there is some loss unless the diet is combined with exercise. Many diets have claimed that the lean component is unaltered with their particular diet, but the simple truth is that regardless of what nutrients may be added to the diet, if caloric restrictions are too severe, there will always be a loss of lean tissue.

Unfortunately, too many people constantly engage in low-calorie diets, and every time they do so the metabolic rate keeps slowing down as more lean tissue is lost. It is not uncommon to find individuals in the forties or older who weigh the same as they did when they were twenty and feel that they are at ideal body weight. Nevertheless, during this span of twenty years or more, they have dieted all too many times without engaging in physical activity. The weight is regained shortly after terminating each diet, but most of that gain is in fat. Perhaps at age twenty they weighed 150 pounds and were only 15 to 16 percent fat. Now at age forty, even though they still weigh 150 pounds, they may be 30 to 40 percent fat. They may feel that they are at ideal body weight and wonder why it is that they are eating very little and still have a difficult time maintaining weight.

Exercise: The Key to Weight Loss

Based on the preceding discussion on weight control, you have probably concluded that exercise is the key to weight loss. If you have done so, you are totally right. Not only will exercise maintain lean tissue, but advocates of the setpoint theory also indicate that it resets your fat thermostat to a new lower level. For a lot of people this change occurs rapidly, but in some instances it may take time. In one particular case, a significantly overweight woman faithfully exercised on an almost daily basis, sixty minutes at a time, for a whole year before significant weight changes started to occur. Those individuals who have a very "sticky" setpoint will need to be patient and persistent.

If you do have a weight problem, the type of exercise that offsets the setpoint has to be aerobic in nature. In addition, you should also engage in a weight training program, since this type of training has the greatest impact in increasing lean body mass. Weight training is especially recommended for those who feel that they are at optimal body weight, but yet the body fat percentage is higher than ideal. The guidelines for weight training programs have already been introduced and are given in Chapter 3.

Keep in mind, however, that the most effective type of exercise to lose weight is aerobic exercise. The number of calories burned following an hour of aerobic exercise is much greater than during an hour of weight training. Due to the high intensity of weight training, frequent rest intervals are required to recover from each set of exercise. The average individual only engages in actual lifting a total of twelve minutes out of every hour of exercise. Weight loss can occur with a regular weight training program, but at a much slower rate.

It is also important to clarify that just doing several sets of daily sit-ups will not help to get rid of fat in the midsection of the body. Research has shown that there is no such thing as spot reducing. When fat comes off, it does so from throughout the entire body, and not just the exercised area. The greatest proportion of fat may come off the largest fat deposits, but the caloric output of a few sets of sit-ups is practically nil to have a real effect on total body fat reduction. The amount of exercise has to be much longer to have a real impact on weight reduction.

Although we now know that a negative caloric balance of 3,500 calories will not always result in an exact loss of one pound of fat, a negative balance, either by exercising more, eating less, or both, is a must to lose weight. Unless there is some type of pathological condition, there simply are no "miracle" diet programs to help you lose weight in a quick and easy way.

Sadly, some individuals claim that the amount of calories burned during exercise is hardly worth the effort. These individuals feel that it is easier to cut the daily intake by some 200 calories, rather than participate in some sort of physical activity that would burn the equivalent amount of calories. The only problem is that the willpower to cut those 200 calories only lasts a few weeks, and then it is right back to the old eating patterns. If you get into the habit of exercising regularly, say three times per week, running three miles per exercise session (about 300 calories burned), this would represent 900 calories in one week, 3,600 in one month, or 43,200 calories per year. This apparently insignificant amount of exercise could mean as many as twelve extra pounds of fat in one year, twenty-four in two, and so on. We tend to forget that our weight creeps up gradually over the years, and not just overnight. Hardly worth the effort? And we have not even taken into consideration the increase in lean tissue, the possible resetting of the setpoint, the benefits to the cardiovascular system, and most important, the improved quality of life! There is very little argument that the fundamental reasons for overfatness and obesity are physical inactivity and sedentary living.

LOSING WEIGHT THE SOUND AND SENSIBLE WAY

Dieting has never been fun and never will be. If you have a weight problem and you are serious about losing weight, you will have to make exercise a regular part of your daily life, along with sensible adjustments in your caloric intake.

What form of exercise is best? For those who are significantly overweight, you should choose an activity where you will not have to support your own body weight, but that will still be effective in burning calories. Joint and muscle injuries are very common among overweight individuals who participate in weight-bearing exercises such as walking, jogging, and aerobic dancing. Swimming may not be a good exercise either. The increased body fat makes the person more buoyant, and most people do not have the skill level to swim fast enough to get the heart rate in the optimal target zone (see Chapter 2). The tendency is to just "float" along, limiting the amount of calories burned, as well as the benefits to the cardiovascular system. Some better alternatives are riding a bicycle (either road or stationary), walking in a shallow pool, or running in place in deep water (treading water). The last exercise is quickly gaining in popularity and has proven to be effective in achieving weight reduction without the "pain" and fear of injuries.

How long should each exercise session last? To develop and maintain cardiovascular fitness, twenty to thirty minutes of exercise at the ideal target rate, three to five times per week is sufficient. For weight loss purposes, many experts recommend exercising for an hour at a time, five to six times per week. Do not try to increase your duration and frequency too fast. Use the exercise prescription given in Chapter 2 (Figure 2.9), and thereafter increase the duration by five minutes each week. This practice will not only insure a high caloric output, but due to the prolonged duration of exercise, the metabolic rate will remain at a higher level long after you have finished the exercise session. In other words, extra calories are still being burned even though you are all done exercising. The longer the duration of exercise in the appropriate target zone, the longer it takes the body to recover. Therefore, a greater number of calories can still be burned in excess of those used during the normal resting state.

One final benefit of exercise as related to weight control is that fat can be burned more efficiently. Since both carbohydrates and fats are sources of energy, when the glucose levels begin to decrease during prolonged exercise, more fat is used as an energy substrate. Equally important is the fact that fat-burning enzymes increase with aerobic training. The role of these enzymes is quite significant, because fat can only be lost by burning it in muscle. As the concentration of the enzymes increases, so does the ability to burn fat.

How To Set Up Your Own Weight Control Program

To write your own weight control program, you will need to determine your typical daily caloric intake, including exercise, required to maintain your current weight (use Figure 6.5). The first step is to estimate your daily caloric requirement without exercise. This requirement is based on typical lifestyle patterns, total body weight, and gender. Individuals who hold jobs that require heavy manual labor burn more calories during the day as opposed to sedentary jobs, such as working behind a desk. To determine your activity level, refer to Table 6.2 and rate yourself accordingly. Since the number given in Table 6.2 is per pound of body weight, multiply your current body weight by that number. For example, the typical caloric requirement to maintain body weight for a moderately active male who weighs 160 pounds would be 2,400 calories (160 lbs. x 15 cal/lb.).

Figure 6.5. *Computation Form for Daily Caloric Intake.*

Name: ______________________________ Sex: ________

A. Date	____	____	____	____
B. Weight	____	____	____	____
C. Caloric requirement per/lb of body weight (Table 6.2)	____	____	____	____
D. Typical daily caloric intake (B × C)	____	____	____	____
E. Selected physical activity	____	____	____	____
F. Number of exercise sessions per/week	____	____	____	____
G. Duration of each exercise session (in minutes)	____	____	____	____
H. Total weekly exercise time in minutes (F × G)	____	____	____	____
I. Average daily exercise time in minutes (H ÷ 7)	____	____	____	____
J. Caloric expenditure per/lb/min of activity (Table 6.3)	____	____	____	____
K. Calories burned per/min of physical activity (B × J)	____	____	____	____
L. Average daily calories burned as a result of exercise (I × K)	____	____	____	____
M. Total daily caloric intake with exercise (D + L)	____	____	____	____
N. Number of calories to subtract from daily intake in order to achieve a negative balance[a]	____	____	____	____
O. Target caloric intake to lose weight (M − N)	____	____	____	____

[a]Subtract 500 if total daily intake with exercise (M) is below 3,000. As many as 1,000 may be subtracted for daily intakes above 3,000.

Table 6.2.
Average Caloric Requirement Per Pound of Body Weight Based on Lifestyle Patterns and Sex

	Calories per pound	
Activity Rating	**Men**	**Women[a]**
Sedentary — Limited physical activity	13.0	12.0
Moderate physical activity	15.0	13.5
Hard labor — Strenuous physical effort	17.0	15.0

[a]Pregnant or lactating women add three calories to these figures.

The second step is to determine the average number of calories that are burned on a daily basis as a result of exercise. To obtain this number, look up the energy expenditure of the activity that you have selected for your exercise program in Table 6.3. Multiply that number by your body weight in pounds. Before you can figure out the average daily expenditure, determine the total number of minutes that you exercise on a weekly basis and divide this number by seven. For instance, if you are cycling at thirteen miles per hour, five times per week, for thirty minutes each time, your total weekly exercise time would be 150 minutes. The average daily exercise time would be twenty-one minutes (150 divided by 7 and round off to the lowest unit). Next, using Table 6.3, determine the energy requirement for the activity (or activities) that you have chosen for your exercise program. In the case of cycling (thirteen miles per hour), the requirement is .071 calories per minute of activity per pound of body weight (cal/min/lb). With a body weight of 160 pounds, each minute this man would burn 11.4 calories (body weight x .071 or 160 x .071). In twenty-one minutes he would burn approximately 240 calories. The total daily caloric intake to maintain his body weight would be the typical intake plus the average calories burned through exercise. In our example, it would be 2,640 calories (2,400 + 240).

Table 6.3.
Caloric Expenditure of Selected Physical Activities (expressed in calories per pound per minute of activity)

Activity	Cal/min/lb	Activity	Cal/min/lb
Archery	0.030	Rowing (vigorous)	0.090
Badminton		Running	
Recreation	0.038	11.0 min/mile	0.070
Competition	0.065	8.5 min/mile	0.090
Baseball	0.031	7.0 min/mile	0.102
Basketball		6.0 min/mile	0.114
Moderate	0.046	Deep water[a]	0.100
Competition	0.063	Skating (moderate)	0.038
Cycling (level)		Skiing	
5.5 mph	0.033	Downhill	0.060
10.0 mph	0.050	Level (5 mph)	0.078
13.0 mph	0.071	Soccer	0.059
Bowling	0.030	Swimming (crawl)	
Calisthenics	0.033	20 yrds/min	0.031
Dance		25 yrds/min	0.040
Moderate	0.030	45 yrds/min	0.057
Vigorous	0.055	50 yrds/min	0.070
Golf	0.030	Table Tennis	0.030
Gymnastics		Tennis	
Light	0.030	Moderate	0.045
Heavy	0.056	Competition	0.064
Handball	0.064	Volleyball	0.030
Hiking	0.040	Walking	
Judo/Karate	0.086	4.5 mph	0.045
Racquetball	0.065	Shallow pool	0.090
Rope Jumping	0.060	Wrestling	0.085

[a]Treading water (estimated value)

Adapted from:

Allsen, P. E., J. M. Harrison, B. Vance. *Fitness for Life: An Individualized Approach.* Dubuque, IA: Wm. C. Brown, 1984.
Bucher, C. A., and W. E. Prentice. *Fitness for College and Life.* St. Louis: Times Mirror/Mosby College Publishing, 1985.
Consolazio, C. F., R. E. Johnson, and L. J. Pecora. *Physiological Measurements of Metabolic Functions in Man.* New York: McGraw-Hill Book Company, 1963.
Hockey, R. V. *Physical Fitness: The Pathway to Healthful Living.* St. Louis: Times Mirror/Mosby College Publishing, 1985.

If this person wanted to lose weight, he would have to consume less than the 2,640 daily calories to achieve his objective. Because of the many different factors that play a role in weight control, the previous number is only an estimated daily requirement. Furthermore, to lose weight, it would be difficult to say that exactly one pound of fat would be lost in one week if daily intake was reduced by 500 calories (500 x 7 = 3,500 calories, or the equivalent of one pound of fat). Nevertheless, the estimated daily caloric figure will at least provide a good guideline for weight control.

The number of calories that you subtract from your daily intake to lose weight will depend on your typical daily requirements. Use Figure 6.5 to compute your own daily caloric needs. Periodic readjustments are necessary because there can be significant differences among individuals, and the estimated daily cost will change as you lose weight and modify your exercise habits. At this point, the best recommendation that can be made is to moderately decrease the daily intake, never below 1,200 calories for women and 1,500 for men. A good rule to follow is to restrict your intake by 500 or fewer calories if the daily requirement is below 3,000 calories. For caloric requirements in excess of 3,000, as many as 1,000 calories per day may be subtracted from your total intake. Most of your calories should come from complex carbohydrates. Your daily caloric distribution should be approximately 60 percent complex carbohydrates, 25 percent fat, and 15 percent protein. To monitor your daily diet, use Figure 6.4, but remember to always give priority to the basic requirements from each food group. The caloric content for each food that you eat is found in Appendix E. Record your information immediately after each meal, since no blanks could be provided in this form to list the actual foods and amounts eaten. Based on your progress, make necessary adjustments in your typical daily caloric intake and/or exercise program.

References

1. Bennett, W., and J. Gurin. "Do Diets Really Work?" *Science* 42-50, March 1982.
2. "Brown Fat is Good Fat." *The Health Letter.* December 11, 1981.
3. "Brown Fat/White Fat." *Aviation Medical Bulletin.* June, 1981.
4. "Dangerous Dieting." *The Health Letter.* July 25, 1980.
5. Girdano, D. A., D. Dusek, and G. S. Everly. *Experiencing Health.* Englewood Cliffs, NJ: Prentice-Hall, 1985.
6. "How to Balance Your Diet." *Fit* 46-47, April 1983.
7. *Interpreting Your Nutritional Analysis.* Lake Geneva, WI: Fitness Monitoring Preventive Medicine Clinic, 1984.
8. Kirschmann, J. D. *Nutrition Almanac.* New York: McGraw-Hill Book Company, 1979.
9. Morgan, B. L. G. *The Lifelong Nutrition Guide.* Englewood Cliffs, NJ: Prentice-Hall, 1983.
10. "Obesity Not Necessarily Related to Overeating." *Aviation Medical Bulletin.* June 1981.
11. Remington, D., A. G. Fisher, and E. A. Parent. *How to Lower Your Fat Thermostat.* Provo, UT: Vitality House International, Inc., 1983.
12. Shephard, R. J. *Alive Man: The Physiology of Physical Activity.* Springfield, IL: Charles C. Thomas Publisher, 1972.
13. "Use a Variety of Fibers." *The Health Letter.* March 1982.
14. "Vitamin Information for Patients." *Medical Times* 35, November 1982.

CHAPTER SEVEN

Cardiovascular Disease Risk Reduction

Cardiovascular disease is the leading cause of death in the United States, accounting for one-half of the total mortality rate in 1984. The disease refers to any pathological condition that affects the heart and the circulatory system (blood vessels). Some examples of cardiovascular diseases are coronary heart disease, peripheral vascular disease, congenital heart disease, rheumatic heart disease, atherosclerosis, strokes, high blood pressure, and congestive heart failure. Although heart and blood vessel disease is still the number one health problem in the country, the incidence has declined by 36 percent in the last twenty years. The primary cause for this dramatic decrease has been health education. More people are now aware of the risk factors for cardiovascular disease and are making significant changes in their lifestyles to lower their own potential risk of suffering from this disease.

The major form of cardiovascular disease is coronary heart disease (CHD), a condition where the arteries that supply the heart muscle with oxygen and nutrients are narrowed by fatty deposits such as cholesterol and triglycerides. The narrowing of the coronary arteries diminishes the blood supply to the heart muscle, which can eventally lead to a heart attack. CHD is the single leading cause of death in the United States, accounting for approximately one-third of all deaths, and more than half of all cardiovascular deaths. Oddly enough, almost all of the risk factors for CHD are preventable and reversible, and risk reduction can be accomplished by the individual himself.

CARDIOVASCULAR RISK FACTOR ANALYSIS

The most important determinant in whether an individual will suffer from CHD is his or her own personal lifestyle. The leading risk factors that contribute to the development of CHD have been identified and are listed in the Self-Assessment Cardiovascular Risk Factor Analysis contained in Figure 7.2. Since the contribution of each factor in the development of the disease differs, a weighing system has been developed, assigning the highest number of risk points to the most significant factors. This weighing system was developed based on current research available in this area, and according to the work done at leading preventive medicine facilities in the United States.

The self-assessment form was constructed in such a way that it can be used by someone who has limited or no medical information concerning his or her state of health, as well as by a person who has had a thorough medical examination. The self-assessment risk factor analysis was developed with two objectives in mind: (a) to screen individuals who may be at high risk for the disease, and (b) to educate regarding the primary risk factors that lead to its development. Since the guidelines for zero risk are outlined for each factor, the form can be used as a valuable tool in cardiovascular risk factor management. For instance, a person who fills out the form would know that he or she needs to exercise aerobically a minimum of three times per week for at least

Figure 7.1. *Anatomy of the coronary arteries*

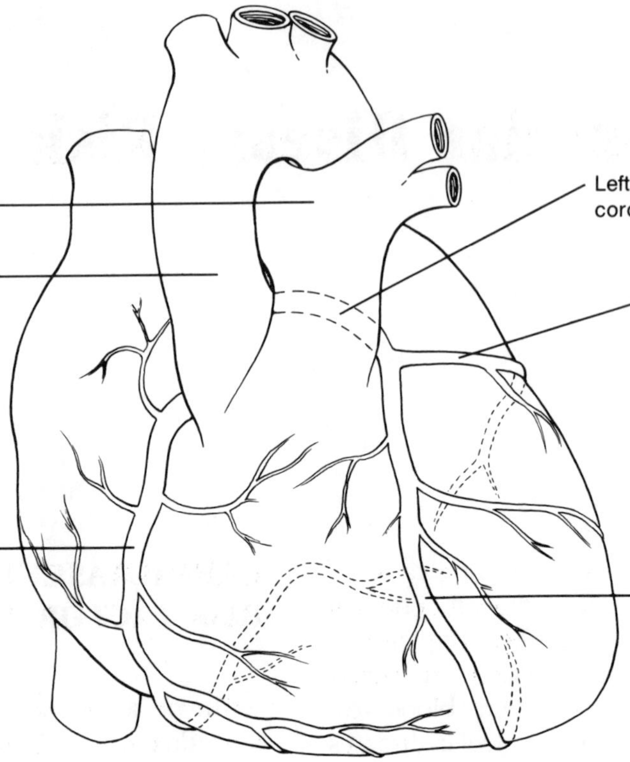

twenty minutes per session, that ideal blood pressure is around 120/80 or less, that total cholesterol-HDL ratio should be 4.5 or lower, and if unknown, basic nutritional guidelines are given (the role of HDL-cholesterol in heart disease protection will be discussed later in this chapter), that risk is reduced by smoking less or quitting altogether, etc. Before proceeding any further, you should fill out the risk factor analysis in Figure 7.2 and record your total number of risk points and respective risk category in the fitness and wellness profile in Appendix A.

INTERPRETATION OF THE CARDIOVASCULAR RISK FACTOR ANALYSIS

When interpreting the results, remember that this is only an estimated risk factor analysis. A high score does not indicate that you will definitely develop heart disease, nor does a low score guarantee absolute protection. More precise testing is required for an accurate prediction. Also note that this risk factor analysis should never take the place of a comprehensive medical examination. Nevertheless, the final score will indicate whether you are taking good care of your cardiovascular health and whether you are practicing appropriate preventive medicine techniques. Furthermore, it provides a guide to identify potential risk and steps that can be taken to lower your overall risk for heart disease.

A score in the "very low" risk category places you in the lowest risk group for developing heart disease based on your age and sex. The "low" risk category indicates that you are taking pretty good care of your cardiovascular health, but small improvements can be made (unless all the risk points came from your age and family history). "Moderate" risk shows that you can make definite improvements in your lifestyle to decrease your risk for cardiovascular disease. If you scored in the "high" category, you should see a physician within

Figure 7.2. *Cardiovascular Risk Factor Analysis: Self-Evaluation Form.*

			Score
1. CARDIOVASCULAR FITNESS	Do you participate in a regular aerobic exercise program (brisk walking, jogging, swimming, bicycling, jazzercise etc.) for more than 20 minutes:		
	Once a week or less	6	
	Two times per week	3	
	Three or more times per week	0	_____
2. BLOOD PRESSURE	Blood pressure reading is (score applies to each reading, e.g. 150/86 score = 5):		
	Systolic / Diastolic		
	161 or higher (4) / 101 or higher (4)	4-8	
	141 - 160 (3) / 91 - 100 (3)	3-6	
	121 - 140 (2) / 81 - 90 (2)	2-4	
	Unknown (1) / Unknown (1)	1-2	
	20 or less (0) / 80 or less (0)	0	_____
3. BODY COMPOSITION	Body Fat Percentage		
	Men / Women		
	28% or higher / 33% or higher	4	
	23% - 27% / 28% - 32%	3	
	18% - 22% / 23% - 27%	2	
	13% - 17% / 18% - 22%	1	
	12% or less / 17% or less	0	_____
4. TOTAL CHOLESTEROL-HDL RATIO	Ratio is 10.0 or higher	10	
	Ratio is between 6.6 - 9.9	7	
	Ratio is between 5.6 - 6.5	4	
	Ratio is between 4.6 - 5.5	2	
	Ratio is less than 4.5	0	
	If unknown answer question 6		_____
5. TRIGLYCERIDES	Level is above 250	2	
	Level between 101 and 249	1	
	Level less than 100	0	
	If unknown answer question 6		_____
6. DIET	Do not answer if 4 and 5 have been answered. Does your normal diet include (high score if all apply):		
	One or more daily servings of red meat, 7 or more eggs/week, daily butter-cheese-whole milk, daily sweets and alcohol	8-12	
	Four to six servings of red meat/week, 4-6 eggs/week, margarine, 1 or 2% milk, some cheese, sweets and alcohol	3-7	
	Fish (no hard-shell), poultry, red meat less than three times/week, less than 3 eggs/week, skim milk and skim milk products, moderate sweets and alcohol	0	_____
7. DIABETES	Are You:		
	Diabetic and blood sugar is out of control	6	
	Diabetic and blood sugar controlled with medication	3	
	Diabetic and blood sugar controlled with diet alone	2	
	Non-diabetic	0	_____
	Sub Total Risk Score		_____

Adapted from Hoeger, W. W. K. "Self Evaluation of Cardiovascular Risk." *Corporate Fitness & Recreation (in press, 1986).*

Figure 7.2. *Cardiovascular Risk Factor Analysis: Self-Evaluation Form.* (continued)

	Subtotal Risk Score (from previous page)		______
8. EKG	Add scores for both EKG's Resting EKG / Stress EKG Abnormal ...... (4) / Abnormal ..... (10)	4-14	
	Equivocal ...... (2) / Equivocal ...... (5)	2-7	
	Normal .... (0) / Normal .... (0)	0	
	Unknown and age 35 or older and never had resting EKG	2	______
9. SMOKING	Smoke 40 or more cigarettes per day	8	
	Smoke 30-39 cigarettes per day	6	
	Smoke 20-29 cigarettes per day	5	
	Smoke 10-19 cigarettes per day	4	
	Smoke 1-9 cigarettes per day	3	
	Smoke less than 1 cigarette per day	1	
	Pipe, cigar smoker or chew tobacco	2	
	Ex-smoker less than one year	1	
	Non-smoker, but live or work in smoking environment	2	
	Ex-smoker over one year	0	
	Lifetime non-smoker	0	______
10. TENSION AND STRESS	Are you: Always tense, uptight, on the run, easily angered	4	
	Nearly always tense, quite impatient, often hurried	3	
	Often tense, impatient when waiting, moody	2	
	Sometimes tense, slight impatience, seldom rushed	1	
	Hardly ever tense, easygoing, not rushed	0	______
11. PERSONAL HISTORY	Have you ever had a heart attack, stroke, coronary bypass surgery or any type of KNOWN heart problem: During the last year	10	
	1-2 years ago	6	
	2-5 years ago	3	
	More than 5 years ago	2	
	Never had heart problems	0	______
12. FAMILY HISTORY	Have any of your blood relatives (parents, uncles, brothers, sisters, grandparents) suffered from cardiovascular disease (heart attack, strokes, bypass surgery): One or more before age 50	4	
	One or more between ages 51 and 60	2	
	One or more after age 61	1	
	None have suffered from cardiovascular disease	0	______
13. AGE	55 or older	4	
	45-54	3	
	35-44	2	
	25-34	1	
	24 or younger	0	______
14. ESTROGEN USE (Birth control pills and certain hormone drugs)	Are you: 35 or older and using estrogen	2	
	Any age and used estrogen for over 5 years	2	
	35 or younger and used estrogen for less than 5 years	1	
	Do not use estrogen	0	______
	Total Risk Score		______

CARDIOVASCULAR RISK CATEGORIES

Very low	5 or less points
Low	Between 6 and 15 points
Moderate	Between 16 and 25 points
High	Between 26 and 35 points
Very High	36 or more points

the next couple of months and start implementing your personal risk reduction program. A score in the "very high" risk category indicates a very strong probability of developing heart disease within the next three to five years. You should have a medical-physical evaluation immediately, including an exercise stress EKG test. Thereafter, you need to implement all of the medical, nutritional, and exercise recommendations made by the professional staff.

Once you have determined your risk score, you should be aware that with the exception of age, family history of heart disease, and some EKG abnormalities, all of the other risk factors are preventable and reversible. To aid you in the implementation of a lifetime risk reduction program, the primary risk factors for coronary heart disease will now be discussed in detail, along with the general recommendations for risk reduction.

CARDIOVASCULAR FITNESS

Cardiovascular fitness has been defined as the ability of the heart, lungs, and blood vessels to deliver adequate amounts of oxygen and nutrients to the cells to meet the demands of prolonged physical activity. Even though cardiovascular endurance is not the most significant factor in terms of the maximal number of risk points assigned (six points for a poor level of fitness, as compared to ten for a very high total cholesterol/HDL ratio — *see* Figure 7.2), this factor has perhaps the greatest impact in overall heart disease risk reduction. While specific recommendations can be followed to improve each individual risk factor, engaging in a regular aerobic exercise program has shown to control most of the major risk factors that lead to heart disease. Aerobic exercise will help with all of the following: (a) increase cardiovascular endurance, (b) decrease and control blood pressure, (c) decrease body fat, (d) decrease blood lipids (cholesterol and triglycerides), (e) improve HDL cholesterol, (f) help control diabetes, (g) increase and maintain good heart function, improving in many cases certain EKG abnormalities, (h) motivate toward smoking cessation, (i) decrease tension and stress, and (j) prevent a personal history of heart disease. In the words of Dr. Kenneth H. Cooper, pioneer of the aerobic movement in the United States, the evidence of the benefits of aerobic exercise in the reduction of heart disease is "far too impressive to be ignored."

Caution should be taken, however, not to ignore the other risk factors. Good cardiovascular fitness by itself is not an absolute guarantee for a lifetime free of cardiovascular problems. Poor lifestyle habits such as smoking, eating excessive fatty/salty/and sweet foods, excess body fat, and high levels of stress increase cardiovascular risk and will not always be completely eliminated through aerobic exercise. Yet, cardiovascular exercise, if carried out as explained in Chapter 2, is one of the most important aspects in the prevention and reduction of coronary disease.

BLOOD PRESSURE

There are some 60,000 miles of blood vessels running through the human body. As the heart forces the blood through these vessels, the fluid is under pressure. Hence, blood pressure is but a measure of the force exerted against the walls of the vessels by the blood flowing through them. Blood pressure is measured in milliliters of mercury and is usually expressed in two numbers. Ideal blood pressure should be 120/80 or below. The higher number reflects the pressure exerted during the forceful contraction of the heart or systole (therefore, the name "systolic" pressure), and the lower pressure is taken during the heart's relaxation or diastolic phase, when no blood is being ejected.

When Is Blood Pressure Considered Too High?

A few years ago, a systolic pressure of 100 plus your age was the acceptable standard. However, this is no longer the case. Hypertension is now viewed as the point where the pressure doubles the mortality risk. This pressure has been determined at about 160/95. Traditionally, the upper limits of normal were established at 140/90, a reading that by today's standards is considered by many as borderline hypertension. Readings between 140/90 and 160/95 (either number being in that range) are classified as mild hypertension.

While the upper limits of normal pressure have been set at 140/90, many experts believe that the lower the blood pressure, the better. Even if the pressure drops to around 90/50, as long as you have no symptoms of low blood pressure or hypotension, you need not be concerned. Typical hypotension symptoms are dizziness, lightheadedness, and fainting.

Blood pressure may also fluctuate during a regular day. Many factors affect blood pressure, and one single reading may not be a true indicator of your real pressure. For example, physical activity and stress increase blood pressure, while rest and relaxation decrease it. Consequently, several measurements should be made before a diagnosis of elevated pressure is suggested.

Based on 1985 estimates, some 38 million Americans are hypertensive (one in every four adults), and another 25 million suffer from mild hypertension. As a disease, hypertension has been referred to as the silent killer. It does not hurt, it does not make you feel sick, and unless you check it, years may go by before you even realize that you have a problem. Elevated blood pressure is a risk factor not only for coronary heart disease, but also for congestive heart failure, strokes, and kidney failure.

What Makes Hypertension A Killer?

All inner walls of arteries are lined by a layer of smooth endothelial cells. These cells are so slippery that fats cannot penetrate them and build up, unless damage is done to the cells. High blood pressure is a leading factor contributing to the destruction of this lining. As blood pressure rises, so does the risk for atherosclerosis or the development of fatty-cholesterol deposits in the walls of the arteries. The higher the pressure, the greater the damage that is done to the arterial wall, allowing a faster occlusion of the vessels, especially if serum cholesterol is also elevated. Occlusion of the coronary vessels decreases the blood supply to the heart muscle and can lead to heart attacks. When brain arteries are involved, strokes may follow.

A clear example of the role of elevated pressure in the development of atherosclerosis is seen in our own bodies. Even when significant atherosclerosis is present throughout major arteries in the body, fatty plaques are rarely seen in the pulmonary artery, which goes from the right heart to the lungs. The pressure in this artery is normally below 40. At such low pressure, signficant deposits do not occur. This is one of the reasons why people with low blood pressure have a lower incidence of cardiovascular disease.

Constantly elevated blood pressure also causes the heart to work much harder. Initially the heart does well, but in time, this constant strain results in a pathologically enlarged heart and subsequent congestive heart failure. Furthermore, high pressure damages blood vessels to the kidneys and eyes, leading to eventual kidney failure and vision loss.

How Can Hypertension Be Controlled?

Ninety percent of all hypertension has no definite cause. This type of hypertension is referred to as essential hypertension and is treatable. Aerobic exercise, weight reduction, a low-sodium/high-potassium diet, stress reduction, smoking cessation, decreasing blood lipids, lowering caffeine and alcohol intake, and antihypertensive medication have all been used effectively in treating essential hypertension. The other 10 percent is caused by such pathological conditions as narrowing of the kidney arteries, glomerulonephritis (a kidney disease), tumors of the adrenal glands, and narrowing of the aorta artery. With this type of hypertension, the pathological cause has to be treated first in order to correct the blood pressure problem.

Antihypertensive medications are many times the first choice of treatment modality, but they also produce multiple side effects. Some of these side effects are lethargy, somnolence, sexual difficulties, increased blood cholesterol and glucose levels, lower potassium levels, and elevated uric acid levels. Oftentimes a physician may find himself treating these side effects as much as the hypertension problem itself. Because of the multiple side effects, approximately 50 percent of the patients will stop taking the medication within the first year of treatment.

Perhaps one of the most significant factors contributing to elevated blood pressure is excessive sodium in the diet (salt is sodium chloride and contains approximately 40 percent sodium). Water retention increases with high sodium intake. As water retention increases, so does the blood volume, which in turn drives the pressure up. On the other hand, high intake of potassium seems to regulate water retention and therefore appears to lower the pressure slightly.

While sodium is essential for normal physiological functions, only 200 mg or one-tenth of a teaspoon of salt is required on a daily basis. Even under the most strenuous conditions, such as jobs and sports participation where heavy sweating is involved, the greatest amount of sodium required by the organism never exceeds 3,000 mg per day. Yet, in the typical American diet, sodium intake ranges between 6,000 and 20,000 mg per day! No wonder hypertension is so prevalent today.

In underdeveloped countries and Indian tribes where no salt is used in cooking nor added at the table, and the only sodium consumed comes from food in its natural form, daily intake seldom exceeds 2,000 mg. Blood pressure among these people does not increase with age, and hypertension is practically unknown. These findings seem to indicate that the human body may be able to handle 2,000 mg per day, but higher intakes than that on a regular basis may cause a gradual rise in blood pressure over the years.

You may ask yourself, where does all the sodium come from? The answer is found in Table 7.1. Most people do not realize the amount of sodium contained in various foods, and the list in Table 7.1 does not include the salt added at the table. Even if you do not have a blood pressure problem now, you need to be concerned about sodium intake — otherwise blood pressure may sneak up on you.

When treating high blood pressure, prior to using medication (unless elevation is extremely high), many sportsmedicine physicians prefer a combination of aerobic exercise, weight loss, and sodium reduction. In most instances this treatment modality will bring blood pressure under control.

The link between hypertension and obesity has been well established. Not only does blood volume increase with excess body fat, but every additional pound of fat requires an estimated extra mile of blood vessels to feed this tissue. Furthermore, blood capillaries are constricted by the adipose tissue as these vessels run through them. As a result, the heart muscle must work harder to pump the blood through a longer and constricted network of blood vessels.

The role of aerobic exercise in the treatment of hypertensive patients is becoming more important each day. On the average, cardiovascularly fit individuals have lower blood pressures than unfit people. Several well-documented studies have shown that nearly 90 percent of hypertensive patients who initiate an aerobic exercise program can expect a significant decrease in blood pressure after only a few months of training. These changes, however, are not maintained if aerobic exercise is discontinued.

The best tip yet, though, is to use a preventive approach. It is a lot easier to keep blood pressure under control than try to bring it down once it is elevated. Blood pressure should be checked regularly, regardless of whether elevation is present or not. Regular physical exercise, weight control, low salt diet, smoking cessation, and stress management are basic guidelines for blood pressure control. If you suffer from hypertension, you should not stop using the medication unless your physician so indicates. Remember — high blood pressure can kill you if not treated properly. Combining the medication with the other treatment modalities may eventually lead to a reduction or a complete elimination of the drug therapy.

BODY COMPOSITION

As discussed in previous chapters, body composition refers to the ratio of lean body weight to fat weight. If too much fat is accumulated, the person is considered to be obese (*see* Chapter 5 for a complete definition and classification of obesity).

Obesity has been long recognized as a primary risk factor for coronary heart disease. But until a few years ago, experts felt that the disease was actually brought on by some of the other risk factors that usually deteriorate with increased body fat (higher cholesterol and triglycerides, hypertension, diabetes, lower level of cardiovascular fitness). Recent evidence, however, suggests that excess body fat, in and of itself, is a serious coronary risk factor. Even when all of the other risk factors are in good range, individuals with body fat percentages higher than the "ideal" standard have a higher incidence of coronary disease. The ideal body fat percentages, based on age and sex, are given in Chapter 5, Table 5.4. Attaining ideal body composition is not only important in decreasing cardiovascular risk, but also to achieve a better state of health and wellness.

The only positive thing that can be said about excess body fat accumulation is that it can be lost through a combination of diet and exercise. Dieting by itself very seldom works. If you have a

Table 7.1.
Sodium and Potassium Levels of Selected Foods

Food	Serving Size	Sodium (mg)	Potassium (mg)
Apple	1 med.	1	182
Asparagus	1 cup	2	330
Avocado	1/2	5	680
Banana	1 med.	1	440
Bologna	3 oz.	1,107	133
Bouillon Cube	1	960	4
Cantaloupe	1/4	17	341
Carrot (raw)	1	38	225
Cheese			
American	2 oz.	614	93
Cheddar	2 oz.	342	56
Muenster	2 oz.	356	77
Parmesan	2 oz.	1,056	53
Swiss	2 oz.	148	64
Chicken (light meat)	6 oz.	108	700
Corn (canned)	1/2 cup	195	80
Corn (natural)	1/2 cup	3	136
Frankfurter	3 oz.	1,003	136
Haddock	6 oz.	300	594
Hamburger	1	500	321
Lamb (leg)	6 oz.	108	700
Milk (whole)	1 cup	120	351
Milk (skim)	1 cup	126	406
Orange	1 med.	1	263
Orange Juice	1 cup	1	200
Peach	1 med.	2	308
Pear	1 med.	2	130
Peas (canned)	1/2 cup	294	82
Peas (boiled — natural)	1/2 cup	1	168
Pizza (cheese — 14" diam.)	1/8	456	85
Potato	1 med.	6	763
Potato Chips	10	200	226
Potato (french fries)	10	5	427
Pork	6 oz.	96	438
Roast Beef	6 oz.	98	448
Salami	3 oz.	1,047	170
Salmon	6 oz.	198	756
Salt	1 tsp.	2,132	—
Soups			
Chicken Noodle	1 cup	979	55
Clam Chowder (Manhattan)	1 cup	938	184
Cream of Mushroom	1 cup	955	98
Vegetable Beef	1 cup	845	162
Soy Sauce	1 tsp.	1,123	22
Spaghetti (tomato sauce and cheese)	6 oz.	648	276
Strawberries	1 cup	1	244
Tomato (raw)	1 med.	5	444
Tuna (drained)	3 oz.	38	225

Adapted from USDA Handbooks, No. 456 and No. 8.

weight problem and you desire to achieve ideal weight, two things must take place: (a) an increase in the level of physical activity, and (b) a moderate reduction in caloric intake that will still provide all of the necessary nutrients to sustain normal physiological body functions.

CHOLESTEROL AND TRIGLYCERIDES

The term blood lipids (fats) is mainly used in reference to cholesterol and triglycerides. These lipids are carried in the bloodstream by molecules of protein known as high-density lipoproteins, low-density lipoproteins, very low-density lipoproteins, and chylomicrons. A significant elevation in blood lipids has long been associated with heart and blood vessel disease.

Cholesterol has received considerable attention in the last few years. This fatty or lipid substance is essential for certain metabolic functions in the body. It is found in different types of food, but the body is also able to manufacture its own cholesterol from saturated fats. These fats are abundant in meats and dairy products. There are individual differences as to how much cholesterol can be manufactured by the body. Some people can have higher than normal intakes of saturated fats and still maintain normal blood levels, while others with a lower intake can have abnormally high levels.

High levels of blood cholesterol contribute to the formation of the atherosclerotic plaque or the buildup of fatty tissue in the walls of the arteries. In the case of the heart, as the plaque builds up, it obstructs the coronary vessels. Since these arteries supply the heart muscle (myocardium) with oxygen and nutrients, when obstruction occurs, a myocardial infarction or heart attack will follow. Unfortunately, the heart disguises its problems quite effectively, and typical symptoms of heart disease, such as angina pectoris or chest pain, do not start until the arteries are about 75 percent

Figure 7.3. *Heart attack: A result of acute reduction in the flow of blood through a coronary vessel.*

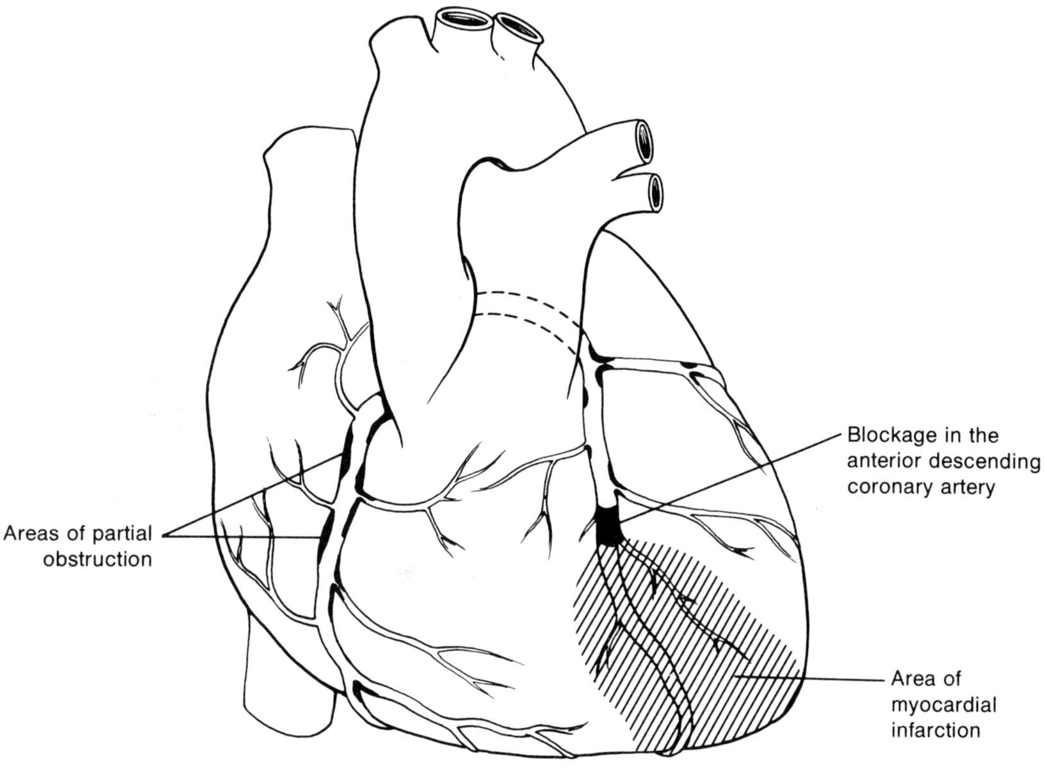

occluded; and in many cases, the first symptom is sudden death.

Only a few years ago the general recommendation was to keep total blood cholesterol levels below 200 mg/dl (milligrams per deciliter). Even though this guideline should still be followed, the crucial factor seems to be the way in which cholesterol is carried in the bloodstream rather than the total amount present.

Cholesterol is primarily transported in the form of high-density lipoprotein cholesterol (HDL-cholesterol) and low-density lipoprotein cholesterol (LDL-cholesterol). The high-density molecules have a high affinity for cholesterol and tend to attract cholesterol, which is then carried to the liver to be metabolized and excreted. In other words, they act as "scavengers," removing cholesterol from the body, thus preventing plaque formation in the arteries. On the other hand, LDL-cholesterol tends to stick to the walls of the arteries, therefore enhancing the process of atherosclerosis.

From the previous discussion, it can easily be seen that the more HDL present, the better. HDL is the so-called "good cholesterol" and offers a certain degree of protection against heart disease. Many authorities now believe that the ratio of total cholesterol to HDL is a better indicator of potential risk for cardiovascular disease than the total value by itself. It is generally accepted that a 4.5 or lower ratio (total cholesterol/HDL cholesterol) is excellent for men, and 4.0 or lower is best for women. For instance, 50 mg/dl of HDL as compared to 200 mg/dl of total cholesterol yields a ratio of 4.0 (200/50 = 4.0). The lower the ratio, the greater the protection. In another instance, a person's total cholesterol could also be 200 mg/dl, but if the HDL is only 20 mg/dl, the ratio could be 10.0. Such a ratio is extremely dangerous and very conducive to atherosclerosis and coronary disease.

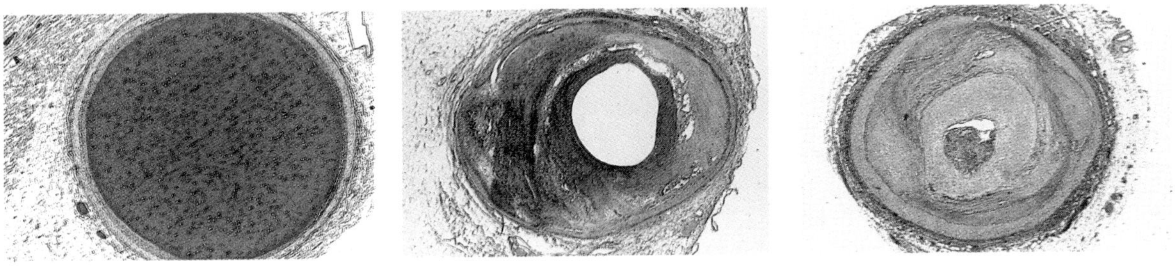

(a) (b) (c)

Figure 7.4. *The atherosclerotic process. (a) = cross-section of normal artery; (b) = lumen is significantly narrowed by fibrous lesion; (c) = progression of lesion shown in (b), with almost complete obstruction of the artery. Reproduced with permission.* The Atherosclerotic Process. *The American Heart Association.*

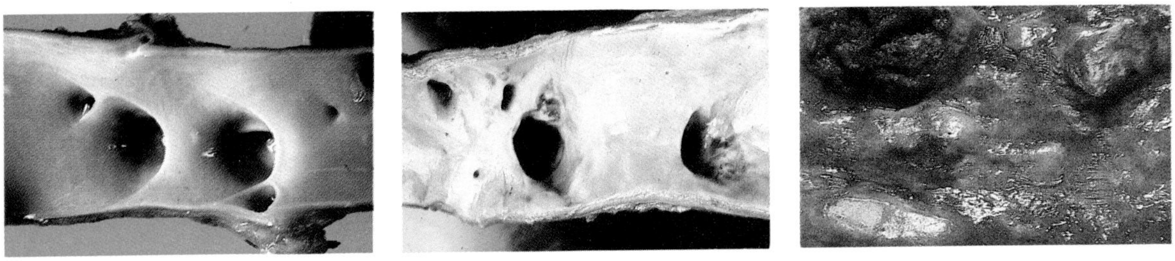

(a) (b) (c)

Figure 7.5. *Comparison of a normal healthy artery (a) and a diseased artery (b) and (c). Illustrations (a) and (b) are reproduced with permission,* The Atherosclerotic Process, *American Heart Association. Illustration (c) reproduced with permission from "If You Smoke" slide show by Gordon Hewlett.*

If the HLD-total cholesterol ratio is higher than ideal, certain guidelines should be followed to lower the ratio. Initially, total cholesterol levels should be lowered. This can be accomplished by lowering the LDL-cholesterol component. This type of cholesterol increases proportionally with the amount of cholesterol and saturated fats eaten in your regular diet. The total daily consumption of cholesterol should never exceed 300 mg, and much less if either the total amount or the ratio are elevated. The cholesterol content of selected foods is found in Table 7.2. LDL-cholesterol can also be lowered by losing excess body fat and with the use of medication. As a general rule of thumb, the following dietary guidelines should be followed to lower LDL-cholesterol levels:

a. Eat less than three eggs a week.
b. Red meats should be consumed less than three times per week. Avoid organ meats (e.g., liver and kidneys), sausage, bacon, hot dogs, and canned meats.
c. Use low-fat milk (1 percent or less preferably) and low-fat low-cholesterol dairy products.
d. Avoid shellfish, coconut oil, palm oil, and cocoa butter.
e. Achieve ideal body weight.

The second factor involved in improving the ratio is increasing the HDL component. HDL-cholesterol is genetically determined, and women have higher values than men. This is probably one of the reasons why heart disease is less common among women. Research has indicated that increases in HDL values are almost completely dependent upon a very regular aerobic exercise program. There seems to be a linear relationship between HDL-cholesterol and aerobic exercise. The greater the amount of exercise, the higher the HDL-cholesterol. Your cardiovascular exercise program, if followed as prescribed, should yield positive results. A combination of adequate nutrition and aerobic exercise is the best prescription for achieving a "zero risk" ratio.

You should also be aware that several other factors can lower the HDL levels. Beta-blocker type medications (used in treating heart disease and hypertension), tobacco usage, and birth control pills all have a negative effect on HDL levels. A combination of two or three of these is even worse.

Table 7.2.
Cholesterol Content (mg) of Selected Foods

Food	Serving Size	Cholesterol (mg)
Bacon	2 slc.	30
Beans (all types)	any	—
Beef		
(lean, fat trimmed off)	8 oz.	200
Beef — Brains (raw)	3 oz.	1,680
Beef — Heart (cooked)	3 oz.	150
Beef — Liver (cooked)	3 oz.	255
Beef — Kidney (cooked)	3 oz.	680
Butter	1 tsp.	12
Cheese		
American	2 oz.	54
Cheddar	2 oz.	60
Cottage (1% fat)	1 cup	10
Cottage (4% fat)	1 cup	31
Cream Cheese	2 oz.	62
Muenster	2 oz.	54
Parmesan	2 oz.	38
Swiss	2 oz.	52
Caviar	1 oz.	85
Chicken (no skin)	8 oz.	119
Chicken — Liver	3 oz.	472
Chicken — Thigh, Wing	8 oz.	184
Egg (yolk)	1	250
Frankfurter	2	90
Fruits	any	—
Grains (all types)	any	—
Halibut, Flounder	3 oz.	43
Ice Cream	½ cup	27
Lamb	8 oz.	160
Lard	1 tsp.	5
Lobster	3 oz.	170
Margarine (all vegetable)	1 tsp.	—
Mayonnaise	1 tbsp.	10
Milk		
Skim	1 cup	5
Low Fat (2%)	1 cup	18
Whole	1 cup	34
Nuts	any	—
Oysters	3 oz.	42
Salmon	3 oz.	30
Scallops	3 oz.	29
Seeds	any	—
Sherbet	1 cup	14
Shrimp	3 oz.	128
Trout	3 oz.	45
Tuna (canned — drained)	3 oz.	55
Turkey — Dark Meat	8 oz.	225
Turkey — Light Meat	8 oz.	175
Vegetables	any	—

Adapted from several sources.

Triglycerides are also known as free fatty acids and, in combination with cholesterol, accelerate the formation of the plaque. Triglycerides are carried in the bloodstream primarily by the very low-density lipoproteins (VLDL) and chylomicrons. These fatty acids are found in poultry skin, lunchmeats, and shellfish. However, they are mainly manufactured in the liver from refined sugars, starches, and alcohol. High intake of alcohol and sugars (honey included) will significantly increase triglyceride levels. Thus, they can be lowered by decreasing the consumption of the above-mentioned foods along with weight reduction (if overweight) and aerobic exercise.

If you have never had a blood chemistry test, you should probably have one done in the near future. An initial test is always useful to establish a baseline for future reference. Make sure that the blood test does include the HDL-cholesterol component, since many clinics and hospitals still do not include this factor in their regular analyses. While no definite guidelines have yet been given, following an initial normal baseline test, and as long as the recommended dietary and exercise guidelines are kept, a blood analysis every two or three years prior to the age of thirty-five should suffice. After the age of thirty-five, a blood lipid test should be conducted every year in conjunction with a regular preventive medicine physical examination.

DIABETES

Diabetes is a condition where the blood glucose is unable to enter the cells because of insufficient insulin production by the pancreas. Several studies have shown that the incidence of cardiovascular disease among diabetic patients is quite high. Cardiovascular disease is also the leading cause of death among these patients.

Individuals with chronically elevated blood glucose levels may also have problems in metabolizing fats. This in turn can increase the susceptibility to atherosclerosis, increasing the risk for coronary disease and other conditions such as vision loss and kidney damage.

Although there is a genetic predisposition to diabetes, adult-onset diabetes is closely related to obesity. In most cases, this type of condition can be corrected by following a special diet, a weight loss program, and exercise. If you do have elevated blood glucose levels, you should consult your physician and let him decide on the best approach to treat this condition.

ABNORMAL ELECTROCARDIOGRAM

The electrocardiogram, or EKG, is a valuable record of the heart's function. It is a record of the electrical impulses that stimulate the heart to contract. In the actual reading of an EKG, five general areas are interpreted: heart rate, the heart's rhythm, the heart's axis, enlargement or hypertrophy of the heart, and myocardial infarction or heart attacks.

On a standard twelve-lead EKG, ten electrodes are placed on your body. From these ten electrodes, twelve "pictures" or leads of the electrical impulses as they travel through the heart muscle (myocardium) are studied from twelve different positions. By looking at the tracings of an EKG, it is possible to identify abnormalities in the functioning of the heart. Based on the findings, the EKG may be interpreted as normal, equivocal, or abnormal. Since not all problems will always be identified by an EKG, a normal tracing is not an absolute problem-free guarantee, nor does an abnormal tracing necessarily mean the presence of a serious condition.

EKGs are taken at rest, during stress of exercise, and during recovery. A stress EKG is also known as a maximal exercise tolerance test. Similar to a high-speed road test on a car, a stress EKG reveals the tolerance of the heart to high-intensity exercise. It is a much better test for the discovery of coronary artery heart disease (as compared to a resting EKG). It is also used to determine cardiovascular fitness levels, to screen persons for preventive and cardiac rehabilitation programs, to detect abnormal blood pressure response during exercise, and to establish actual or functional maximal heart rate for exercise prescription purposes. The recovery EKG also becomes an important diagnostic tool in the monitoring of the return of the heart's activity to normal conditions.

Experts in the field of preventive medicine recommend that every person should have at least a baseline resting EKG and possibly a stress EKG prior to the age of thirty-five. While not everyone needs a stress EKG prior to initiating an exercise program, and controversy still exists as to when

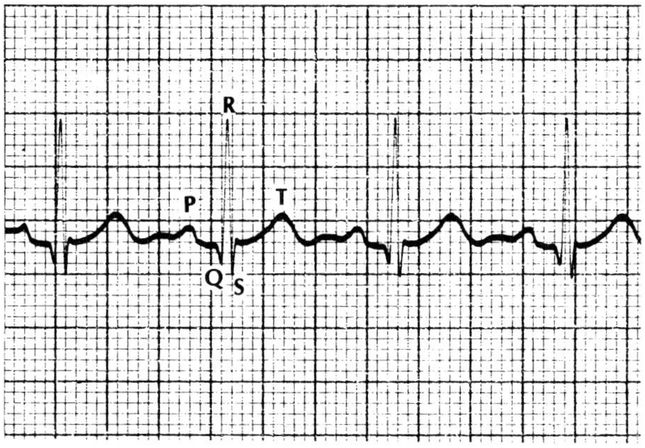

Figure 7.6. *Normal electrocardiogram (P wave =* artrial depolarization, QRS = ventricular depolarization, T wave = ventricular repolarization)

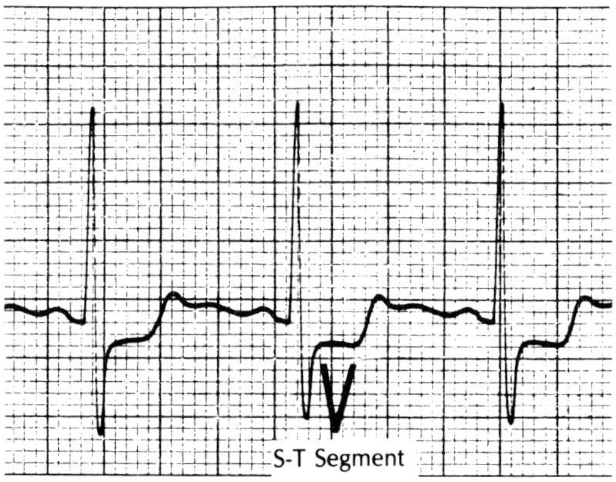

Figure 7.7. *Abnormal electrocardiogram showing a depressed S-T segment (commonly seen during exercise in patients with coronary disease).*

this test should be given, many authorities feel that the test should be administered if any of the following conditions are present:

1. Adults thirty-five years or older
2. A total cholesterol level above 200 mg/dl, or a total cholesterol/HDL ratio above 4.0 for women and 4.5 for men
3. Hypertensive and diabetic patients
4. Cigarette smokers
5. Those individuals with a family history of coronary heart disease, syncope, or sudden death before age sixty
6. All individuals with symptoms of chest discomfort, dysrrhythmias, syncope, or chronotropic incompetence (a heart rate that increases slowly during exercise and never reaches maximum)

Although the predictive value of a stress EKG has been at times questioned, it must be remembered that at present it is the most practical, inexpensive, noninvasive procedure available in diagnosing latent coronary heart disease. The sensitivity of the test is increased as the severity of the disease increases. Test protocols, number of leads, electrocardiographic criteria, and the quality of the technicians administering the test further increase its sensitivity. It therefore still remains a very useful tool in identifying those who are suffering from coronary disease and are at high risk for exercise-related sudden death.

SMOKING

Cigarette smoking is the single largest preventable cause of illness and premature death in the United States. Smoking has been linked to cardiovascular disease, cancer, bronchitis, emphysema, and peptic ulcers. In relation to coronary disease, not only does it speed up the process of atherosclerosis, but there is also a threefold increase in the risk of sudden death following a myocardial infarction.

Smoking causes the release of nicotine and some other 1,200 toxic compounds into the bloodstream. Similar to hypertension, many of these substances are destructive to the inner membrane that protects the walls of the arteries. As mentioned before, once the lining is damaged, cholesterol and triglycerides can be readily deposited in the arterial wall. As the plaque builds up, blood flow is significantly decreased as obstruction of the arteries occurs. Furthermore, smoking enhances the formation of blood clots, which can completely obstruct an already narrowed artery due to atherosclerosis. In addition, carbon monoxide, a byproduct of cigarette smoke, significantly decreases the oxygen-carrying capacity of the blood. A combination of obstructed arteries, decreased oxygen, and the presence of nicotine itself in the heart muscle greatly increases the risk for a serious heart problem.

Smoking also increases heart rate, blood pressure, and the irritability of the heart, which can trigger fatal cardiac arrhythmias. Another harmful effect that has been shown is a decrease in HDL cholesterol, or the "good type" that helps control your blood lipids. There is no question that

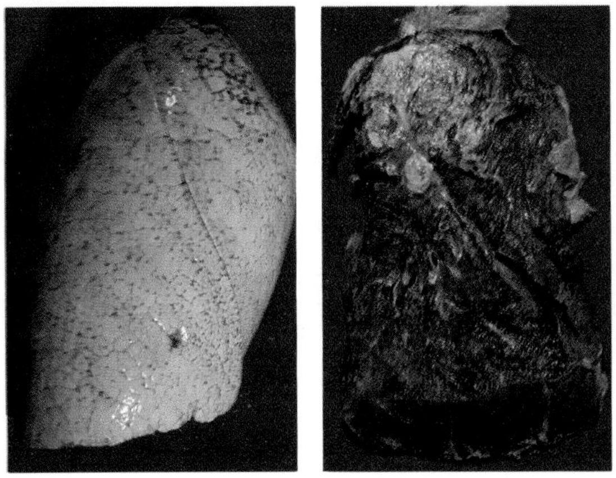

Figure 7.8. *Normal healthy lung to the left. Diseased lung to the right: The white growth near the top is cancer; the dark appearance on the bottom half is emphysema. Reproduced with permission from "If You Smoke" slide show by Gordon Hewlett.*

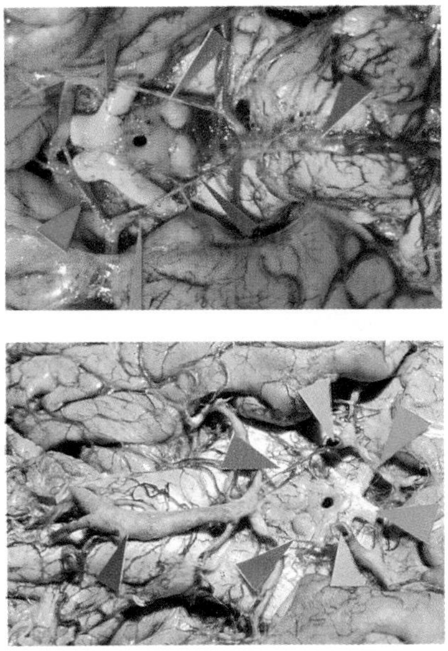

Figure 7.9. *Comparison of normal and atherosclerotic arteries at the base of the brain. Top: a healthy artery. Bottom: obstruction of the same artery by fatty substances (cholesterol and triglycerides). Reproduced with permission from "If You Smoke" slide show by Gordon Hewlett.*

smoking actually causes a much greater risk of death from heart disease than from lung cancer.

Pipe and/or cigar smoking and chewing tobacco also increase risk for heart disease. Even if no smoke is inhaled, certain amounts of toxic substances can be absorbed through the mouth membranes and end up in the bloodstream. Individuals who use tobacco in any of these three forms also have a much greater risk for cancer of the oral cavity.

Cigarette smoking along with a poor total cholesterol/HDL ratio and high blood pressure are the three most significant risk factors for coronary disease. Nevertheless, the risk for both cardiovascular disease and cancer starts to *decrease* the moment you quit. The risk approaches that of a lifetime nonsmoker ten and fifteen years, respectively, following cessation. If you smoke, for the sake of your own health, you should strongly consider smoking cessation. A more thorough discussion of the harmful effects of cigarette smoking, the benefits of quitting, and a complete program for smoking cessation are outlined in Chapter 10.

TENSION AND STRESS

Tension and stress have become a normal part of every person's life. Everyone has to deal with goals, objectives, responsibilities, pressures, etc. in daily life. Almost everything in life (whether positive or negative) is a source of stress. However, it is not the stressor itself that creates the health hazard, but rather the individual's response to it that may pose a health problem.

There are basically two types of behavior. Type A behavior is typical of a person who is hard-driving, high-strung, overly competitive, and easily irritated. Type B behavior, on the contrary, is characteristic of a relaxed, easy-going, casual person, who sometimes even appears apathetic toward life. A person exhibiting Type A behavior (high stress) is at higher risk for coronary disease than Type B. Such individuals actually become ill due to their inability to deal with increasing quantities of stress.

The way in which the human body responds to stress is by increasing the amount of catecholamines (hormones) to prepare the body for the so-called "fight or flight" mechanism. These hormones increase heart rate, blood pressure, and blood glucose levels, preparing the individual to take action. If the person "fights or flees," the increased levels of catecholamines are metabolized and the body is able to return to a "normal" state. However, if a person is under constant stress and unable to take action (such as is the case in the death of a close relative or friend, loss of a job, trouble at work, financial security, etc.), the catecholamines will remain elevated in the bloodstream. The person cannot relax and will experience a constant low-level strain on the cardiovascular system which could manifest itself in the form of heart disease. Additionally, when a person is in a stressful situation, the coronary arteries that feed the heart muscle constrict (clamp down), reducing oxygen supply to the heart. If significant arterial occlusion due to atherosclerosis is present, abnormal rhythms of the heart or a heart attack itself may follow.

If you are mostly of the Type A behavior and feel that you are under a lot of stress, and do not cope well with it, you need to begin to take appropriate measures to reduce the effects of stress in your life. Type A behavior is mostly a learned behavior. One of the best recommendations is to identify the sources of stress and learn how to cope with those events. Even slight changes in behavioral responses can slide you along the continuum so that you become more Type B and less Type A. You need to take control of yourself and examine and act upon the things of greatest importance in your life. Less significant or meaningless details should be ignored. If you feel stress to be a serious concern in your life, excellent stress management choices are available. Some of these choices are introduced in Chapter 9.

One of the best ways to relieve stress has been found to be physical exercise. When you engage in physical activity, excess catecholamines are metabolized, and the body is able to return to a normal state. Exercise also increases muscular activity, which causes muscular relaxation upon completion of physical activity. Many executives in large cities are choosing the evening hours for their physical activity programs, stopping right after work at the health or fitness club. This way they are able to "burn up" the excess tension built up during the day and better enjoy the evening hours. This has proven to be one of the best stress management techniques.

PERSONAL AND FAMILY HISTORY

Individuals who have suffered from cardiovascular problems are at higher risk over someone who has never had a problem. If you have a personal history, you are strongly encouraged to maintain the other risk factors as low as possible. Since most risk factors are reversible, this practice significantly decreases the risk for future problems. The longer it has been since the incidence of the cardiovascular problem, the lower the risk for recurrence.

The genetic predisposition toward heart disease has been clearly demonstrated and seems to be gaining in importance each day. All other factors being equal, a person who has had blood relatives who suffered from heart disease prior to age sixty runs a greater risk than someone who has no such history. The younger the age at which the incident happened to the relative, the greater the risk for the disease.

In many cases, there is no way of knowing whether there is a true genetic predisposition or simply poor lifestyle habits that led to a particular problem. It is quite possible that a person may have been physically inactive, overweight, had smoked, had bad dietary habits, etc., leading to a heart attack and therefore you now have such a family history. Since there is no definite way of telling them apart, a person with a family history should keep a close watch on all other factors and maintain them at as low a risk level as possible. In addition, an annual blood chemistry analysis is strongly recommended to make sure that blood lipids are being handled properly.

AGE

Age has also become a risk factor because of the greater incidence of heart disease among older people. This tendency may be partly induced by an increased risk among the other factors due to changes in lifestyle as we get older (less physical activity, poor nutrition, obesity, etc.).

Young people, however, should not feel that heart disease will not affect them. The disease process begins early in life. This was clearly shown among American soldiers who died during the Korean and Vietnam conflicts. Autopsies conducted on soldiers killed at twenty-two years old and younger revealed that approximately 70 percent of them showed early stages of atherosclerosis. Other studies have found elevated blood cholesterol levels in children as young as ten years old.

While the aging process cannot be stopped, it can certainly be slowed down. It has often been said that certain individuals in their sixties or older possess the bodies of twenty-year-olds. The opposite also holds true: twenty-year-olds often are in such poor condition and health that they almost seem to have the bodies of sixty-year-olds. Adequate risk factor management and positive lifestyle habits are the best ways to slow down the natural aging process.

ESTROGEN USE

Only recently were estrogens (found in oral contraceptives and certain other drugs) added to the list of risk factors for coronary disease. Estrogens cause an increase in blood pressure, enhance the clotting mechanism of the blood, and also decrease HDL-cholsterol (the "good guys"). High blood pressure by itself will increase the susceptibility to atherosclerosis. If in addition to that HDL-cholesterol is reduced, a greater amount of fats can be deposited in the arteries (even worse among women smokers, as this also decreases HDL-cholesterol). As the plaque builds up, complete obstruction may occur from a blood clot enhanced by the use of estrogen. It is therefore recommended that women at moderate or high risk for heart disease either decrease the dosage or seek an alternate method of birth control. Your personal physician should be consulted in this regard.

A FINAL WORD ON CORONARY RISK REDUCTION

As was mentioned at the beginning of this chapter, most of the risk factors for coronary heart disease are reversible and preventable. The fact that you may have a family history of heart disease and possibly some of the other risk factors because of neglect in your present lifestyle does not signify by any means that you are doomed. The objective of this chapter was to provide the guidelines and recommendations to decrease your own risk. As you have learned, a healthier lifestyle — free of cardiovascular problems — is something that you can pretty much control by yourself. You are encouraged to be persistent. It requires willpower and commitment to develop positive patterns that will eventually turn into healthy habits conducive to total well-being. Only you can act on it by taking control of your lifestyle and thereby reaping the benefits of wellness.

References

1. *American Heart Association Coronary Risk Handbook: Estimating Risk of Coronary Heart Disease in Daily Practice.* Dallas, TX: The Association, 1973.
2. American Heart Association. *Heart Facts.* Dallas, TX: The Association, 1985.
3. Blair, S. N., N. N. Goodyear, L. W. Gibbons, and K. H. Cooper. "Physical Fitness and Incidence of Hypertension in Healthy Normotensive Men and Women." *JAMA* 252:487-490, 1984.
4. Blair, S. N., K. H. Cooper, L. W. Gibbons, L. R. Gettman, S. Lewis, and N. N. Goodyear. "Changes in Coronary Heart Disease Risk Factors Associated with Increased Treadmill Time in 753 Men." *American Journal of Epidemiology* 3:352-359, 1983.
5. Cooper, K. H. *Running Without Fear.* New York: Mount Evans and Co., 1985.
6. Cooper, K. H. The Aerobics Way. New York: Mount Evans and Co., 1977.
7. Cooper, K. H. The Aerobics Program for Total Well-Being. New York: Mount Evans and Co., 1982.
8. Diethrich, E. B. The Arizona Heart Institute's Heart Test. New York: International Heart Foundation, 1981.
9. Gibbons, L. W., S. Blair, K. H. Cooper, and M. Smith. "Association Between Coronary Heart Disease Risk Factors and Physical Fitness in Healthy Adult Women." *Circulation* 5:977-983, 1983.
10. Guss, S. B. *Heart Attack Risk Score.* Cardiac Alert, 1983.
11. Hoeger, W. W. K. *Ejercicio, Salud y Vida* [*Exercise, Health and Life*]. Caracas, Venezuela: Editorial Arte, 1980.
12. Hoeger, W. W. K. U. T. Permian Basin Wellness Center: Coronary Heart Disease Risk Factor Analysis Interpretation. Odessa, TX: U. T. Permian Basin, 1984.
13. "How Good Is "Good" Cholesterol." *The Health Letter,* April 9, 1982.
14. Hubert, H. B., M. Feinleib, P. M. MacNamara, and W. P. Castelli. "Obesity As An Independent Risk Factor for Cardiovascular Disease: A 26-year Follow-Up of Participants in the Framingham Heart Study." *Circulation* 5:968-977, 1983.
15. Johnson, L. C. *Interpreting Your Test Results.* Lake Geneva, WI: Fitness Monitoring Preventive Medicine Clinic, 1981.
16. Kannel, W. B., D. McGee, and T. Gordon. "A General Cardiovascular Risk Profile: The Framingham Study." *The American Journal of Cardiology* 7:46-51, 1976.
17. "Multiple Risk Factor Intervention Trial. Risk Factor Changes and Mortality Results. Multiple Risk Factor Intervention Trial Research Group." *JAMA* 248-1465-1477, 1982.
18. Neufeld, H. N., and U. Gouldbourt. "Coronary Heart Disease: Genetic Aspects." *Circulation* 5:943-954, 1983.
19. Page, L. B. "On Making Sense of Salt and Your Blood Pressure." *Executive Health,* August 1982.
20. Van Camp, S. P. "The Fixx Tragedy: A Cardiologist's Perspective." *Physician and Sportsmedicine* 12:153-155, 1984.
21. Wiley, J. A., and T. C. Camacho. "Lifestyle and Future Health: Evidence from the Alameda County Study." *Preventive Medicine* 9:1-21, 1980.

CHAPTER EIGHT

Cancer Prevention

WHAT IS CANCER?

There are approximately 100 trillion cells in the human body, and under normal conditions these cells reproduce themselves in an orderly manner. The growth of cells occurs so that old, worn-out tissues can be replaced and injuries can be repaired. Every second, 15 million cells are replaced in the human body. However, in some instances certain cells grow in an uncontrolled and abnormal manner. Some cells will grow into a mass of tissue called a tumor, which can be either benign or malignant. A malignant tumor is considered to be a "cancer." These tumors compress, invade, and destroy normal tissue. Through metastasis (the movement of bacteria or body cells from one part of the body to another), cells break away from a malignant tumor and migrate to other parts of the body where they can cause new cancer. Benign tumors do not invade other tissue. They can interfere with normal body functions but rarely cause death.

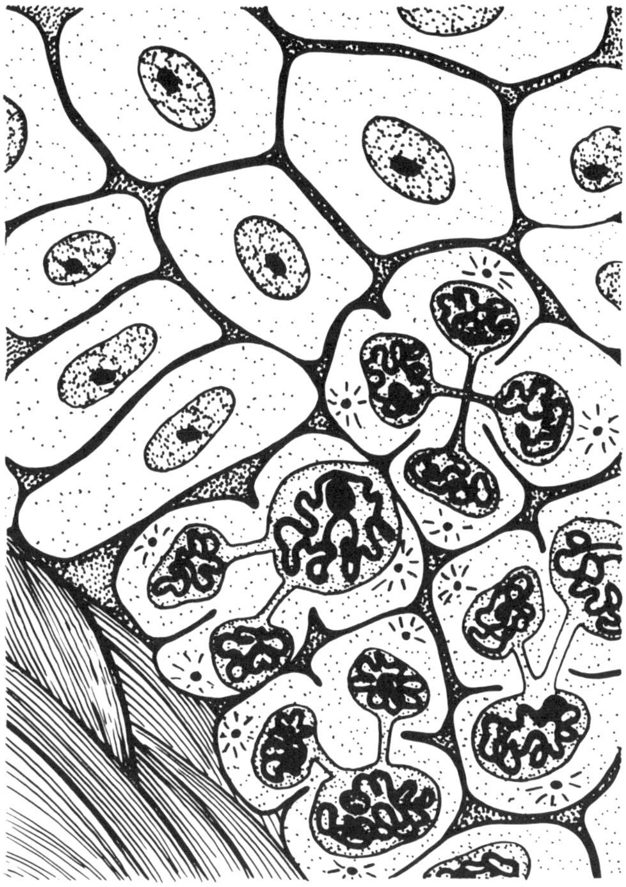

Figure 8.1. *Cancer cells divide erratically and crowd out normal cells. Illustration courtesy of American Cancer Society (contained in* Youth Looks at Cancer. *New York: American Cancer Society, p. 4, 1982).*

CANCER RISK

Approximately 20 percent of all deaths in the United States are caused by cancer. It is the second leading cause of death in the country and the leading cause among children between the ages of three and fourteen. About 462,000 people died of the disease in 1985, and approximately 910,000 new cases were expected the same year. There are now over 5 million Americans alive who have a history of cancer, and close to 3 million of them are considered cured. In fact, cancer is now the most curable of all chronic diseases. Over half of all cancers are curable.

According to the American Cancer Society*, the following were the 1985 statistical estimates of cancer incidence and deaths by sex and site for the United States (excluding nonmelanoma skin cancer and carcinoma in situ):

Men

Cancer	Incidence	Deaths
Lung	22%	35%
Prostate	19%	10%
Colon & Rectum	15%	12%
Urinary	9%	5%
Leukemia & Lymphomas	8%	8%
Oral	4%	3%
Pancreas	3%	5%
Skin	2%	2%
Others	18%	20%

Women

Cancer	Incidence	Deaths
Breast	26%	18%
Colon & Rectum	16%	15%
Uterus	11%	5%
Lung	10%	18%
Leukemia & Lymphomas	7%	9%
Ovary	4%	5%
Urinary	4%	3%
Pancreas	3%	5%
Skin	2%	1%
Oral	2%	1%
Others	15%	20%

Estimates also indicate that of the present population, 67 million Americans will suffer from cancer in their lifetime, striking approximately three out of every four families. However, as in coronary heart disease, cancer is largely a preventable disease. It is very encouraging to note that as much as 80 percent of all human cancers could be prevented, and the biggest factor in fighting cancer is health education. People need to be informed regarding the risk factors for cancer and the guidelines for early detection.

CANCER PREVENTION

The American Cancer Society* has issued the following recommendations in regard to cancer prevention:

1. **Dietary changes.** Fundamentally, a diet low in fat, high in fiber, and with ample amounts of vitamins A and C from natural sources. Cruciferous vegetables are encouraged in the diet, alcohol should be used in moderation, and obesity should be avoided.

   High fat intake has been linked primarily to breast, colon, and prostate cancer. Low fiber intake seems to increase the risk of colon cancer. Foods high in vitamins A and C may help decrease the incidence of larynx, esophagus, and lung cancers.

   Additionally, salt-cured, smoked, and nitrite-cured foods should be avoided. These foods have been linked to cancer of the esophagus and stomach. Cruciferous vegetables (cauliflower, broccoli, Brussels sprouts, and kohlrabi) should be included in the diet, since they seem to decrease the risk for the development of certain cancers.

   Alcohol should be used in moderation. Alcoholism increases the risk of certain cancers, especially when combined with tobacco smoking or smokeless tobacco. In combination, they significantly increase the risk of mouth, larynx, throat, esophagus, and liver cancers. According to some research, the synergistic action of heavy use of alcohol and tobacco yield a fifteen-fold increase in cancer of the oral cavity.

   Maintenance of ideal body weight is also recommended. Obesity has been associated with colon, rectum, breast, prostate, gallbladder, ovary, and uterine cancers.

2. **Abstinence from cigarette smoking.** It has been reported that 83 percent of all lung cancer and 30 percent of all cancers are attributed to smoking. Smokeless tobacco also increases the risk of mouth, larynx, throat, and

*From *1985 Cancer Facts and Figures.* New York: American Cancer Society, 1985.

esophagus cancers. About 138,600 annual cancer deaths are attributed to the use of tobacco. However, cigarette smoking by itself is a major health hazard. When considering all related deaths, cigarette smoking is responsible for 450,000 unnecessary deaths per year. The average life expectancy for a chronic smoker is seven years less than for a nonsmoker.

3. **Avoid sun exposure.** Sunlight exposure is a major factor in the development of skin cancer. Almost 100 percent of the 400,000 non-melanoma skin cancer cases reported annually in the United States are related to sun exposure. Sunscreen lotion should be used at all times when the skin is going to be exposed to sunlight for extended periods of time. Tanning of the skin is the body's natural reaction to cell damage taking place as a result of excessive sun exposure.

4. **Avoid estrogen use, radiation exposure, and occupational hazard exposure.** Estrogen use has been linked to endometrial cancer but can be taken safely under careful physician supervision. Radiation exposure also increases cancer risk. Many times, however, the benefits of X-ray use outweigh the risk involved, and most medical facilities use the lowest dose possible to decrease the risk to a minimum. Occupational hazards, such as asbestos fibers, nickel and uranium dusts, chromium compounds, vinyl chloride, bischlormethyl ether, etc., increase cancer risk. The risk of occupational hazards is significantly magnified by the use of cigarette smoking.

The contribution of many of the other much publicized factors are not as significant as the above factors. The contribution to total cancer incidence of intentional food additives, saccharin, processing agents, pesticides, and packaging materials in current use in the United States and other developed countries appears to be minimal.

Genetics plays a role in susceptibility in only 2 percent of all cancers. Most of it is seen in early childhood years. Some cancer can be seen as a combination of genetic and environmental liability. Genetics may act to enhance environmental risks of certain types of cancers. The biggest carcinogenic exposure in the work place is cigarette smoke. However, environment means more than pollution, smoke, etc. It includes diet, lifestyle-related events, viruses, and physical agents such as X-rays and sun exposure.

Equally important is the fact that through early detection, many cancers can be controlled or cured. The real problem is the spreading of cancerous cells. Once spreading occurs, it becomes very difficult to wipe the cancer out. It is therefore crucial to practice effective prevention or at least catch cancer when the possibility of cure is greatest. Herein lies the importance of proper periodic screening for prevention and/or early detection.

The following are the seven warning signals for cancer. Every individual should familiarize himself with these warning signals and bring them to the attention of a physician if any of them are present:

1. Change in bowel or bladder habits
2. A sore that does not heal
3. Unusual bleeding or discharge
4. Thickening or lump in breast or elsewhere
5. Indigestion or difficulty in swallowing
6. Obvious change in wart or mole
7. Nagging cough or hoarseness

In addition to these warning signals, the Guidelines for Screening Recommendations by the American Cancer Society outlined in Table 8.1 should be included in regular physical examinations as a part of a cancer prevention program.

There is also growing evidence that the body's auto-immune system may play a role in preventing cancer. Studies have indicated that exercise improves the auto-immune system. On the other hand, high levels of tension and stress and/or poor coping may have a negative effect on this system and consequently reduce the body's effectiveness in dealing with the various cancers.

Scientific evidence and testing procedures for prevention and/or early detection of cancer do change. Results of current clinical and epidemiologic studies provide constant new information about cancer prevention and detection. The purpose of cancer prevention programs is to educate and guide individuals toward a lifestyle that will aid them in the prevention and/or early detection of malignancy. Treatment of cancer should always be left to specialized physicians and cancer clinics.

Table 8.1.
Guidelines for Cancer Screening

Test	Patient age	Frequency
Breast physical examination	20-40 Over 40	Every 3 yr Annually
Breast self-examination	Over 20	Monthly
Chest X-ray	No specific recommendation	No specific recommendation
Digital rectal examination	Over 40	Annually
Endometrial tissue examination	At menopause[a]	At menopause
Mammography	35-40 40-49 Over 50	One baseline Every 1-2 yr Annually
Pap smear	20-65 and sexually active teenagers	2 consecutive yr, then every 3 yr
Pelvic examination	20-40 Over 40 At menopause[b]	Every 3 yr Annually
Sigmoidoscopy	Over 50	2 consecutive yr, then every 3-5 yr
Sputum cytology	No specific recommendation	No specific recommendation
Stool guaiac	Over 50	Annually
Health counseling and cancer check-up	Over 20 Over 40	Every 3 yr Every yr

From *Guidelines for the Cancer-Related Checkup: Recommendations and Rationale.* New York: American Cancer Society, July/August 1980. Reproduced with permission.

[a]Recommended for obese women with a history of involuntary infertility, failure of ovulation, abnormal uterine bleeding, or estrogen therapy.

[b]To include examinations for cancers of the thyroid, testicles, prostate, ovaries, lymph nodes, oral region, and skin.

CANCER QUESTIONNAIRE: ASSESSING YOUR RISKS**

This simple self-testing method is designed by the Texas Division of the American Cancer Society to help you assess your risk for cancer. Some people may have more than the average risk of developing certain cancers. These people will be identified by risk factors for certain common types of cancer. These are the major risk factors and by no means represent the only ones that might be involved.

**Cancer Questionnaire: Assessing Your Risks obtained from the Texas Division of the American Cancer Society and reproduced with permission. (NOTE: This questionnaire is not available nationwide, and distribution is limited for Texas residents only). Reproduced with permission.

Read each question concerning each site and its specific risk factors. Be honest in your responses. Place the number in parentheses (risk points) in the correct space on your score panel to the left. For example, Question #2 on lung cancer: If you are fifty-three years old (age fifty to fifty-nine) then enter five (risk points) as your score on the left. At the end of each site, total your number of points for that particular site. The final number of points should also be recorded in Figure 8.2.

Men should complete the score panel for lung, colon-rectum, and skin cancer. Additionally, three major cancer sites for women are included with space to enter the score totals.

Check your own risks with the answers contained on this questionnaire. Individual numbers for specific questions are not to be interpreted as a precise measure of relative risk, but the totals for a given site should give you a general indication

Figure 8.2. *Cancer Profile.*

Name: ____________________ Date: ____________

Cancer Site	Total Points		Risk Category
	Men	Women	
Lung Cancer	______	______	______
Colon-Rectum Cancer	______	______	______
Skin Cancer	______	______	Not Applicable
Breast Cancer		______	______
Cervical Cancer		______	______
Endometrial Cancer		______	______

of your risk. An explanation of the different risk factors for each type of cancer follows the questionnaire. You are advised to discuss the results with your physician if you are at higher risk.

Lung Cancer

_____ 1. **Sex**
- a. Male (2)
- b. Female (1)

_____ 2. **Age**
- a. 39 or less (1)
- b. 40 - 49 (2)
- c. 50 - 59 (5)
- d. 60 + (7)

_____ 3. **Smoking status**
- a. Smoker (8)
- b. Nonsmoker (1)

_____ 4. **Type of smoking**
- a. Current cigarettes or little cigars (10)
- b. Pipé and/or cigar, but not cigarettes (3)
- c. Ex-cigarette smoker (2)

_____ 5. **Amount of cigarettes smoked per day**
- a. 0 (1)
- b. Less than ½ pack per day (5)
- c. ½ - 1 pack (9)
- d. 1 - 2 packs (15)
- e. 2 + packs (20)

_____ 6. **Type of cigarette**
- a. High tar/nicotine (10)*
- b. Medium T/N (9)
- c. Low T/N (7)
- d. Nonsmoker (1)

_____ 7. **Duration of smoking**
- a. Never smoked (1)
- b. Ex-smoker (3)
- c. Up to 15 years (5)
- d. 15 - 25 years (10)
- e. 25 + years (20)

_____ 8. **Type of industrial work**
- a. Mining (3)
- b. Asbestos (7)
- c. Uranium & radioactive products (5)

_____
Total

*High T/N	20 mg + Tar/1.3 + mg. nicotine
Medium T/N	16 - 19 mg. Tar/1.1 - 1.2 nicotine
Low T/N	15 mg. or less Tar/1.0 mg. or less nicotine

Colon-Rectum Cancer

_____ 1. **Age**
- a. 39 or less (10)
- b. 40 - 59 (20)
- c. 60 and over (50)

_____ 2. **Has anyone in your immediate family ever had:**
a. Colon cancer (20)
b. One or more polyps of the colon (10)
c. Neither (1)

_____ 3. **Have you ever had:**
a. Colon cancer (100)
b. One or more polyps of the colon (40)
c. Ulcerative colitis (20)
d. Cancer of the breast or uterus (10)
e. None (1)

_____ 4. **Bleeding from the rectum** (other than obvious hemorrhoids or piles)
a. Yes (75)
b. No (1)

_____
Total

Skin Cancer

_____ 1. **Frequent work or play in the sun:**
a. Yes (10)
b. No (1)

_____ 2. **Work in mines, around coal tars, or around radioactivity:**
a. Yes (10)
b. No (1)

_____ 3. **Complexion** - Fair and/or light skin:
a. Yes (10)
b. No (1)

_____
Total

Breast Cancer

_____ 1. **Age group**
a. 20 - 34 (10)
b. 35 - 49 (40)
c. 50 and over (90)

_____ 2. **Race group**
a. Oriental (5)
b. Black (20)
c. White (25)
d. Mexican American (10)

_____ 3. **Family history**
a. Mother, sister, aunt, or grandmother with breast cancer (30)
b. None (10)

_____ 4. **Your history**
a. Previous lumps or cysts (25)
b. No breast disease (10)
c. Previous breast cancer (100)

_____ 5. **Maternity**
a. 1st pregnancy before 25 (10)
b. 1st pregnancy after 25 (15)
c. No pregnancies (20)

_____
Total

Cervical Cancer

(Lower Portion of Uterus. These questions would not apply to a woman who has had a total hysterectomy.)

_____ 1. **Age group**
a. Less than 25 (10)
b. 25 - 39 (20)
c. 40 - 54 (30)
d. 55 & over (30)

_____ 2. **Race**
a. Oriental (10)
b. Puerto Rican (20)
c. Black (20)
d. White (10)
e. Mexican American (20)

_____ 3. **Number of pregnancies**
a. 0 (10)
b. 1 to 3 (20)
c. 4 and over (30)

_____ 4. **Viral infections**
a. Herpes and other viral infections or ulcer formations on the vagina (10)
b. Never (1)

_____ 5. **Age at first intercourse**
a. Before 15 (40)
b. 15 - 19 (30)
c. 20 - 24 (20)
d. 25 and over (10)
e. Never (5)

_____ 6. **Bleeding between periods or after intercourse**
a. Yes (40)
b. No (1)

_____
Total

Endometrial Cancer

(Body of Uterus. These questions would not apply to a woman who has had a total hysterectomy.)

_____ 1. **Age group**
a. 39 or less (5)
b. 40 - 49 (20)
c. 50 and over (60)

_____ 2. **Race**
a. Oriental (10)
b. Black (10)
c. White (20)
d. Mexican American (10)

_____ 3. **Births**
a. None (15)
b. 1 to 4 (7)
c. 5 or more (5)

_____ 4. **Weight**
a. 50 or more pounds overweight (50)
b. 20 - 49 pounds overweight (15)
c. Underweight for height (10)
d. Normal (10)

_____ 5. **Diabetes** (elevated blood sugar)
a. Yes (3)
b. No (1)

_____ 6. **Estrogen hormone intake**
a. Yes, regularly (15)
b. Yes, occasionally (12)
c. None (10)

_____ 7. **Abnormal uterine bleeding**
a. Yes (40)
b. No (1)

_____ 8. **Hypertension** (high blood pressure)
a. Yes (3)
b. No (1)

_____
Total

CANCER QUESTIONNAIRE INTERPRETATION

The following interpretation of the cancer questionnaire is to summarize, explain new evidence, and provide valuable information on the individual risk that a person may have for each type of cancer. Potential cancer risk is based on individual lifestyle and medical history.

Lung Cancer

1. **Sex.** Men have a higher risk of lung cancer than women, equating them for type, amount, and duration of smoking. Since more women are smoking cigarettes for a longer duration than previously, their incidence of lung and upper respiratory tract (mouth, tongue, and larynx) cancer is increasing.
2. **Age.** The occurrence of lung and upper respiratory tract cancer increases with age.
3. **Smoking status.** Cigarette smokers have up to twenty times or even greater risk than nonsmokers. However, the rates of ex-smokers who have not smoked for ten years approach those of nonsmokers.
4. **Type of smoking.** Pipe and cigar smokers are at a higher risk for lung cancer than nonsmokers. Cigarette smokers are at a much higher risk than nonsmokers or pipe and cigar smokers. All forms of tobacco, including chewing, markedly increase the user's risk of developing cancer of the mouth.
5. **Amount of cigarettes smoked per day.** Male smokers of less than one-half pack per day have five times higher lung cancer rates than nonsmokers. Male smokers of one to two packs per day have fifteen times higher lung

cancer rates than nonsmokers. Smokers of more than two packs per day are twenty times more likely to develop lung cancer than nonsmokers.

6. **Type of cigarette.** Smokers of low-tar/nicotine cigarettes have slightly lower lung cancer rates.
7. **Duration of smoking.** The frequency of lung and upper respiratory tract cancer increases with the duration of smoking.
8. **Type of industrial work.** Exposures to materials used in the industries mentioned in the questionnaire have been demonstrated to be associated with lung cancer. Smokers who work in these industries may have greatly increased risks. Exposures to material in other industries may also carry a higher risk.

If your total is:

24 or less ...	You have a low risk for lung cancer (low risk category).
25 - 29......	You may be a light smoker and would have a good chance of kicking the habit (light risk).
50 - 74......	As a moderate smoker, your risks of lung and upper respiratory tract cancer are increased. If you stop smoking now, these risks will decrease (moderate risk).
75 - over	As a heavy cigarette smoker, your chances of getting lung and upper respiratory tract cancer are greatly increased. Your best bet is to stop smoking now — for the health of it. See your doctor if you have a nagging cough, hoarseness, persistent pain, or a sore in the mouth or throat (high risk).

Colon-Rectum Cancer

1. **Age.** Colon cancer occurs more frequently after the age of fifty.
2. **Family predisposition.** Colon cancer is more common in families with a previous history of this disease.
3. **Personal history.** Polyps and bowel diseases are associated with colon cancer.
4. **Rectal bleeding.** Rectal bleeding may be a sign of colorectal cancer.

If your total is:

29 or less ...	You are at a low risk for colon-rectum cancer.
30 - 69......	This is a moderate risk category. Testing by your physician may be indicated.
70 - over	This is a high-risk category. You should see your physician for the following tests: digital rectal exam, guaiac slide test, and protoscopic exam.

Skin Cancer

1. **Sun exposure.** Excessive ultraviolet light causes cancer of the skin. Protect yourself with a sunscreen medication.
2. **Work environment.** Working in mines, around coal tar, or radioactive materials can cause cancer of the skin.
3. **Complexion.** Persons with light complexions need more protection than others.

Total risk:

Numerical risks for skin cancer are difficult to state. For instance, a person with a dark complexion can work longer in the sun and be less likely to develop cancer than a light-complected person. Furthermore, a person wearing a long-sleeve shirt and wide-brimmed hat may work in the sun and be less at risk than a person who wears a bathing suit for only a short period. The risk greatly increases with age.

If you answer "yes" to any question, you need to protect your skin from the sun or any other toxic material. Changes in moles, warts, or skin sores are very important and need to be seen by your doctor.

Breast Cancer

If your total is:

Under 100 ...... Low-risk women should practice monthly breast self-examination (BSE) and have their breasts examined by a doctor as a part of a cancer-related checkup.

100 - 199 .... Moderate-risk women should practice monthly BSE and have their breasts examined by a doctor as part of a cancer-related checkup. Periodic breast X-rays should be included as your doctor may advise.

200 or higher ... High-risk women should practice monthly BSE and have the above examinations more often. See your doctor for the recommended (frequency of breast physical examinations and X-ray) examinations related to you.

Cervical Cancer

1. **Age.** The highest occurrence is in the forty and over age group. The numbers represent the relative rates of cancer for different age groups. A forty-five-year-old woman has a risk three times higher than a twenty-year-old.
2. **Race.** Puerto Ricans, Blacks, and Mexican Americans have higher rates of cervical cancer.
3. **Number of pregnancies.** Women who have delivered more children have a higher occurrence.
4. **Viral infections.** Viral infections of the cervix and vagina are associated with cervical cancer.
5. **Age at first intercourse.** Women with earlier intercourse and with more sexual partners are at a higher risk.
6. **Bleeding.** Irregular bleeding may be a sign of uterine cancer.

If your total is:

40 - 69 .... This is a low-risk group. Ask your doctor for a pap test. You will be advised how often you should be tested after your first test.

70 - 99 .... In this moderate risk group, more frequent pap tests may be required.

100 or more ... You are in a high-risk group and should have a pap test (and pelvic exam) as advised by your doctor.

Endometrial Cancer

1. **Age.** Endometrial cancer is seen in older age groups. The numbers by the age groups represent relative rates of endometrial cancer at different ages. A fifty-year-old woman has a risk twelve times higher than a thirty-five-old woman.
2. **Race.** Caucasians have a higher occurrence.
3. **Births.** The fewer children one has delivered, the greater the risk of endometrial cancer.
4. **Weight.** Women who are overweight are at greater risk.
5. **Diabetes.** Cancer of the endometrium is associated with diabetes.
6. **Estrogen use.** Cancer of the endometrium may be associated with prolonged continuous estrogen hormone intake. This occurs in only a small number of women. You should consult your physician before starting or stopping any estrogen medication.
7. **Abnormal bleeding.** Women who do not have cyclic regular menstrual periods are at greater risk.
8. **Hypertension.** Cancer of the endometrium is associated with high blood pressure.

If your total is:

45 - 59 .... You are at low risk for developing endometrial cancer.

60 - 99 .... Your risks are slightly higher (moderate risk). Report any abnormal bleeding immediately to your doctor. Tissue sampling at menopause is recommended.

100 and over ... Your risks are much greater (high risk). See your doctor for tests as appropriate.

WHAT CAN YOU DO?

If you are at high risk for any of the cancer sites, you are advised to discuss the results with your physician. An ounce of prevention is worth a pound of cure. Although cardiovascular disease is the number one killer in the country, cancer is the number one fear. Keep in mind that close to 80 percent of all cancers are preventable and about 50 percent are curable. Since most cancers are lifestyle related, awareness of the risk factors and implementation of the screening guidelines (Table 8.1), along with the basic recommendations for cancer prevention, will significantly decrease your personal risk for cancer. The main purpose of the information provided in this chapter is to educate and help you initiate your own fight against cancer.

References

1. American Cancer Society, Texas Division. *Cancer: Assessing Your Risk.* Dallas, TX: The Society, 1982.
2. American Cancer Society. *1985 Cancer Facts and Figures.* New York: The Society, 1985.
3. American Cancer Society. *Guidelines for the Cancer-Related Checkup: Recommendations and Rationale.* New York: The Society, 1980.
4. Greenwald, P. "Assessment of Risk Factors for Cancer." *Preventive Medicine* 9:260-263, 1980.
5. Hammond, E. C., and H. Seidman. "Smoking and Cancer in the United States." *Preventive Medicine* 9:169-173, 1980.
6. Higginson, J. "Proportion of Cancers Due to Occupation." *Preventive Medicine* 9:180-188, 1980.
7. Rothman, K. J. "The Proportion of Cancer Attributable to Alcohol Consumption." *Preventive Medicine* 9:174-179, 1980.
8. Weisburger, J. H., D. M. Hegsted, G. B. Gori, and B. Lewis. "Extending the Prudent Diet to Cancer Prevention." *Preventive Medicine* 9:297-304, 1980.
9. Williams, C. L. "Primary Prevention of Cancer Beginning in Childhood." *Preventive Medicine* 9:275-280, 1980.
10. Williams, P. A. "A Productive History and Physical Examination in the Prevention and Early Detection of Cancer." *Cancer* 47:1146-1150, 1981.

CHAPTER NINE

Stress Assessment and Management Techniques

Learning to live and get ahead today is practically impossible without stress. To work under pressure has become the rule rather than the exception for most people to succeed in an unpredictable world that changes with every new day. As a result, stress has become one of the most common problems that we face. While excessive stress is one of the factors related to twentieth-century patterns of life that is detrimental to human health, it is also a factor that can be self-controlled. Most people have accepted stress as a normal part of their daily life, and even though everyone has to deal with it, few seem to understand it and know how to cope effectively. On the other hand, stress should not be completely avoided, since a certain amount is necessary for an optimal level of performance and well-being. It is difficult to succeed and have fun in life without "hits, runs, and errors."

Just what is stress? Dr. Hans Selye, one of the foremost authorities on stress, defined stress as the nonspecific response of the human organism to any demand that is placed upon it. The term "nonspecific" indicates that the body will react in a similar fashion, regardless of the nature of the event that led to the stress response. In simpler terms, stress is the mental, emotional, and physiological response of the body to any situation that is new, threatening, frightening, or exciting.

STRESS: EUSTRESS VERSUS DISTRESS

The response of the human body to stress has been the same ever since man was first put on the earth. Stress prepares the organism to react to the stress-causing event (also referred to as stressor). The problem, though, is the manner in which we react to stress. Many people thrive under stress, while others under similar circumstances are unable to handle it. The individual's reaction to the particular stress-causing agent will determine whether stress is positive or negative.

The way in which we react to stress has been defined by Dr. Selye as either "eustress" or "distress." In both cases, the nonspecific response is almost the same, but in the case of eustress, health and performance continue to improve, even as stress increases. Distress, on the other hand, refers to the unpleasant or harmful stress under which health and performance begin to deteriorate.

Every person needs an optimal stress level that is most conducive to adequate performance. However, when stress levels reach the mental, emotional, and physiological limits, stress becomes distress and the person no longer functions effectively. Chronic distress increases the risk for many health disorders, including coronary heart disease, hypertension, ulcers, diabetes, asthma, depression, migraine headaches, and chronic fatigue. Recognizing this turning point, and overcoming the problem quickly and efficiently, are crucial in maintaining emotional and physiological stability.

SOURCES OF STRESS

During recent years, several instruments have been developed to assess sources of stress in life. One of the most common instruments used is the

Life Experiences Survey (*see* Figure 9.1), which identifies life changes within the last twelve months that may have an impact on a person's physical and psychological well-being. The survey contains forty-seven questions for all respondents and an additional ten designed for students only.

The format of the survey requires the subjects to rate the extent to which the life events that they experienced had a positive or negative impact on their life at the time they occurred. The ratings are on a seven-point scale. A rating of negative three (–3) indicates an extremely undesirable impact. A rating of zero (0) suggests neither a positive nor a negative impact. A rating of positive three (+3) indicates an extremely desirable impact. After determining the life events that have taken place, sum the negative and the positive points separately. Both scores should be expressed as positive numbers (e.g., positive ratings: 2, 1, 3, 3=9 points positive score; negative ratings: –3, –2, –2, –1, –2 = 10 points negative score). A final "total life change" score can be obtained by adding both the positive and negative scores together as positive numbers (e.g., total life change score: 9 + 10=19 points).

Since negative as well as positive changes can produce a nonspecific response, the total life change score gives a good indication of total life stress. However, most research in this area indicates that the negative change score is a better predictor for potential physical and/or psychological illness than the total change score. More research is necessary before the role of total change and the role of the ratio of positive to negative stress can be established. Therefore, only the negative score will be used as a part of your stress profile. To evaluate your results, refer to Table 9.1, which presents the various stress categories established for college students. Report your total number of negative points and the stress category in Figure 9.4 and Appendix A.

Table 9.1.
Stress Ratings for the Life Experiences Survey

Category	Negative Score		Total Score	
	Men	Women	Men	Women
Very Poor	13+	15+	27+	27+
Poor	7-12	8-14	17-26	18-26
Average	6	7	16	17
Good	1-5	1-6	5-15	6-15
Excellent	0	0	1-4	1-5

Adapted from Sarason, I. G., et al. "Assessing the Impact of Life Changes: Development of the Life Experiences Survey." *Journal of Consulting and Clinical Psychology* 46:932-946, 1978.

TYPE A BEHAVIOR

Common life events are not the only source of stress in life. All too often, stress is brought on by the individual as a result of behavior patterns. In Chapter 7, it was briefly mentioned that individuals can be categorized as having one of two types of behavior patterns: Type A or Type B. Each type has several characteristics that are used in classifying people into one of these behavior patterns. Even though several attempts have been made to develop an objective scale to properly identify the Type A individuals, these questionnaires are not as valid and reliable as researchers would like them to be. Consequently, the primary assessment tool used to determine behavior type has been the Structured Interview method.

During the Structured Interview, a person is asked to reply to different questions that describe Type A and Type B behavior patterns. The interviewer notes not only the responses to the questions, but also mental, emotional, and physical behaviors exhibited as the individual replies to each question. Based on the answers and the behaviors exhibited, the interviewer actually rates the person along a continuum, ranging from Type A to Type B. Along this continuum, behavior patterns are classified into five categories: A-1, A-2, X (a mix of Type A and Type B), B-3, and B-4. The Type A-1 exhibits all of the Type A characteristics, while a relative absence of the Type A behaviors is observed in the Type B-4. The Type A-2 does not exhibit a complete Type A pattern, and the Type B-3 only exhibits a few Type A characteristics.

The Type A behavior is primarily charateristic of a hard-driving, overambitious, aggressive, at times hostile, and overly competitive person. These individuals often set their own goals, are self-motivated, try to accomplish many tasks at the same time, are excessively achievement-oriented, and have a high degree of time urgency. In contrast, the Type B behavior is characteristic of a calmed, casual, relaxed, and easy-going individual. The Type B person takes one thing at a time, does not feel pressured nor hurried, and seldom sets his own deadlines.

Over the years, research studies indicated that individuals classified as Type A are under much more stress and have a significantly higher incidence of coronary heart disease. Based on these findings, Type A individuals have been counseled to decrease their stress level by modifying many

Figure 9.1. *The Life Experiences Survey*

Listed below are a number of events that sometimes bring about change in the lives of those who experience them and that necessitate social readjustment. Please check events that you have experienced in the past twelve months. Be sure that all check marks are directly across from the items to which they correspond (only check those that apply).

Also, for each item checked below, please indicate the extent to which you viewed the event as having either a positive or negative impact on your life at the time the event occurred. That is, indicate the type and extent of impact that the event had. A rating of –3 would indicate an extremely negative impact. A rating of 0 suggests no impact either positive or negative. A rating of +3 would indicate an extremely positive impact.

Section 1

1. Marriage	–3	–2	–1	0	+1	+2	+3
2. Detention in jail or comparable institution	–3	–2	–1	0	+1	+2	+3
3. Death of spouse	–3	–2	–1	0	+1	+2	+3
4. Major change in sleeping habits (much more or much less sleep)	–3	–2	–1	0	+1	+2	+3
5. Death of close family member:							
a. mother	–3	–2	–1	0	+1	+2	+3
b. father	–3	–2	–1	0	+1	+2	+3
c. brother	–3	–2	–1	0	+1	+2	+3
d. sister	–3	–2	–1	0	+1	+2	+3
e. grandmother	–3	–2	–1	0	+1	+2	+3
f. grandfather	–3	–2	–1	0	+1	+2	+3
g. other (specify)	–3	–2	–1	0	+1	+2	+3
6. Major change in eating habits (much more or less food intake)	–3	–2	–1	0	+1	+2	+3
7. Foreclosure on mortgage or loan	–3	–2	–1	0	+1	+2	+3
8. Death of close friend	–3	–2	–1	0	+1	+2	+3
9. Outstanding personal achievement	–3	–2	–1	0	+1	+2	+3
10. Minor law violations (traffic tickets, disturbing the peace, etc.)	–3	–2	–1	0	+1	+2	+3
11. Male: Wife/girlfriend's pregnancy	–3	–2	–1	0	+1	+2	+3
12. Female: Pregnancy	–3	–2	–1	0	+1	+2	+3
13. Changed work situation (different work responsibility, major change in working conditions, working hours, etc.)	–3	–2	–1	0	+1	+2	+3
14. New job	–3	–2	–1	0	+1	+2	+3
15. Serious illness or injury or close family member:							
a. father	–3	–2	–1	0	+1	+2	+3
b. mother	–3	–2	–1	0	+1	+2	+3
c. sister	–3	–2	–1	0	+1	+2	+3
d. brother	–3	–2	–1	0	+1	+2	+3
e. grandfather	–3	–2	–1	0	+1	+2	+3
f. grandmother	–3	–2	–1	0	+1	+2	+3
g. spouse	–3	–2	–1	0	+1	+2	+3
h. other (specify)	–3	–2	–1	0	+1	+2	+3
16. Sexual difficulties	–3	–2	–1	0	+1	+2	+3
17. Trouble with employer (in danger of losing job, being suspended, demoted, etc.)	–3	–2	–1	0	+1	+2	+3
18. Trouble with in-laws	–3	–2	–1	0	+1	+2	+3
19. Major change in financial status (a lot better off or a lot worse off)	–3	–2	–1	0	+1	+2	+3

(Continued)

From Sarason, I. G., et al. Assessing the impact of life changes: Development of the Life Experiences Survey. Journal of Consulting and Clinical Psychology 46:932-946, 1978.

Figure 9.1. *The Life Experiences Survey (continued)*

20. Major change in closeness of family members (increased or decreased closeness)	−3	−2	−1	0	+1	+2	+3
21. Gaining a new family member (through birth, adoption, family member moving in, etc.)	−3	−2	−1	0	+1	+2	+3
22. Change of residence	−3	−2	−1	0	+1	+2	+3
23. Marital separation from mate (due to conflict)	−3	−2	−1	0	+1	+2	+3
24. Major change in church activities (increased or decreased attendance)	−3	−2	−1	0	+1	+2	+3
25. Marital reconciliation with mate	−3	−2	−1	0	+1	+2	+3
26. Major change in number of arguments with spouse (a lot more or a lot less arguments)	−3	−2	−1	0	+1	+2	+3
27. Married Male: Change in wife's work outside the home (beginning work, ceasing work, changing to a new job, etc.)	−3	−2	−1	0	+1	+2	+3
28. Married female: Change in husband's work (loss of job, beginning new job, retirement etc.)	−3	−2	−1	0	+1	+2	+3
29. Major change in usual type and/or amount of recreation	−3	−2	−1	0	+1	+2	+3
30. Borrowing more than $10,000 (buying home, business, etc.)	−3	−2	−1	0	+1	+2	+3
31. Borrowing less than $10,000 (buying car, TV, getting school loan, etc.)	−3	−2	−1	0	+1	+2	+3
32. Being fired from job	−3	−2	−1	0	+1	+2	+3
33. Male: Wife/girlfriend having abortion	−3	−2	−1	0	+1	+2	+3
34. Female: Having abortion	−3	−2	−1	0	+1	+2	+3
35. Major personal illness or injury	−3	−2	−1	0	+1	+2	+3
36. Major change in social activities, e.g., parties, movies, visiting (increased or decreased participation)	−3	−2	−1	0	+1	+2	+3
37. Major change in living conditions of family (building new home, remodeling, deterioration of home, neighborhood, etc.)	−3	−2	−1	0	+1	+2	+3
38. Divorce	−3	−2	−1	0	+1	+2	+3
39. Serious injury or illness of close friend	−3	−2	−1	0	+1	+2	+3
40. Retirement from work	−3	−2	−1	0	+1	+2	+3
41. Son or daughter leaving home (due to marriage, college, etc.)	−3	−2	−1	0	+1	+2	+3
42. Ending of formal schooling	−3	−2	−1	0	+1	+2	+3
43. Separation from spouse (due to work, travel, etc.)	−3	−2	−1	0	+1	+2	+3
44. Engagement	−3	−2	−1	0	+1	+2	+3
45. Breaking up with boyfriend/girlfriend	−3	−2	−1	0	+1	+2	+3
46. Leaving home for the first time	−3	−2	−1	0	+1	+2	+3
47. Reconciliation with boyfriend/girlfriend	−3	−2	−1	0	+1	+2	+3
48. Others ____________________	−3	−2	−1	0	+1	+2	+3
49. ____________________	−3	−2	−1	0	+1	+2	+3
50. ____________________	−3	−2	−1	0	+1	+2	+3
51. Beginning a new school experience at a higher academic level (college, graduate school, professional school, etc.)	−3	−2	−1	0	+1	+2	+3
52. Changing to a new school at the same academic level (undergraduate, graduate, etc.)	−3	−2	−1	0	+1	+2	+3
53. Academic probation	−3	−2	−1	0	+1	+2	+3
54. Being dismissed from dormitory or other residence	−3	−2	−1	0	+1	+2	+3
55. Failing an important exam	−3	−2	−1	0	+1	+2	+3
56. Changing a major	−3	−2	−1	0	+1	+2	+3
57. Failing a course	−3	−2	−1	0	+1	+2	+3
58. Dropping a course	−3	−2	−1	0	+1	+2	+3
59. Joining a fraternity/sorority	−3	−2	−1	0	+1	+2	+3
60. Financial problems concerning school (in danger of not having sufficient money to continue)	−3	−2	−1	0	+1	+2	+3

of their Type A behaviors. Most experts agree that Type A behavior is a learned behavior. Consequently, if people can learn to identify the sources of stress and make changes in behavioral responses, they can move down along the continuum and respond more like the Type B. The debate, however, has been centered around which Type A behaviors should be changed, since not all of them are undesirable.

Although experts have known that individuals exhibiting the Type A behavior were more coronary prone and that behavioral changes were needed to decrease the risk for disease, new scientific evidence indicates that not all of the typical Type A people are at a higher risk for disease. It seems that mainly the Type A individual who commonly exhibits behaviors of anger and hostility is at higher risk for disease. Therefore, many behavioral modification counselors now work primarily on changing the latter behaviors to prevent the incidence of disease.

For years it has also been known that there are many individuals who perform well under pressure. They are typically classified as Type A but never exhibit any of the detrimental effects of stress. These people have recently been referred to by Drs. Robert and Marilyn Kriegel as exhibiting Type C behavior. The Type C individuals are just as highly stressed as the Type A but do not seem to be at higher risk for disease than the Type B. The keys to successful Type C performance seem to be commitment, confidence, and control. These people are highly committed to what they are doing, have a great deal of confidence in their ability to do their work, and can be in constant control of their actions. In addition, Type C people love and enjoy their work and maintain themselves in top physical condition to be able to meet the mental and physical demands of their work.

STRESS VULNERABILITY

Researchers have now been able to identify a number of factors that can affect the way in which people handle stress. How they deal with these factors can actually increase or decrease their vulnerability to stress. The questionnaire found in Figure 9.2 contains a list of these factors and has been designed to help you determine your vulnerability quotient. The questionnaire will also help you identify particular areas where improvements can be made to help you cope more efficiently. As you take this test, you will notice that most of the items describe situations and behaviors that are within your own control. On the test you will rate yourself on a scale from 1 (almost always) to 5 (never), according to how each particular statement applies to you. To make yourself less vulnerable to stress, modify the behaviors on which you gave yourself a score of 3 or higher. It is also recommended that you start by modifying those behaviors that are easiest to change before undertaking some of the most difficult ones. After completing the questionnaire, be sure to record the results in Figure 9.4 and in Appendix A.

STRESS MANAGEMENT TECHNIQUES

It is obvious that the ability to handle stress varies among individuals. If you feel that stress is definitely a problem in your life and that it is interfering with your optimal health and performance, several stress management techniques have been developed to help you cope better.

The initial step, of course, is to recognize that you have a problem. Many people either do not want to accept the fact that they are under too much stress and/or fail to recognize some of the typical symptoms of distress. Noting some of the stress-related symptoms will help you respond more objectively and initiate an adequate coping response. A list of different symptoms that people experience when stress becomes distress is given in Figure 9.3. By going through this list, you will probably recognize some of your own bodily responses when confronted with a stressful event.

If you are experiencing stress-related symptoms, initially you should try to identify and remove the stressor or stress-causing agent. This is not as simple as it may seem, because in some situations, elimination of the stressor is impossible, or perhaps you do not know the exact causing agent. If you do not know the cause, it may be helpful to keep a log of the time and days when the symptoms occur, as well as the events that transpire before and after the onset of symptoms. For instance, a couple had noted that every afternoon around six o'clock, the wife became very nauseated and experienced a significant amount of abdominal pain. After seeking professional help, the

Figure 9.2. *Stress Vulnerability Scale*

The following scale has been designed to rate your vulnerability to stress. Rate each item from 1 (almost always) to 5 (never), according to how each particular statement applies to you. Make sure to mark each item. If a particular item doesn't apply to you, circle a 1 (for example, if you don't smoke, circle 1).

Item		Score				
1.	I eat at least one hot, balanced meal a day.	1	2	3	4	5
2.	I get seven to eight hours of sleep at least four nights a week.	1	2	3	4	5
3.	I give and receive affection regularly.	1	2	3	4	5
4.	I have at least one relative within fifty miles on whom I can rely.	1	2	3	4	5
5.	I exercise to the point of perspiration at least twice a week.	1	2	3	4	5
6.	I limit myself to less than half a pack of cigarettes a day.	1	2	3	4	5
7.	I take fewer than five alcoholic drinks a week.	1	2	3	4	5
8.	I am at the appropriate weight for my height.	1	2	3	4	5
9.	I have an income adequate to meet basic expenses.	1	2	3	4	5
10.	I get strength from my religious beliefs.	1	2	3	4	5
11.	I regularly attend club or social activities.	1	2	3	4	5
12.	I have a network of friends and acquaintances.	1	2	3	4	5
13.	I have one or more friends to confide in about personal matters.	1	2	3	4	5
14.	I am in good health (including eyesight, hearing, teeth).	1	2	3	4	5
15.	I am able to speak openly about my feelings when angry or worried.	1	2	3	4	5
16.	I have regular conversations with the people I live with about domestic problems — for example, chores and money.	1	2	3	4	5
17.	I do something for fun at least once a week.	1	2	3	4	5
18.	I am able to organize my time effectively.	1	2	3	4	5
19.	I drink fewer than three cups of coffee (or other caffeine-rich drinks) a day.	1	2	3	4	5
20.	I take some quiet time for myself during the day.	1	2	3	4	5

To obtain your final score, add up all of the numbers that you circled and subtract 20.

Total Score: ________ - 20 = ________ Points

Stress Vulnerability Rating

0-10 Points .... Excellent. Excellent resistance to stress
11-30 Points .... Good. Very little vulnerability to stress
31-50 Points .... Fair. Some vulnerability to stress
51-80 Points .... Poor. Seriously vulnerable to stress

From "Vulnerability Scale." *Stress Audit,* developed by Lyle H. Miller and Alma Dell Smith. Boston University Medical Center.

Figure 9.3. *Typical Symptoms of Stress*

_______ Headache

_______ Muscular aches (mainly neck, shoulders, and back)

_______ Grinding teeth

_______ Nervous tick, finger tapping, toe tapping

_______ Increased sweating

_______ Increase or loss of appetite

_______ Insomnia

_______ Nightmares

_______ Fatigue

_______ Dry mouth

_______ Stuttering

_______ High blood pressure

_______ Tightness or pain in the chest

_______ Impotence

_______ Hives

_______ Others that you experience (list):

_______ Dizziness

_______ Depression

_______ Irritation

_______ Anger

_______ Frustration

_______ Hostility

_______ Fear, panic, anxiety

_______ Stomach pain, flutters

_______ Nausea

_______ Cold, clammy hands

_______ Poor concentration

_______ Pacing

_______ Restlessness

_______ Rapid heart rate

_______ Low-grade infection

_______ Loss of sex drive

_______ Rash or acne

____

____

Figure 9.4. *Stress Profile*

Name: ______________________________

Date	______	______	______
Life Event Survey			
Score (negative)	______	______	______
Stress Rating	______	______	______
Stress Vulnerability			
Final Score	______	______	______
Rating	______	______	______
Stress Management Technique(s) to be used	______	______	______

couple was instructed to keep a log of daily events. It soon beame clear that the symptoms did not occur on weekends, but always started just before the husband came home from work. Following some personal interviews with the couple, it was determined that the wife felt a lack of attention from her husband and subconsciously responded by becoming ill to the point where it required personal care and affection from her husband.

In other instances where the stressor cannot be removed (e.g., death of a close family member, first year in college, an intolerable professor, final exams, etc.), stress can be decreased or eliminated through the use of relaxation techniques.

When the body responds to stress by activating the "fight or flight" mechanism, it prepares you to take action by stimulating your vital defense systems. This stimulation originates in the hypothalamus and the pituitary gland in the brain. The hypothalamus activates the sympathetic nervous system, and the pituitary activates the release of catecholamines (hormones) from the adrenal glands. These changes increase heart rate, blood pressure, blood flow to active muscles, glucose levels, oxygen consumption, and strength — all necessary for the body to "fight or flee." In order for the body to relax, action must take place. If you "fight or flee," the body relaxes and the stress is dissipated. If you cannot take action, tension and tightening of the muscles increase. In the latter case, the increased tension and tightening can be effectively dissipated with adequate relaxation techniques.

Several relaxation techniques will now be discussed. Although benefits are reaped immediately after performing a given technique, several months of regular practice may be necessary for complete mastery. Keep in mind that relaxation exercises are not a cure-all panacea. If the exercises outlined in this chapter do not prove effective, you should refer to a more specialized textbook or seek professional help. It is also possible that in some instances the symptoms that you are experiencing may not be caused by stress, but rather related to a different medical disorder.

Physical Exercise as a Means for Stress Reduction

Physical exercise is one of the simplest tools used to control stress. The value of exercise in reducing stress is related to several factors. The principal factor is a decrease in muscular tension. If you are distressed because you are having problems with your boss, or if you are driving home after a long day and the car in front of you is going much slower than the speed limit, you may not be able to dissipate your stress by hitting your boss or the car in front of you, but you can certainly "hit" the tennis ball, the weights, the swimming pool, or the jogging trail. By engaging in physical activity, you are able to reduce the muscle tension and metabolize the increased catecholamines that brought about the physiological changes that triggered the "fight-or-flight" mechanism.

A point of interest is that the early evening hours are becoming the most popular time to exercise for a lot of highly stressed executives. On the way home from work, they will stop at the health club or the fitness center. Exercising at this hour helps them dissipate the excessive stress accumulated during the day. Perhaps you will remember how good the shower felt the last time you concluded a good strenuous exercise session after a hard day at the office. For this reason, many individuals have said that "the best part of exercise is the shower afterwards." Not only will exercise help get rid of the stress, but it will also provide an opportunity to enjoy a better evening. At home, the family will appreciate the fact that you come home more relaxed (leaving your work problems behind), and that you have more energy to dedicate to family activities.

The same thing can be said about students. If you have had a hard day at school, exercising in the evening hours will help dissipate your stress and allow you to better concentrate on your work and assignments for the next school day.

Another way that exercise helps in reducing stress is by deliberately diverting stress to various body systems. Dr. Hans Selye explains in his book *Stress Without Distress* that when the accomplishment of one specific task becomes difficult, a change in activity can be as good or better than rest itself. For example, if you are having a difficult time writing a term paper, it is better to go jogging or swimming for a while, rather than sitting around and getting frustrated. In this manner, the mental strain is diverted to the working muscles, and the one system helps the other relax. Another psychologist, Dr. William James, has indicated that when muscular tension is removed from the emotional strain, the emotional strain disappears. In many cases, the change of activity will suddenly clear the mind and help put the pieces together.

Other researchers have found that physical exercise gives people a psychological boost because exercise: (a) reduces feelings of anxiety, depression, frustration, aggression, anger, and hostility, (b) decreases insomnia, (c) provides an opportunity to meet social needs and develop new friendships, (d) allows the person to share common interests and problems, (e) develops discipline, and (f) provides the opportunity to do something enjoyable and constructive that will lead to better health and total well-being.

Progressive Muscle Relaxation

Progressive muscle relaxation was developed by Dr. Edmund Jacobsen in the 1930s. This technique enables individuals to relearn the sensation of deep relaxation. The technique involves progressive contraction and relaxation of muscle groups throughout the body. Since chronic stress leads to high levels of muscular tension, being closely aware of how it feels to progressively tighten and relax the muscles will release the tension on the muscles and teach the body to relax at will. Being aware of the tension felt during the exercises also helps the person be more alert to signs of distress, since similar feelings are experienced in stressful situations. In everyday life, such feelings can then be used as a cue to implement adequate relaxation exercises.

Relaxation exercises should be conducted in a quiet, warm, and well-ventilated room. The recommended exercises and the duration of the routine vary from one author to the next. However, the important consideration is that you pay attention to the sensation felt each time you tense and relax. The exercises should also include all muscle groups of the body. An example of a sequence of progressive muscle relaxation exercises is given below. The instructions outlined for these exercises can be either read to you, memorized, or recorded on a tape. Allow yourself about twenty minutes to perform the entire sequence. Doing them any faster will defeat the purpose of the exercises. Ideally, the sequence should be performed twice a day.

Instructions: Stretch out comfortably on the floor (with your back against the floor), place a pillow under your knees, and allow yourself to relax as much as possible. Contract each muscle group in sequence, taking care to avoid any strain. You should only tighten to about 70 percent of the total possible tension to avoid cramping or some type of injury to the muscle itself. Pay attention to the sensation of tensing up and relaxing. Hold each contraction for about five seconds, then allow the muscles to go totally limp. Make sure that you allow sufficient time to contract and relax before the next statement is given.

1. Point your feet, curling the toes downward, and study the tension in the arches and the top of the feet. Hold it and continue to note the tension, then relax. Repeat a second time.
2. Flex the feet upwards toward the face and note the tension in your feet and calves. Hold it . . ., and relax . . . Repeat again.
3. Push your heels down against the floor as if burying them in the sand. Hold it and note the tension on the back of the thigh; relax. Repeat one more time.
4. Contract the right thigh by straightening the leg, gently raising the leg off the floor. Hold it and study the tension; relax . . . Repeat with the left leg; hold and relax. Repeat both legs again.
5. Tense the buttocks by raising your hips ever so slightly off the floor. Hold it and note the tension, and relax . . . Repeat again.
6. Contract the abdominal muscles. Hold them tight and note the tension; relax . . . Repeat one more time.
7. Suck in your stomach — try to make it reach your spine. Flatten your lower back to the floor; hold it and feel the tension in the stomach and lower back; relax . . . Repeat again.
8. Take a deep breath and hold it . . ., and exhale. Repeat again. Note your breathing becoming slower and more relaxed.
9. Place your arms on the side of your body and clench both fists. Hold it . . ., study the tension, and relax . . . Repeat a second time.
10. Flex the elbow by bringing both hands to the shoulders. Hold it tight and study the tension in the biceps; relax . . . Repeat again.
11. Place your arms flat on the floor, palms up, and push the forearm hard against the floor. Note the tension on the triceps; hold it . . ., and relax . . . Repeat the exercise.

12. Shrug your shoulders, raising them as high as possible. Hold it and note the tension; relax . . . Repeat again.
13. Gently push your head backward; note the tension in the back of the neck. Hold it . . ., relax . . . Repeat one more time.
14. Gently bring the head against the chest, push forward, hold, and note the tension in the neck. Relax . . . Repeat a second time.
15. Press your tongue toward the roof of your mouth. Hold it . . .; study the tension; relax . . . Do it again.
16. Press your teeth together. Hold it and study the tension; relax . . . Repeat again.
17. Close your eyes tightly. Hold them closed and note the tension. Relax, leaving your eyes closed. Repeat again.
18. Wrinkle your forehead. Note the tension; hold it . . ., and relax . . . Repeat one more time.

In some instances during your daily routine when time is a factor, you may not be able to do the entire sequence. In such cases, perform only the exercises specific to the area where you feel muscle tension. Even a short exercise is better than none at all. But remember, the complete sequence produces better results.

Breathing Techniques For Relaxation

Breathing exercises can also be used as an antidote to stress. Such exercises have been used for centuries in the Orient and India as a means to develop better mental, physical, and emotional stamina. In breathing exercises, the person concentrates on "breathing away" the tension and inhaling fresh oxygen to the entire body.

Breathing exercises can be learned in only a few minutes and require considerably less time than the progressive muscle relaxation exercises. As with any other relaxation technique, you will need to find a quiet, pleasant, and well-ventilated room. Three examples of breathing exercises will now be presented. You can conduct any one of these exercises whenever you feel that you are tensing up.

1. **Deep breathing:** Lie with your back flat against the floor, place a pillow under your knees, feet slightly separated, and toes pointing outward (the exercise may also be conducted sitting up in a chair or standing straight up). Place one hand on your abdomen and the other one on your chest. Slowly breathe in and out so that the hand on your abdomen rises when you inhale and falls as you exhale. The hand on the chest should not move much at all. Repeat the exercise about ten times. Next, scan your body for tension, and compare your present tension with that felt at the beginning of the exercise. Repeat the entire process once or twice more.
2. **Sighing:** Using the abdominal breathing technique, breathe in through your nose to a specific count (i.e., 4, 5, 6, etc.). Now exhale through pursed lips to double the intake count (i.e., 8, 10, 12, etc.). Repeat the exercise eight to ten times whenever you feel tense.
3. **Complete natural breathing:** Sit in an upright position or stand straight up. Breathe through your nose and gradually fill up your lungs from the bottom up. Hold your breath for several seconds. Now exhale slowly by allowing complete relaxation of the chest and abdomen. Repeat the exercise eight to ten times.

Autogenic Training

Autogenic training is basically a form of self-suggestion, where an individual is able to place himself in an autohypnotic state by repeating and concentrating on feelings of heaviness and warmth in the extremities. This technique was developed by Johannes H. Schultz, a German psychiatrist who noted that hypnotized individuals developed sensations of warmth and heaviness in the limbs and torso. The sensation of warmth is caused by dilation of blood vessels, which increases blood flow to the limbs. The heaviness is felt as a result of muscle relaxation.

When using this technique, the person lies or sits down in a comfortable position with eyes closed and progressively concentrates on six fundamental stages:

1. **Heaviness**
   My right (left) arm is heavy
   Both arms are heavy
   My right (left) leg is heavy
   Both legs are heavy
   My arms and legs are heavy

2. **Warmth**
   My right (left) arm is warm
   Both arms are warm
   My right (left) leg is warm
   Both legs are warm
   My arms and legs are warm

3. **Heart**
   My heartbeat is calm and regular (repeat four or five times)

4. **Respiration**
   My body breathes itself (repeat four or five times)

5. **Abdomen**
   My abdomen is warm (repeat four or five times)

6. **Forehead**
   My forehead is cool (repeat four or five times)

The autogenic training technique is more difficult to master than any of those previously mentioned. Do not move too fast through the entire exercise, since this practice may actually interfere with the learning and relaxation process. Master each stage before you conduct the next one.

Meditation

Meditation is a mental exercise that can bring about psychological and physical benefits. The objective of meditation is to gain control over your attention, clearing the mind and blocking out the stressor(s) responsible for the increased tension. This technique can also be learned rather quickly and be used frequently during periods of increased tension and stress.

Initially, the person who is trying to learn to meditate should choose a room that is comfortable, quiet, and free of all disturbances (including telephones). Nevertheless, once the technique is learned, the person will be able to meditate just about anywhere. Set aside approximately fifteen minutes, twice a day, and practice the following exercises:

1. Sit in a chair in an upright position with the hands resting either in your lap or on the arms of the chair. Close your eyes and focus on your breathing. Allow your body to relax as much as possible. Do not try to consciously relax, since trying means work. Rather, assume a passive attitude and concentrate on your breathing.

2. Allow the body to breathe regularly, at its own rhythm, and repeat in your mind the word "one" everytime you inhale, and the word "two" everytime you exhale. Paying attention to these two words keeps distressing thoughts from entering into your mind.

3. Continue to breathe for about fifteen minutes. Since the objective of meditating is to bring about a hypometabolic state, leading to body relaxation, do not use an alarm clock to remind you that the fifteen minutes have expired. The alarm will only trigger your stress response again, defeating the purpose of the exercise. It is fine to open your eyes once in a while to keep track of the time. But remember not to "rush" or anticipate the end of the fifteen minutes. This time has been set aside for meditation and you need to relax, take your time, and enjoy the exercise.

Which Technique is Best

It does not really matter which technique you select, as long as it works. You may want to experiment with all of them or use a combination of two or more. All of these techniques will help block out the stressor(s) and lead to mental and physical relaxation by diverting your attention to a different, nonthreatening action. Some of the techniques are easier to learn and may take less time per session. Regardless of which technique you use, if stress is a significant problem in your life, the time that you spend doing these exercises is well worth the effort. "Relax" and take your time. It is not stress that makes you ill, but rather the way in which you react to the particular stress-causing agent. Being diligent and taking control of yourself will provide you with a better, happier, and healthier life.

References

1. Blue Cross Association. *Stress.* Chicago: The Association, 1974.
2. Chesney, M. A., J. R. Eagleston, and R. H. Rosenman. "Type A Assessment and Intervention." In *Medical Psychology: Contributions to Behavioral Medicine.* Edited by C. K. Prokop and L. A. Bradley. New York: Academic Press, 1981.
3. Gauron, E. F. *Mental Training For Peak Performance.* Lansing, NY: Sport Science Associates, 1984.
4. Girdano, D., and G. Everly. *Controlling Stress and Tension.* Englewood Cliffs, NJ: Prentice-Hall, Inc., 1979.
5. Greenberg, J. S. *Comprehensive Stress Management.* Dubuque, IA: Wm. C. Brown Company Publishers, 1983.
6. Kriegel, R. J., and M. H. Kriegel. *The C Zone: Peak Performance Under Stress.* Garden City, NY: Anchor Press/Doubleday, 1984.
7. Luthe, W. "Autogenic Training: Method, Research and Application in Medicine." *American Journal of Psychotherapy* 17:174-195, 1963.
8. McKay, M., M. Davis, and P. Fanning. *Thoughts and Feelings: The Act of Cognitive Stress Intervention.* Richmond, CA: New Harbinger Publications, 1981.
9. Miller, L. H., and A. D. Smith. "Vulnerability Scale." Stress Audit, 1983.
10. Sarason, I. G., J. H. Johnson, and J. M. Siegel. "Assessing the Impact of Life Changes: Development of the Life Experiences Survey." *Journal of Consulting and Clinical Psychology* 46:932-946, 1978.
11. Selye, H. *Stress Without Distress.* New York: Signet, 1974.
12. Selye, H. *The Stress of Life.* New York: McGraw-Hill Book Co., 1978.

CHAPTER TEN

Smoking Cessation

Tobacco has been used throughout the world for hundreds of years. Prior to the eighteenth century, it was smoked primarily in the form of pipes or cigars. Cigarette smoking per se did not become popular until the mid-1800s, and its use started to increase dramatically at the turn of the century. In 1915, 18 billion cigarettes were consumed in the United States, as compared to 640 billion in 1981. There are now more than 53 million Americans over the age of seventeen who smoke an average of one and one-half packs of cigarettes per day.

The harmful effects of cigarette smoking and tobacco usage in general were not exactly known until the early 1960s, when researchers began to show a positive link between tobacco use and disease. In 1964, the United States Surgeon General issued the first major report presenting scientific evidence that cigarettes were indeed a major health hazard in our society.

The use of tobacco in all forms is now considered a significant threat to life. Cigarette smoking is the largest preventable cause of illness and premature death in the United States. When considering all related deaths, smoking is responsible for 450,000 unnecessary deaths each year. There is a definite increase in death rates from heart disease, cancer, stroke, aortic aneurysm, chronic bronchitis, emphysema, and peptic ulcers. Maternal cigarette smoking has been linked to retarded fetal growth, increased risk for spontaneous abortion, and prenatal death. Smoking is also the most common cause of fire deaths and injuries. The average life expectancy for a chronic smoker is seven years less than a nonsmoker, and the death rate among chronic smokers during the most productive years of life, between the ages of twenty-five and sixty-five is twice that of the national average.

According to American Heart Association estimates, over 30 percent or 120,000 fatal heart attacks annually are due to smoking. Heart attack risk is 50 to 100 percent greater for smokers as compared to nonsmokers. There is also an increased mortality rate following heart attacks, since they are usually more severe and the risk for deadly arrhythmias is much greater. Cigarette smoking affects the cardiovascular system by increasing heart rate, blood pressure, susceptibility to atherosclerosis, and blood clots. Evidence also indicates that it decreases high-density lipoprotein (HDL) cholesterol, or the so-called "good" cholesterol, which decreases the risk for heart disease. Finally, carbon monoxide found in smoke decreases the oxygen delivery capacity of the blood to the tissues of the body.

Also known is the fact that the biggest carcinogenic exposure in the work place is cigarette smoke. The American Cancer Society reports that 83 percent of lung cancer and 30 percent of all cancers are due to smoking. It kills about 138,000 people each year. Lung cancer is the leading cancer killer and is responsible for 35 percent of all cancer deaths. While it is encouraging to note that over 50 percent of all cancers are now curable, the five-year survival rate for lung cancer is less than 10 percent. Tobacco use also increases cancer risk of the oral cavity, larynx, esophagus, bladder, pancreas, and kidneys.

While most tobacco users are aware of the health consequences of cigarette smoking, many fail to realize the risk of pipe smoking, cigar smoking, and chewing tobacco. As a group in

Figure 10.1. *Emphysema. Normal-looking alveoli (air cells) are shown on the left side. To the right, an obstructed airway and enlarged alveoli as a result of mucus and pus accumulation seen in emphysemic patients.*

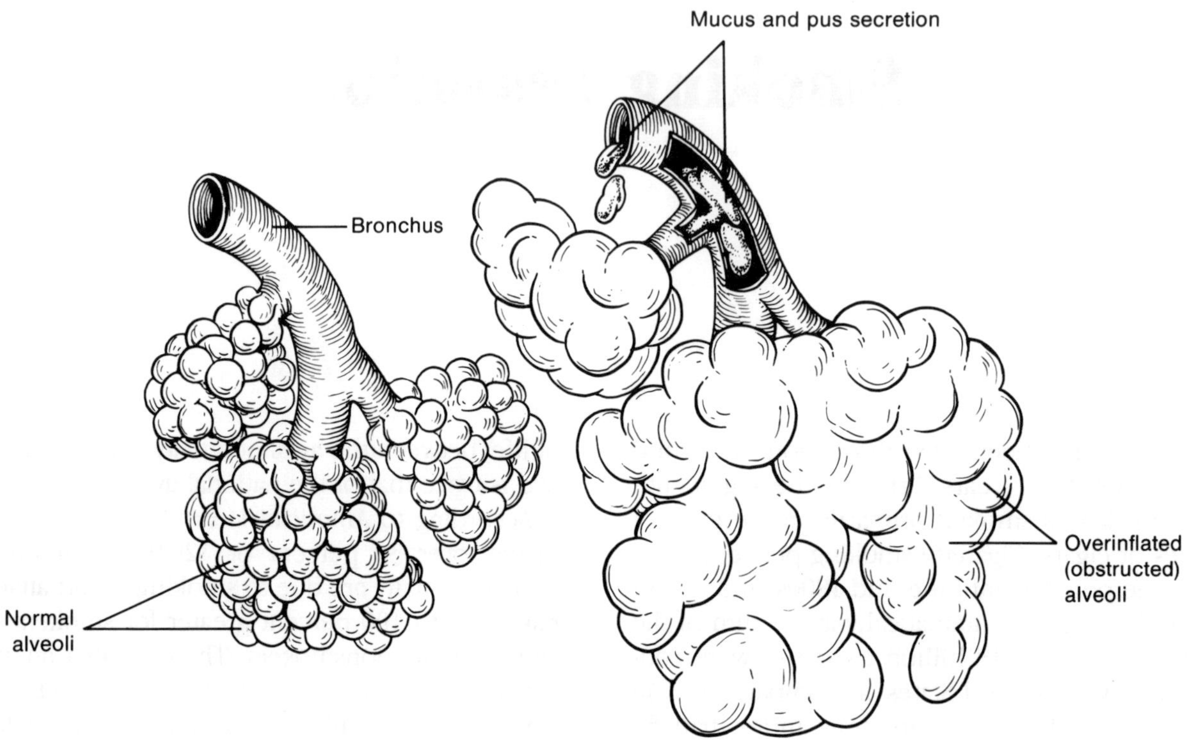

general, the risk for heart disease and lung cancer is lower than for cigarette smokers. However, blood nicotine levels in pipe and cigar smokers have been shown to approach those of cigarette smokers, since nicotine is still absorbed through the mouth membranes. Therefore, there is still a higher risk for heart disease as compared to nonsmokers. Cigarette smokers who substitute pipe or cigar smoking for cigarettes usually continue to inhale the smoke, which actually results in a greater amount of nicotine and tar being brought into the lungs. Consequently, the risk for disease is even greater if pipe or cigar smoke is inhaled. The risk and mortality rates for lip, mouth, and larynx cancer for pipe smoking, cigar smoking, or chewing tobacco are actually higher than for cigarette smokers.

The economical impact of cigarette smoking among American business and industry is also staggering. Companies pay in excess of $16 billion each year as a direct result of smoking at the work place and another $37 billion in lost productivity and earnings because of illness, disability, and death. Heavy smokers have been shown to use the health care system, especially hospitals, over 50 percent more than nonsmokers. The yearly cost to a given company has been estimated between $624 and $4,611 per smoking employee. These costs include employee health care, absenteeism, additional health insurance, morbidity/disability and early mortality, on-the-job lost time, property damage/maintenance and depreciation, Workmen's Compensation, and involuntary smoking impact.

In spite of the fact that the ill effects of tobacco have been well documented, not enough is being done to decrease and eradicate its use. Consider the following example. In the summer of 1985, over 1,500 people died around the world in major airplane accidents. These accidents resulted in a tremendous amount of worldwide media attention, and planes were grounded for safety reasons. Now imagine what the coverage and concern would be if 450,000 people each year died in the United States alone because of airplane accidents. People would not even consider flying anymore. Most individuals would think of it as a form of suicide.

Similarly, think of the public outrage if close to half a million Americans were to die annually in a meaningless war, or if a single nonprescription drug would cause over 138,000 cancer deaths and 120,000 fatal heart attacks. The American public would never tolerate such situations. We would probably mount a very intense fight to prevent these deaths. Yet, are we not committing a form of slow suicide by smoking cigarettes? Isn't tobacco a nonprescription drug available to most anyone who wishes to smoke, killing in excess of 450,000 people each year?

We may ask ourselves, why isn't there a greater campaign against all forms of tobacco use? There are primarily two reasons. First, it is extremely difficult to fight an industry that has as great a financial and political influence in a country as the tobacco industry has in the United States. The tobacco industry produces 2.5 percent of the gross national product and has cleverly influenced elections by emphasizing the individual's right to smoke, avoiding the fact that so many people die because of its use. Second, tobacco had been socially accepted for so many years that many people just learned to live with it. However, for the first time, in the 1980s, cigarette smoking is no longer acceptable in many social circles. Nonsmokers and ex-smokers alike are fighting for their right to clean air and health. Estimates have indicated that if every smoker gave up cigarettes, in one year alone, sick time would be decreased by approximately 90 million days, there would be 280,000 fewer heart conditions and 1 million fewer cases of chronic bronchitis and emphysema, and total death rates from cardiovascular disease, cancer, and peptic ulcers would drastically decrease.

It is also interesting to note that many smokers are really unaware or simply do not care to realize how much cigarette smoke bothers nonsmokers. These smokers feel that it is not really that bad, and if they can put up with it, it should not bother nonsmokers that much. In most instances, they think that blowing the smoke off to the side is sufficient to get it out of the way. As a matter of fact, it is not enough. Smokers do not comprehend this until they quit and later find themselves in such situations. At times, ex-smokers are even bothered by someone else smoking several yards away and all of a sudden come to realize why cigarette smoke is so unpleasant and undesirable to most people.

WHY DO PEOPLE SMOKE?

In most instances, people begin to smoke without realizing the detrimental effects of tobacco on their health and life in general. While there are many different reasons why people start to smoke, the three fundamental causes are peer pressure, to appear "grown up," and rebellion against authority. Unfortunately, it only takes three packs of cigarettes to develop the physiological addiction, turning it into a "nasty" habit that has become the most widespread example of drug dependency in the country.

When tobacco leaves are burned, hot air and gases containing nicotine and tar (chemical compounds) are released in the smoke. Over 1,200 toxic chemicals have been found in tobacco smoke. Tar contains about thirty chemical compounds that are proven carcinogens. The drug nicotine has strong addictive properties. Within seconds of inhalation, nicotine affects the central nervous system and can act both as a tranquilizer and a stimulant. The stimulating effect produces strong physiological and psychological dependency. The addiction to nicotine is six to eight times greater than alcohol and most likely greater than some of the hard drugs currently used around the world. The psychological dependency is developed over a longer period of time. Not only do people smoke to help them relax, but there is also a certain amount of pleasure involved with the ritual of smoking. There are many activities in daily life that smokers automatically associate with cigarettes. Events such as drinking coffee, drinking alcohol, social gatherings, after a meal, talking on the telephone, driving, reading, watching television, etc., make habitual smokers crave for cigarettes. In many cases, the social rituals of smoking are the most difficult to eliminate. This psychological dependency is so strong that even years after individuals have stopped smoking, they still crave cigarettes when engaged in some of the aforementioned activities.

Most people smoke for a variety of reasons. In order to find out why people smoke, a simple test was developed by the National Clearinghouse for Smoking and Health (Figure 10.2). The scores obtained on this test will give an indication on each of six factors that describe people's feelings when they smoke. The first three factors point out the positive feelings that people get from smoking. The fourth factor aids them in tension reduction and relaxation. The fifth shows their dependence on cigarettes. The last factor indicates habit smoking or purely automatic smoking.

WHY DO YOU SMOKE TEST

In the test contained in Figure 10.2 are some statements made by people to describe what they get out of smoking cigarettes. As a smoker, indicate how often you feel this way when smoking. Circle one number for each statement. It is important that you answer every question.

INTERPRETING THE RESULTS OF THE WHY DO YOU SMOKE TEST

In this test that examines reasons why you smoke, a score of eleven or above on any factor indicates that it is an important source of satisfaction for you. The higher you score (fifteen is the highest), the more important a particular factor is in your smoking and the more useful the discussion of that factor can be in your attempt to quit.

If you do not score high on any of the six factors, chances are that you do not smoke very much or have not been smoking for very many years. If so, giving up smoking — and staying off — should be easy.

1. Stimulation. If you score high or fairly high on this factor, it means that you are one of those smokers who is stimulated by the cigarette — you feel that it helps wake you up, organize your energies, and keep you going. If you try to give up smoking, you may want a safe substitute — a brisk walk or moderate exercise, for example — whenever you feel the urge to smoke.
2. Handling. Handling things can be satisfying, but there are many ways to keep your hands busy without lighting up or playing with a cigarette. Why not toy with a pen or pencil? Or try doodling. Or play with a coin, a piece of jewelry, or some other harmless object.
3. Accentuation of pleasure — pleasurable relaxation. It is not always easy to find out whether you use the cigarette to feel good, that is, get real, honest pleasure out of smoking (Factor 3) or to keep from feeling bad (Factor 4). About two-thirds of smokers score high or fairly high on accentuation of pleasure, and about half of those also score as high or higher on reduction of negative feelings.

   Those who do get real pleasure out of smoking often find that an honest consideration of the harmful effects of their habit is enough to help them quit. They substitute social and physical activities and find that they do not seriously miss their cigarettes.
4. Reduction of negative feelings, or "crutch". Many smokers use the cigarette as a kind of crutch in moments of stress or discomfort. But the heavy smoker, the person who tries to handle severe personal problems by smoking many times a day, is apt to discover that cigarettes do not help in dealing with problems effectively.

   When it comes to quitting, this kind of smoker may find it easy to stop when everything is going well but may be tempted to start again in a time of crisis. Again, physical exertion or social activity may serve as useful substitutes for cigarettes, even in times of tension.
5. "Craving" or dependence. Quitting smoking is difficult for the person who scores high on this factor, that of dependence. For the addicted smoker, the craving for a cigarette begins to build up the moment the cigarette is put out, so tapering off is not likely to work. This smoker must go "cold turkey."

   If you are dependent on cigarettes, it may be helpful for you to smoke more than usual for a day or two, so that the taste for cigarettes is spoiled, and then isolate yourself completely from cigarettes until the craving is gone.
6. Habit. If you are smoking out of habit, you no longer get much satisfaction from your cigarettes. You just light them frequently without

Figure 10.2. *Why-Do-You-Smoke Test*

	Always	Fre- quently	Occa- sionally	Seldom	Never
A. I smoke cigarettes in order to keep myself from slowing down.	5	4	3	2	1
B. Handling a cigarette is part of the enjoyment of smoking it.	5	4	3	2	1
C. Smoking cigarettes is pleasant and relaxing.	5	4	3	2	1
D. I light up a cigarette when I feel angry about something.	5	4	3	2	1
E. When I have run out of cigarettes I find it almost unbearable until I can get them.	5	4	3	2	1
F. I smoke cigarettes automatically without even being aware of it.	5	4	3	2	1
G. I smoke cigarettes to stimulate me, to perk myself up.	5	4	3	2	1
H. Part of the enjoyment of smoking a cigarette comes from the steps I take to light up.	5	4	3	2	1
I. I find cigarettes pleasurable.	5	4	3	2	1
J. When I feel uncomfortable or upset about something, I light up a cigarette.	5	4	3	2	1
K. I am very much aware of the fact when I am not smoking a cigarette.	5	4	3	2	1
L. I light up a cigarette without realizing I still have one burning in the ashtray.	5	4	3	2	1
M. I smoke cigarettes to give me a "lift."	5	4	3	2	1
N. When I smoke a cigarette, part of the enjoyment is watching the smoke as I exhale it.	5	4	3	2	1
O. I want a cigarette most when I am comfortable and relaxed.	5	4	3	2	1
P. When I feel "blue" or want to take my mind off cares and worries, I smoke cigarettes.	5	4	3	2	1
Q. I get a real gnawing hunger for a cigarette when I haven't smoked for a while.	5	4	3	2	1
R. I've found a cigarette in my mouth and didn't remember putting it there.	5	4	3	2	1

Scoring Your Test:

Enter the numbers you have circled on the test questions in the spaces provided below, putting the number you have circled to question A on line A, to question B on line B, etc. Add the three scores on each line to get a total for each factor, For example, the sum of you scores over lines A, G, and M gives you your score on "Stimulation," lines B, H, and N give the score on "Handling," etc. Scores can vary from 3 to 15. Any score 11 and above is high; any score 7 and below is low.

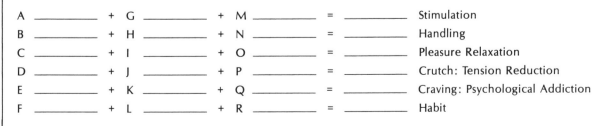

A ________ + G ________ + M ________ = ________ Stimulation

B ________ + H ________ + N ________ = ________ Handling

C ________ + I ________ + O ________ = ________ Pleasure Relaxation

D ________ + J ________ + P ________ = ________ Crutch: Tension Reduction

E ________ + K ________ + Q ________ = ________ Craving: Psychological Addiction

F ________ + L ________ + R ________ = ________ Habit

From *A Self-Test for Smokers.* U.S. Department of Health and Human Services, 1983.

even realizing you are doing so. You may find it easy to quit and stay off if you can break the habit patterns that you have built up. Cutting down gradually may be quite effective if there is a change in the way the cigarettes are smoked and the conditions under which they are smoked. The key to success is becoming aware of each cigarette you smoke. This can be done by asking yourself, "Do I really want this cigarette?" You may be surprised at how many you do not want.

SMOKING CESSATION

Quitting cigarette smoking is no easy task. Only about 20 percent of smokers who try to quit for the first time each year succeed. The addictive properties of nicotine and smoke make it very difficult to quit. The American Psychiatric Association and the National Institute on Drug Abuse have indicated that nicotine is perhaps the most addictive drug known to man. Smokers develop tolerance to nicotine and smoke. They become dependent on both and experience physical and psychological withdrawal symptoms when they stop smoking. While giving up smoking can be extremely difficult, cessation is by no means an impossible task.

Recent sureys have shown that between 75 and 90 percent of all smokers would like to quit. There are now over 36 million Americans who have given up cigarettes. An additional 2 million quit each year. More than 95 percent of the successful ex-smokers have been able to do it on their own, either by quitting cold turkey or using self-help kits available from organizations such as the American Cancer Society, the American Heart Association and the American Lung Association. Only 3 percent of ex-smokers have done so as a result of formal cessation programs. Smoker's Information and Treatment Centers are commonly listed in the yellow pages of the telephone book. Cigarette smoking is now a declining habit in the country. During the last several years, there has been a gradual decrease among smokers of all ages with the exception of young women.

The most important factor in quitting cigarette smoking is the person's sincere desire to do so. Although some smokers can simply quit, in most instances such is not the case. Those who can easily quit are primarily light or casual smokers. They realize that the pleasure of an occasional cigarette is not worth the added risk for disease and premature death. For heavy smokers, cessation will most likely be a difficult battle. While many do not succeed the first time around, the odds of quitting are much greater for those who repeatedly try to stop. To find out a smoker's preparedness to initiate a cessation program, the test contained in Figure 10.3, also developed by the National Clearinghouse for Smoking and Health, will measure a person's attitude toward the four primary reasons why people want to quit smoking. The results will give an indication of whether the person is really ready to start the program.

INTERPRETING THE RESULTS OF THE DO YOU WANT TO QUIT TEST

On this test, the higher you score on any category, say health, the more important that reason is to you. A score of nine or above in one of these categories indicates that this is one of the most important reasons why you may want to quit.

1. Health. Knowing the harmful consequences of cigarettes, many people have stopped smoking and many others are considering it. If your score on the health factor is nine or above, the health hazards of smoking may be enough to make you want to quit now.

   If your score on this factor is low (six or less), look over the hazards of smoking. You may be lacking important information or may even have incorrect information. If so, health considerations are not playing the important role that they should in your decision to keep on smoking or to quit.

2. Example. Some people stop smoking because they want to set a good example for others. Parents quit to make it easier for their children to resist starting to smoke; doctors to influence their patients; teachers to help their students; sports stars to set an example for their young fans; husbands to influence their wives, and vice versa.

Figure 10.3. *Do You Want To Quit Test.*

	Strongly Agree	Mildly Agree	Mildly Disagree	Strongly Disagree
A. Cigarette smoking might give me a serious illness.	4	3	2	1
B. My cigarette smoking sets a bad example for others.	4	3	2	1
C. I find cigarette smoking to be a messy kind of habit.	4	3	2	1
D. Controlling my cigarette smoking is a challenge to me.	4	3	2	1
E. Smoking causes shortness of breath.	4	3	2	1
F. If I quit smoking cigarettes it might influence others to stop.	4	3	2	1
G. Cigarettes cause damage to clothing and other personal property.	4	3	2	1
H. Quitting smoking would show that I have willpower.	4	3	2	1
I. My cigarette smoking will have a harmful effect on my health.	4	3	2	1
J. My cigarette smoking influences others close to me to take up or continue smoking.	4	3	2	1
K. If I quit smoking, my sense of taste or smell would improve.	4	3	2	1
L. I do not like the idea of feeling dependent on smoking.	4	3	2	1

Scoring Your Test:

Write the number you have circled after each statement on the test in the corresponding space to the right. Add the scores on each line to get your totals. For example, the sum of your scores A, E, I gives you your score for the health factor. Scores can vary from 3 to 12. Any score of 9 or over is high; and score 6 or under is low.

A ________ + E ________ + I ________ = ________ Health

B ________ + F ________ + J ________ = ________ Example

C ________ + G ________ + K ________ = ________ Aesthetics

D ________ + H ________ + L ________ = ________ Mastery

From *A Self-Test for Smokers.* U.S. Department of Health and Human Services, 1983.

Such examples are an important influence on our behavior. Research shows that almost twice as many high school students smoke if both parents are smokers compared to those whose parents are nonsmokers or former smokers.

If your score is low (six or less), it may mean that you are not interested in giving up smoking in order to set an example for others. Perhaps you do not appreciate how important your example could be.

3. Aesthetics (the unpleasant aspects). People who score high, that is, nine or above, in this category, recognize and are disturbed by some of the unpleasant aspects of smoking. The smell of stale smoke on their clothing, bad breath, and stains on their fingers and teeth might be reason enough to consider breaking the habit.

4. Mastery (self-control). If you score nine or above on this factor, you are bothered by the knowledge that you cannot control your desire to smoke. You are not your own master. Awareness of this challenge to your self-control may make you want to quit.

BREAKING THE HABIT

The following seven-step plan has been developed as a guide to help you quit smoking. The total program should be completed in four weeks or less. Steps one through four should take no longer than two weeks. A maximum of two additional weeks are allowed for the rest of the program.

Step One. The first step in breaking the habit is to decide positively that you want to quit. Avoid negative thoughts of how difficult this can be. Think positive. You can do it. Now prepare a list of the reasons why you smoke and why you want to quit (use Figure 10.4). Make several copies of the list and keep them in places where you commonly smoke. The reasons for quitting should be reviewed frequently, as this will motivate and psychologically prepare you for cessation. When the reasons for quitting outweigh the reasons for smoking, it will become a lot easier to quit. At this time you should also try to read as much information as possible on the detrimental effects of tobacco and the benefits of quitting.

Figure 10.4. *Smoking versus Quitting Reasons*

Name: ______________________ Date: ______________

Reasons for Smoking Cigarettes

1. ______________________
2. ______________________
3. ______________________
4. ______________________
5. ______________________
6. ______________________
7. ______________________
8. ______________________

Reasons for Quitting Cigarette Smoking

1. ______________________
2. ______________________
3. ______________________
4. ______________________
5. ______________________
6. ______________________
7. ______________________
8. ______________________

Step Two. Initiate a personal diet and exercise program. About one-third of the people who quit smoking gain weight. This could be caused by one or a combination of several reasons: (a) food becomes a substitute for cigarettes, (b) there may be an increased appetite, and (c) basal metabolism may slow down. If the person initiates an exercise and weight control program prior to smoking cessation, weight gain should not be a problem. If anything, exercise and decreased body weight cause a greater awareness of healthy living and increase motivation for giving up cigarettes. Even if some weight is gained, the harmful effects of cigarette smoking are much more detrimental to human health than a few extra pounds of body weight. Experts have indicated that as far as the extra load on the heart is concerned, giving up one pack of cigarettes is the equivalent of losing between fifty and seventy-five pounds of excess body fat!

Step Three. Decide on the approach that you will use to stop smoking. You may quit cold turkey or gradually decrease the number of cigarettes smoked daily. Your decision should be based on the scores obtained on the "why do you smoke test." If you scored eleven points or higher in either the "Crutch: Tension Reduction" or the "Craving: Psychological Addiction" categories, your best chance for success is quitting cold turkey. For any of the other four categories, you may choose either approach.

There is still argument as to which approach may be more effective. Quitting cold turkey may cause less withdrawal symptoms than gradually tapering off. When cutting down, the fewer the cigarettes smoked, the more important each one becomes. Therefore, there is a greater chance for relapse and returning to the original amount smoked. However, when the cutting down approach is used with a definite target date for quitting, the technique has shown to be quite effective. Smokers who taper off without a target date for quitting are the most likely to relapse.

Step Four. For a few days, keep a daily log of your smoking habit. This will help you understand the situations under which you smoke. To assist you in doing so, make copies of Figure 10.5 or develop your own form. Keep this form with you and every time you smoke, record the required information. You should keep track of the number of cigarettes smoked, time of day when smoked, event associated with smoking, the amount of cigarette smoked, and a rating of how badly you needed that cigarette. Rate each cigarette from one to three. A number one means desperately needed, a two means moderately needed, and a three means no real need. This daily log will assist you in three ways. First, you will get you to know your habit. Second, it will help you eliminate cigarettes that you really do not need. Third, it will aid you in finding positive substitutes for situations that trigger your desire to smoke.

Step Five. Set the target date for quitting. If you are going to taper off gradually, read the instructions under the cutting down section of this chapter before you proceed to Step 6. In setting the target date, choosing a special date may add a little extra incentive. An upcoming birthday, anniversary, vacation, graduation, family reunion, etc. are all examples of good dates to free yourself from smoking. Dates when you are going to be away from events that trigger your desire to smoke may be especially helpful. Once you have set the date, do not change it. Do not let anyone or anything interfere with this date. Let your friends and relatives know of your intentions and ask for their support. You may also consider asking someone else to quit with you. This way you can support each other in your efforts to stop. Also, avoid anyone who will not support you in your effort to quit. It is unfortunate, but in many cases other people can be a prime obstacle when attempting to quit. Since many smokers can get quite "intolerable" when they first stop smoking, some friends and relatives prefer that the individual continue to smoke rather than make the extra effort and show increased patience for a few days.

Step Six. Stock up on low-calorie foods. Carrots, broccoli, cauliflower, celery, popcorn (butter and salt free), fruits, sunflower seeds, sugarless gum, and plenty of water. Keep such food handy on the day you stop and the first few days following cessation. Replace such food for cigarettes when you want one.

Step Seven. On your quit day and the first few days thereafter, do not keep cigarettes handy. Stay away from friends and events that trigger your desire to smoke, and drink large amounts of water and fruit juices. An important factor in breaking the habit is to replace the old behavior with new behavior. You will need to replace smoking time with new positive substitutes that will make smoking difficult or impossible. When you desire a cigarette, take a few deep breaths and then occupy yourself by doing a number of things such as talking to someone else, washing your hands, brushing your teeth, eating a healthy snack, chewing on a straw, doing dishes, playing sports, going for a walk or bike ride, going swimming, and so on. Engage in activities that will necessitate the use of your hands. Try gardening, sewing, writing letters, drawing, doing household chores, washing the car. Visit nonsmoking places like libraries, museums, stores, theaters. Plan an outing or a trip away from home. Record your choice of activity or substitute under the remarks/substitute column in Figure 10.5. All these activities have shown to keep your mind away from cigarettes.

Quitting Cold Turkey

Many people have found that quitting all at once is the easiest way to do it. Most smokers have tried this approach at least once. While it may not work the first time, they do not allow themselves to get discouraged and eventually succeed. Many times after several attempts, all of a sudden they are able to overcome the habit without too much difficulty. On the average, as few as three smokeless days are sufficient to break the physiological addiction to nicotine. The psychological addiction may linger on for years but will get weaker as time goes by.

Cutting Down Gradually

Tapering off cigarettes can be done in several ways. You may start by eliminating cigarettes that you do not necessarily need (those ranked as number three and two on your daily log); you can switch to a brand lower in nicotine and/or tar every couple of days; you can smoke less off each cigarette; or you can simply decrease the total number of cigarettes smoked each day.

Most people prefer using a combination of the four methods. When planning your strategy, it is important that you set a target date for quitting before you start cutting down. Remember — once the date is set, it is not to be changed. The total process until your quit date should not take longer than two weeks. You should reduce the total number of cigarettes smoked each day by 10 to 25 percent. As the number is decreased, be careful not to take more puffs or inhale more deeply as you smoke. This would offset the principle of cutting down.

As an aid in tapering off, make several copies of Figure 10.5 (by now you should have already completed the initial daily log of your smoking habit — see Step Four under breaking the habit). Start a new daily log, and every night review your data and set goals for the following day. You will need to decide which cigarettes will be easiest to give up, what brand you will smoke, the total number of cigarettes to be smoked, and how much of each you will smoke. You may also write down any comments or situations that you may want to avoid, as well as any substitutes that you could use to help you in the program. For example, if you always smoke with coffee, substitute juice for coffee. If you smoke while driving, arrange for a ride or take a bus to work. If you smoke with a given friend at lunch, avoid having lunch with that friend for a week or so. Continue using this log until you have completely stopped smoking.

LIFE AFTER CIGARETTES

When you first quit smoking, you can expect to experience a series of withdrawal symptoms. Among the physiological and psychological reactions that you will experience the first few days are a decrease in heart rate and blood pressure; and most likely headaches, gastrointestinal discomfort, changes in mood, irritability, aggressiveness, and difficulty in sleeping. The physiological addiction to nicotine is broken only three days following your last cigarette. As a result, you should not crave cigarettes as much on a regular basis. However, for the habitual smoker, the psychological dependency could be the most difficult to break. The first few days may not be as difficult as the first few months. Any of the activities in daily life that have been associated with smoking, either stress or relaxation, joy or unhappiness, may cause a relapse even months or at times years after cessation.

Ex-smokers should realize that even though some harm may have already been done, it is never too late to quit. The greatest early benefit is

Figure 10.5. *Daily Cigarette Smoking Log*

Today's Date: ____________ Quit Date: ____________ Decision Date: ____________

Cigarettes to be Smoked Today: ____________ Brand: ____________

No.	Time	Activity	Rating[a]	Amount Smoked[b]	Remarks/Substitutes
1.					
2.					
3.					
4.					
5.					
6.					
7.					
8.					
9.					
10.					
11.					
12.					
13.					
14.					
15.					
16.					
17.					
18.					
19.					
20.					

Additional comments, list of friends and/or activities to avoid

[a]Rating: 1 = desperately needed, 2 = moderately needed, 3 = no real need
[b]Amount Smoked: entire cigarette, two-thirds, half, etc.

a decrease in the risk of sudden death. Furthermore, the risk for illness starts to decrease the moment you stop smoking. You will experence a decrease in sore throats, sores in the mouth, hoarseness, cigarette cough, and peptic ulcer risk. There also will be an improvement in blood circulation to the hands and feet, improved gastrointestinal function, and improved kidney and bladder function. In addition, everything will taste and smell better, you will have more energy, and you will experience a sense of freedom, pride, and well-being. You will no longer have to worry whether you have enough cigarettes to last you through a day, a party, a meeting, a weekend, a trip, etc. When you first quit, and you think how tough it is and how miserable you feel because you cannot have a cigarette, try the opposite — think of the benefits and how great it is not to smoke! A final note of encouragement is that the ex-smoker's risk for heart disease approaches that of a lifetime nonsmoker ten years following cessation, and cancer fifteen years after cessation.

If you have been successful and stopped smoking, remember that there are a lot of events that can still trigger your urge to smoke. When confronted with such events, people rationalize and think, "one will not hurt, I have been off for months (years in some cases)" or "I can handle it, I will just smoke today." It will not work! Before you know, you will be back to the regular nasty habit. Therefore, be prepared to take action in those situations. Find adequate substitutes. In addition to the many things that have already been discussed in this chapter, the list of tips given in Figure 10.6 should aid you in retraining yourself to live without cigarettes. You have to start thinking of yourself as a nonsmoker. There are no "buts." Remind yourself of how difficult it has been and how long it has taken you to get to this point. If you have come this far, you can certainly resist "but" small moments of temptation. Remember that it will only get easier rather than worse as time goes on.

References

1. American Cancer Society. *1985 Cancer Facts and Figures.* New York: The Society, 1985.
2. American Cancer Society. *Fifty Most Often Asked Questions About Smoking and Health . . . and the Answers.* New York: The Society, 1982.
3. American Cancer Society. *Quitter's Guide: Seven-Day Plan to Help You Stop Smoking Cigarettes.* New York: The Society, 1978.
4. American Cancer Society. *Why Quit Quiz* (VHS tape). New York: The Society, 1979.
5. American Heart Association. *Heart at Work: Smoking Reduction Program-Coordinator's Guide.* Dallas, TX: The Association, 1984.
6. American Heart Association. *How to Quit.* Dallas, TX: The Association, 1984.
7. American Heart Association. *Smoking and Heart Disease.* Dallas, TX: The Association, 1981.
8. American Heart Association. *The Good Life: A Guide to Becoming a Nonsmoker.* Dallas, TX: The Association, 1984.
9. Carroll, C. R. *Drugs in Modern Society.* Dubuque, IA: Wm. C. Brown, 1985.
10. Channing L. Bete Co., Inc. *Smoking and Your Heart.* South Deerfield, MA: The Author, 1982.
11. Girdano, D. A., D. Dusek, and G. S. Everly. *Experiencing Health.* Englewood Cliffs, NJ: Prentice-Hall, 1985.
12. Halper, M. S. *How to Stop Smoking: A Preventive Medicine Institute/ Strang Clinic Health Action Plan.* New York: Holt Rinehart and Winston, 1980.
13. Hodgson, R. J., and P. Miller. *Self-watching: Addictions, Habits, Compulsions, What to Do.* New York: Facts on File, 1982.
14. National Cancer Institute. *Clearing the Air: A Guide to Quitting Smoking.* Bethesda, MD: The Institute, 1979.
15. Public Health Service. *A Self-Test for Smokers.* Rockville, MD: U.S. Department of Health and Human Services, 1983.
16. Public Health Service. *Chronic Obstructive Lung Disease: A Report of the Surgeon General.* Rockville, MD: U.S. Department of Health and Human Services, 1984.
17. Public Health Service. *Why People Smoke Cigarettes.* Rockville, MD: U.S. Department of Health and Human Services, 1982.
18. Public Health Service. *Smoking Tobacco and Health: A Fact Book.* Rockville, MD: U.S. Department of Health and Human Services, 1981.
19. U.S. Office on Smoking and Health. *Smoking and Health: A Report of the Surgeon General.* Washington, D.C.: U.S. Department of Health, Education and Welfare, 1979.

Figure 10.6. *Tips for Smoking Cessation*

The following are different way smokers retrained themselves to live without cigarettes. Any one or several of these methods in combination might be helpful to you. Check the ones you like and from these develop your own retraining program.

1. Before you quit smoking, try wrapping your cigarettes with a sheet of paper like a Christmas present. Every time you want a cigarette, unwrap the pack and write down what you are doing, how you feel, and how important this cigarette is to you. Do this for two weeks and you'll have cut down as well as developed new insights into your smoking.
2. If cigarettes give you an energy boost, try gum, modest exercise, a brisk walk, or a new hobby. Avoid eating new foods that are high in calories.
3. If cigarettes help you relax, try eating, drinking new beverages, or social activities within reasonable bounds.
4. When you crave cigarettes, you must quit suddenly. Try smoking an excess of cigarettes for a day or two before you quit so that the taste of cigarettes is spoiled. Or, an opportune time to quit is when you are ill with a cold or influenza, and have lost your taste for cigarettes.
5. On a 3" x 5" card, make a list of what you like and dislike about smoking. Add to it and read it daily.
6. Make up a short list of luxuries you have wanted or items you would like to purchase for a loved one. Next to each item write down the cost. Now convert the cost to "packs of cigarettes." If you save the money each day from packs of cigarettes, you will be able to purchase these items. Use a special "piggy" bank for saving your money or start a "Christmas Club" account at your bank.
7. Never smoke after you get a craving for a cigarette until three minutes have passed since you got the urge. During those three minutes, change your thinking or activity. Telephone an ex-smoker or somebody you can talk to until the craving subsides.
8. Plan a memorable date for stopping. You might choose your vacation, New Year's Day, your birthday, a holiday, the birthday of your child, your anniversary. But, don't make the date so distant that you lose momentum.
9. If you smoke under stress at work, pick a date for stopping when you will be away from your work.
10. Decide whether you are going to stop suddenly or gradually. If it is to be gradual, work out a tapering system so that you have intermediate goals on your way to an "I.Q." day.
11. Don't store up cigarettes. Never buy a carton. Wait until one pack is finished before you buy another.
12. Never carry cigarettes about with you at home or at work. Keep your cigarettes as far from you as possible. Leave them with someone or lock them up.
13. Until you quit, make yourself a "smoking corner" that is far from anything interesting. If you like to smoke with others, always smoke alone. If you like to smoke alone, always smoke with others, preferably if they are nonsmokers. Never smoke while watching television.
14. Never carry matches or a lighter with you.
15. Put away your ashtrays or fill them with objects so they cannot be used for ashes. Plant flowers in them or fill them with walnuts. The latter will give you something to do with your hands.
16. Change your brand of cigarettes weekly so that you are always smoking a brand of lower tar and nicotine content than the week before.
17. Never say, "I quit smoking," because your resolution is broken if you have a cigarette. Better to say, "I don't want to smoke." This way you maintain your resolution even if you accidentally have a cigarette.
18. Try to help someone else quit smoking, particularly your spouse.
19. Always ask yourself, "Do I need this cigarette or is this just a reflex!"

Figure 10.6. *Tips for Smoking Cessation (continued)*

20. Each day try to put off lighting your first cigarette.

21. Decide arbitrarily that you will smoke only on even- or odd-numbered hours of the clock.

22. Try going to bed early and rising a half hour earlier than usual to avoid hurrying through breakfast and rushing to work.

23. Keep your hands occupied. Try playing a musical instrument, knitting, or fiddling with hand puzzles.

24. Take a shower. You cannot smoke in the shower.

25. Brush your teeth frequently to get rid of the tobacco taste and stains.

26. If you have a sudden craving for a cigarette, take ten deep breaths, holding the last breath while you strike a match. Exhale slowly, blowing out the match. Pretend the match was a cigarette by crushing it out in an ashtray. Now immediately get busy on some work or activity.

27. Only smoke half a cigarette.

28. After you quit, start using your lungs. Increase your activities and indulge in moderate exercise, such as short walks before or after a meal.

29. Bet with someone that you can quit. Put the cigarette money in a jar each morning and forfeit it if you smoke. You keep the money if you don't smoke by the end of the week. Try to extend this period to a month.

30. If you gain weight because you are not smoking, wait until you get over the craving before you diet. Dieting is easier then.

31. If you are depressed or have physical symptoms that might be related to your smoking, relieve your mind by discussing this with your physician. It is easier to quit when you know your health status.

32. Visit your dentist after you quit and have your teeth cleaned to get rid of the tobacco stains.

33. If the cost of cigarettes is your motivation for quitting, try purchasing a money order equivalent to a year's supply of cigarettes. Give it to a friend. If you smoke in the next year, he cashes the money order and keeps the money. If you don't smoke, he gives back the money order at the end of the year.

34. After you have quit, never face the confusion of "craving a cigarette" alone. Find someone who you can call or visit at this critical time.

35. When you feel irritable or tense, shut your eyes and count backward from ten to zero as you imagine yourself descending a flight of stairs, or imagine that you are looking at the horizon as the sun sets in the west.

36. Get out of your old habits. Seek new activities or perform old activities in a new way. Don't rely on the old ways of solving problems. Do things differently.

37. If you are a "kitchen smoker" in the morning, volunteer your services to schools or nonprofit organizations to get you out of the house.

38. Stock up on light reading materials, crossword puzzles, and vacation brochures that you can read during your coffee breaks.

39. Frequent places where you can't smoke, such as libraries, buses, theatres, swimming pools, department stores, or just going to bed during the first weeks you are off cigarettes.

40. Give yourself time to think and get fit by walking one-half hour each day. If you have a dog, take him for a walk with you.

From *TIPS*. American Cancer Society, Texas Division, Inc., with permission.

CHAPTER ELEVEN

Relevant Questions Related to Fitness and Wellness . . . and the Answers

The purpose of this last chapter is to answer some of the most frequently asked questions that people have regarding different aspects of physical fitness and wellness. The answers to many of the questions will help clarify to an even greater extent different concepts discussed throughout the book, as well as put to rest several myths that serve to misinform fitness and wellness participants.

1. **Can aerobic exercise make a person immune to heart and blood vessel disease?**

   Although aerobically fit individuals have a very low incidence of cardiovascular disease, a regular aerobic exercise program by itself is not an absolute guarantee against cardiovascular disease. There are many other factors that increase the person's risk, including a genetic predisposition. Overall risk factor management is the best guideline to minimize the risk for cardiovascular disease. However, your chances of surviving a heart attack are much greater if you have been exercising regularly.

2. **What is the optimal amount of aerobic exercise recommended to significantly decrease the risk for cardiovascular disease?**

   The basic principles of cardiovascular exercise prescription were introduced in Chapter 2. The required amount of exercise to maintain cardiovascular endurance is a training session every forty-eight hours for twenty to thirty minutes in the appropriate target zone.

   Nevertheless, some researchers indicate that to obtain a certain degree of protection against cardiovascular disease, approximately 300 calories should be expended on a daily basis through aerobic exercise. Dr. Thomas K. Cureton, in his book *The Physiological Effects of Exercise Programs Upon Adults,* reports that 300 calories per exercise session provide the necessary stimuli to control blood fats (cholesterol and triglycerides), which are a primary risk factor for atherosclerosis, coronary disease, and strokes. Dr. Ralph Paffenbarger and co-researchers in their study "Cause-Specific Death Rates per 10,000 Man-Years of Observation Among 16,936 Harvard Alumni, 1962 to 1978, by Physical Activity Index" showed that 2,000 calories expended per week as a result of physical activity yielded the lowest risk for cardiovascular disease among this group of almost 17,000 Harvard alumni (see Chapter 1, Table 1.3). Two thousand calories per week represents about 300 calories per daily exercise session.

3. **At what age should I start concerning myself with heart disease?**

   The disease process, not only for cardiovascular disease, but also cancer, starts early in life as a result of poor lifestyle habits. Studies have shown beginning stages of atherosclerosis and elevated blood lipids in children as young as ten years old. Many positive lifestyle habits can be established early in life within the walls of your own home. If children are taught at a young age that they should avoid excessive calories, sweets, salt, tobacco, alcohol, and participate in physical activity, their chances of leading a healthier life are much greater than the present generation. And remember some of the best advice given to mankind when it comes to teaching: "come and follow me." If you practice positive health habits in your own life, your children will be more likely to follow.

4. **How can I tell if I am exceeding the safe limits for exercise participation?**

The best method to determine whether you are exercising too strenuously is by checking your heart rate and making sure that it does not exceed the limits of your target zone. Exercising above the target zone may not be safe for unconditioned or high-risk individuals. Keep in mind that you do not need to exercise beyond your target zone to provide the desired benefits for the cardiovascular system.

In addition, there are several physiological signs that will tell you when you are exceeding functional limitations. A very rapid or irregular heart rate, labored breathing, nausea, vomiting, lightheadedness, headaches, dizziness, pale skin, flushness, excessive weakness, lack of energy, shakiness, sore muscles, cramps, and tightness in the chest are all signs of exercise intolerance. One of the basic things that you will need to learn is to listen to your body. If you experience any of these signs, you should seek medical attention before continuing your exercise program.

5. **How fast should heart rate decrease following aerobic exercise?**

To a certain extent, recovery heart rate is related to fitness level. The higher your cardiovascular fitness level, the faster your heart rate will decrease following exercise. As a general rule of thumb, heart rate should be below 120 beats per minute five minutes into recovery. If your heart rate is above 120, you have most likely overexerted yourself or could possibly have some other cardiac abnormality. If you decrease the intensity and/or duration of exercise and you still experience a fast heart rate five minutes into recovery, you should consult a physician regarding this condition.

6. **Do people really experience a "physical high" during aerobic exercise?**

During vigorous exercise, morphine-like substances referred to as endorphines are released from the pituitary gland in the brain. These act not only as a pain killer, but can also induce feelings of euphoria and natural well-being. Increased levels of endorphines are commonly seen as a result of aerobic endurance activities and may remain elevated for as long as thirty to sixty minutes following exercise. Many experts now feel that these higher levels explain the so-called "physical high" that people experience during and after prolonged exercise participation.

Endorphine levels have also been shown to be elevated during pregnancy and delivery. Since endorphines act as pain killers, these higher levels could explain a woman's increased tolerance to the pain and discomfort experienced during natural childbirth and the pleasant feelings experienced shortly after the birth of the baby. Since several surveys have shown shorter and easier labor among well-conditioned women, it is very possible that these women may achieve higher endorphine levels during delivery, therefore making childbirth less traumatic as compared to untrained women.

7. **What causes muscle soreness and stiffness?**

Muscle soreness and stiffness is very common among individuals who initiate an exercise program or participate after a prolonged layoff from exercise. The acute soreness experienced the first few hours after exercise is thought to be related to a lack of blood (oxygen) flow and general fatigue of the exercised muscles. The delayed soreness that appears several hours after exercise (usually twelve hours later) and lasts for two to four days may be related to actual minute tears in muscle tissue, muscle spasms that increase fluid retention stimulating the pain nerve endings, and overstretching or tearing of connective tissue in and around muscles and joints. The best way to prevent soreness and stiffness is by stretching adequately before and after exercise, and using a gradual progression into your exercise program. Do not attempt to do too much too quickly. If you experience soreness and stiffness, mild stretching, low-intensity exercise to stimulate blood flow, and a warm bath can help relieve the pain.

8. **How should acute sports injuries be treated?**

The best treatment has always been prevention itself. If a given activity is causing unusual discomfort or chronic irritation, you need to treat the cause by decreasing the intensity, switching activities, or using better equipment such as adequate and proper-fitting shoes.

If an acute injury has occurred, the standard method of treatment is cold application, compression and/or splinting, and elevation of the affected body part. Cold should be applied three to five times a day for fifteen to twenty minutes at a time during the first twenty-four to thirty-six hours. Cold can be applied by either submerging the injured area in cold water, using an ice bag, or applying ice massage to the affected part. Compression can be applied with an elastic bandage or wrap. Elevation, whenever possible, is used to decrease blood flow to the injured part. The purpose of these three treatment modalities is to minimize swelling in the area, which significantly increases the time of recovery. After the initial twenty-four to thirty-six hours, heat can be used if there is no further swelling or inflammation. However, if you have doubts regarding the nature or seriousness of the injury (such as suspected fracture), you should seek a medical evaluation.

Whenever there is obvious deformity, such as in fractures, dislocations, or partial dislocations, splinting, cold application with an ice bag, and medical attention are required. Never try to reset any of these conditions by yourself, as greater damage to muscles, ligaments, and nerves is possible. The treatment of these injuries should always be left to specialized medical personnel.

9. **How should I care for shin splints?**

Shin splints or pain and irritation in the shin region of the leg is a frequent sports injury encountered by participants in fitness programs. Shin splints are usually the result of one or more of the following: (a) lack of proper and gradual conditioning, (b) conducting physical activities on hard surfaces (wooden floors, hard tracks, cement, and asphalt), (c) fallen arches, (d) chronic overuse, (e) muscle fatigue, (f) faulty posture, (g) inadequate shoes, and (h) being excessively overweight and participating in weight-bearing activities.

Shin splints may be managed by: (a) removing or reducing the causing agent (exercising on softer surfaces, wearing better shoes and/or arch supports, or completely stopping exercise until the shin splints heal), (b) doing mild stretching exercises before and after physical activity, (c) use of ice massage for ten to twenty minutes prior to and following physical participation, and (d) active heat (whirlpool and hot baths) for fifteen minutes, two to three times a day. In addition, supportive taping during physical activity is helpful (the proper taping technique can be easily learned from a qualified athletic trainer).

10. **What causes side stitch?**

The exact cause of this sharp pain that sometimes occurs during exercise is unknown. Some experts have suggested that it could be related to a lack of blood flow to the respiratory muscles during strenuous physical exertion. This stitch only seems to occur in unconditioned beginners or trained individuals when they exercise at higher intensities than usual. As you improve your physical condition, this problem will disappear unless you start training at a higher intensity. Whenever you experience this problem, you need to slow down, and if it still persists, stop altogether.

11. **What causes muscle cramps, and what should be done when they occur?**

Muscle cramps are caused by the body's depletion of essential electrolites or a breakdown in the coordination between opposing muscle groups. If you have a muscle cramp, initially you should attempt to stretch the muscles involved. For example, in the case of the calf muscle, pull your toes up toward the knees. After stretching the muscles, gently rub them down, and finally do some mild exercises that require the use of those particular muscles.

In pregnant and lactating women, muscle cramps are often related to a lack of calcium. If women experience cramps during these periods, calcium supplements usually relieve the problem. Tight clothing can also cause cramps because of decreased blood flow to active muscle tissue.

12. **Is it safe to exercise during pregnancy?**

There is no reason why women should not exercise during pregnancy. If anything, it is desirable that women do so to strengthen the body and prepare for delivery. Physically fit women experience shorter labor, easier delivery, and faster recovery as compared to unfit women. Among Indian tribes it is commonly observed that pregnant women continue to carry out all of their hard labor chores up to the very day of delivery, and a few hours after the birth of the baby they resume their normal activities. There have also been several women athletes who have competed in different sports during the early stages of pregnancy. At the 1952 Olympic Games, a bronze medal in track and field was won by a pregnant woman. Nevertheless, the final decision for exercise participation should be made by the woman and her personal physician.

Experts have recommended that if a woman has been exercising regularly, the same activity level can be carried out through the fifth month of pregnancy. Thereafter, walking and/or moderate swimming are indicated in conjunction with some light strengthening exercises. For women who have not exercised regularly, twenty to thirty minutes of daily walking and light strengthening exercises are recommended throughout the entire pregnancy.

13. **Does exercise help relieve dysmenorrhea (painful menstruation)?**

Exercise has not been shown to either cure or aggravate painful menstruation, but it has been shown to relieve menstrual cramps because of improved circulation to the uterus. The decrease in menstrual cramps could also be related to increased levels of endorphines produced during prolonged physical activity that may counteract pain.

14. **Does exercise participation hinder menstruation?**

Although, on the average, women experience a decrease in physical capacity during menstruation, medical surveys at the Olympic Games have shown that women have broken Olympic and world records at all stages of the menstrual cycle. Menstruation should not keep a woman from participating in athletics, nor will it necessarily have a negative impact on performance.

In some instances, highly trained athletes may develop amenorrhea (cessation of menstruation) during training and competition. This condition is primarily seen in extremely lean athletes who also engage in sports that require very strenuous physical effort over a sustained period of time, but it is by no means irreversible. At present, it is unknown whether the condition is caused by physical and/or emotional stress related to a high-intensity training, excessively low body fat, or other factors.

15. **What is osteoporosis and how can it be prevented?**

Osteoporosis has been defined as the softening, deterioration, or loss of total body bone. Bones become so weak and brittle that fractures, primarily of the hip, wrist, and spine, occur very readily. About 1.3 million fractures are attributed to this condition each year. Osteoporosis slowly begins in the third and fourth decade of life, and women are especially susceptible after menopause. This is primarily due to estrogen loss following menopause, which increases the rate at which bone mass is broken down.

The prevention of osteoporosis begins early in life by providing adequate amounts of calcium in the diet (follow the recommended daily allowance of 800 to 1200 mg) and regularly participating in an exercise program. Weight-bearing activities such as walking, jogging, and weight training are especially helpful, because not only do they tone up muscles, but also develop stronger and thicker bones. Following menopause, maintenance of calcium intake, adequate physical exercise, and personal evaluation by your physician for possible estrogen therapy are recommended to prevent osteoporosis. In conjunction with adequate calcium intake, there may be a need for an additional amount of vitamin D, which is necessary for optimal calcium absorption.

16. **What time of the day is best for exercise?**

Just about any time of the day is fine with the exception of the noon and early afternoon hours on hot and humid days. Many people enjoy exercising early in the morning because it gives them a good boost to start the day. Others prefer the lunch hour for weight control reasons. By exercising at noon they do not eat as big a lunch, which helps keep daily caloric intake down. Highly stressed people seem to like the evening hours because of the relaxation effects of exercise.

17. **What type of clothing should I wear when I exercise?**

The type of clothing to be used during exercise should fit you comfortably and allow for free movement of the different body parts. You should also select your clothes according to ambient temperature and humidity. Avoid nylon and rubberized materials and tight clothes that will interfere with the cooling mechanism of the human body and/or obstruct normal blood flow. Proper-fitting shoes, manufactured specifically for your choice of activity, are also recommended to prevent lower limb injuries.

18. **Why is it unsafe to exercise in hot and humid conditions?**

When you exercise, only 30 to 40 percent of the energy produced in the body is used for mechanical work or movement. The rest of the energy (60 to 70 percent) is converted into heat. If this heat cannot be properly dissipated because it is either too hot or the relative humidity is too high, body temperatures will increase, and in extreme cases even death can occur.

The specific heat of body tissue (the heat required to raise the temperature of the body by one degree Centigrade) is .38 calories per pound of body weight per one degree Centigrade (.38 cal/1b/°C). This indicates that if no body heat is dissipated, a 150-pound person would only need to burn 58.5 calories (150 x .38) to increase total body temperature by one degree Centigrade. If this person conducted an exercise session that required 300 calories (about three miles running) without any heat dissipation, inner body temperature would increase by 5.1 degrees Centigrade, or the equivalent of going from 98.6 to 107.8 degrees Fahrenheit!

The above example clearly illustrates why caution should be used when exercising in hot or humid weather. If the relative humidity is too high, body heat cannot be lost through evaporation because the atmosphere is already saturated with water vapor. In one specific instance, a football casualty occurred at a temperature of only sixty-four degrees Fahrenheit, but at a relative humidity of 100 percent. Caution must be taken when air temperature is above ninety degrees and the relative humidity is above 60 percent.

Perhaps the best recommendation is to watch for typical heat-related symptoms. These symptoms usually include cramping, weakness, headaches, dizziness, confusion, hyperventilation, and nausea or vomiting. The sweating mechanism usually stops before severe symptoms occur. If you notice any of these changes when you exercise, stop your workout and allow yourself to recover in a cool environment, providing adequate fluid replacement.

The American College of Sports Medicine has recommended that individuals should not engage in strenuous physical activity when the readings of a wet bulb globe thermometer exceed 82.4 degrees Fahrenheit. With this type of thermometer, the wet bulb is cooled by evaporation and on dry days will show a lower temperature than the regular (dry) thermometer. On humid days, the cooling effect is less because of decreased evaporation; hence, the difference between the wet and dry readings is not as great.

19. **What precautions must be taken when exercising in the cold?**

Exercising in the cold usually does not pose a threat to the individual's health, mainly because adequate clothing for heat conservation can be worn, and exercise by itself will increase body heat production. The popular belief that exercising in cold temperatures (thirty-two degrees Fahrenheit and less) freezes the lungs is totally false, because the air is properly warmed in the air passages before it ever reaches the lungs. It is not cold that poses a threat, but rather the velocity of the wind which has a great effect on the chill factor. For example, exercising at a temperature of twenty-five degrees Fahrenheit with adequate clothing is not too cold, but if the wind is blowing at twenty-five miles per hour, the chill factor reduces the actual temperature to minus five degrees Fahrenheit. This effect is even worse if you are wet and exhausted.

When exercising in the cold, it is important that you protect the face, head, hands, and feet, as they may be subject to frostbite even when the lungs are under no risk. In cold temperatures, about 30 percent of the body's heat is lost through the head's surface area if unprotected. Wearing several layers of lightweight clothing is also preferable over one single thick layer, because warm air is trapped between layers of clothes, allowing for greater heat conservation.

20. **Are rubberized sweatsuits and steam baths an effective way to lose weight?**

The answer to this question is simply no! If you use a sweatsuit or step into a sauna, there is a significant amount of water loss but not fat. Sure, it looks nice immediately after when you step on the scale, but it is just a false loss of weight. As soon as you replace body fluids, the weight is quickly gained back. Wearing rubberized sweatsuits not only increases the rate of body fluid loss, which is vital during prolonged exercise, but also increases core temperature. Dehydration through these methods leads to impaired cellular function and in extreme cases even death.

21. **If fad diets do not work, how can they guarantee that a person will indeed lose weight?**

The diet industry is a multimillion-dollar industry that tries to capitalize on the idea that weight can be lost quickly, without taking into consideration the long-term consequences of fast weight loss.

There are several reasons why fad diets continue to deceive people and can claim that weight will indeed be lost if "all" instructions are followed. Most diets are quite low in calories and/or deprive the body of certain nutrients, creating a metabolic imbalance that can even cause death. Under such conditions, a lot of the weight loss is in the form of water and protein and not fat. When you crash diet, close to 50 percent of the weight loss is in lean (protein) tissue. When the body uses protein instead of a combination of fats and carbohydrates as a source of energy, weight is lost as much as ten times faster. A gram of protein yields half the amount of energy that fat does. In the case of muscle protein, one-fifth of protein is mixed with four-fifths water. In other words, each pound of muscle yields only one-tenth the amount of energy of a pound of fat. So you can clearly see that most of the weight loss is in the form of water, which on the scale, of course, looks good. Nevertheless, when a normal diet is resumed, most of the lost weight comes right back.

Some diets encourage you to eat only certain foods. If people would only realize that there are no "magic" foods that will provide all of the necessary nutrients, and that you have to eat a variety of foods to be well-nourished, the diet industry would not be as successful. The unfortunate thing about most of these diets is that they create a nutritional deficiency which at times can be fatal. The reason why some of these diets succeed is because in due time you become tired of eating the same thing day in and day out, and eventually start eating less. If you happen to achieve the lower weight, once you go back to your old diet without implementing permanent dietary changes, weight is quickly gained back again.

A few diets recommend exercise along with caloric restrictions, which of course is the best method for weight reduction. A lot of the weight lost is due to exercise; hence, the diet has achieved its purpose. Unfortunately, once you discontinue the diet and the exercise program, the weight will also come right back.

22. **Are mechanical vibrators useful in losing weight?**

This type of equipment is worthless in a weight control program. Vibrating belts and turning rollers may feel good but require no effort whatsoever on the part of the muscles. Fat can not be "shaken off" — it has to be burned off in muscle tissue.

23. **When on a diet, does it matter at what time of day I consume most of my calories?**

Theoretically, if daily caloric input equals the output, weight should not be gained or lost regardless of the time of day when the calories are consumed. Nevertheless, evidence indicates that such is not the case. In a research project conducted at the Aerobics Research Center in Dallas, Texas, the results indicated that when on a diet, weight is lost most effectively if the majority of the calories are consumed before 1:00 P.M. and not during the evening meal. The recommendation made at this center's is that when attempting to lose weight, a minimum of 25 percent of the total daily calories should be consumed for breakfast, 50 percent for lunch, and 25 percent or less at dinner.

Other experts have indicated that if most of your daily calories are consumed during one meal, the body may perceive that something is wrong and will slow down your metabolism so that it can store a greater amount of calories in the form of fat. Also, eating most of the calories in one meal causes you to go hungry most of the day, making it more difficult to adhere to the diet.

The principle of consuming most of the calories earlier in the day not only seems to be helpful in losing weight, but also in the management of atherosclerosis. According to one research study, the time of day when most of the fats and cholesterol are consumed can have an impact on blood lipids and coronary heart disease. Peak digestion time following a heavy meal takes place about seven hours after that meal. If most lipids are consumed during the evening meal, digestion peaks while the person is sound asleep, at a time when the metabolism is at its lowest rate. Consequently, the body may not be able to metabolize fats and cholesterol as effectively, leading to higher blood lipids and increasing the risk for atherosclerosis and coronary heart disease.

24. **How long should a person wait after a meal before engaging in strenuous physical exercise?**

The length of time that an individual should wait before exercising after a meal depends on the amount of food consumed. On the average, after a regular meal, the person should wait about two hours before participating in strenuous physical activity. However, there is no reason why the individual should not be able to take a walk or do some other light physical activity following a meal. If anything, such practice helps burn extra calories and may help the body metabolize fats more effectively.

25. **What is the difference between a calorie and a kilocalorie (kcal)?**

A calorie is a unit of measure used to indicate the energy value of food and cost of physical activity. Technically, a kcal or large calorie is the amount of heat necessary to raise the temperature of one kilogram of water from 14.5 to 15.5 degrees Centigrade, but for the purpose of simplicity, people refer to it as a calorie rather than kcal. For example, if the caloric value of a given food is 100 calories (kcal), the energy contained in this food could raise the temperature of 100 kilograms of water by one degree Centigrade.

26. **Why do some people gain rather than lose weight when they initiate an exercise program?**

Physical exercise leads to an increase in lean body mass. Therefore, it is not uncommon for body weight to remain the same or increase when you initiate an exercise program, while inches and percent body fat decrease. The increase in lean tissue results in an increased functional capacity of the human body. With exercise, most of the weight (fat) comes off after a few weeks of training, when the lean component has stabilized.

"Skinny" people should also realize that the only healthy manner to increase body weight is through exercise, primarily strength-training exercises. Attempting to gain weight by just overeating will increase the fat component and not the lean component, which is not conducive to better health. Consequently, exercise is the best solution to weight (fat) reduction as well as weight (lean) gain.

27. **Does cooking affect the amount of calories contained in food?**

Cooking does not significantly alter the caloric content of food. The only exception would be meat, where broiling and barbecuing drains off some of the fat and decreases the caloric content. On the other hand, frying will significantly increase the caloric content of food.

28. **Can cellulite be decreased with special exercises?**

Cellulite is nothing but plain fat storage. As previously discussed, there is no such thing as spot reducing. Since the body draws its energy from all fat stores simultaneously, and not just the parts exercised, there are no special exercises that will help decrease fat in a specific body area. Nevertheless, if you engage in long-duration aerobic exercise, a greater proportion of fat can be drawn from the larger fat stores because of the high caloric requirement of the activity.

The only effective way to decrease body fat is through a combined lifetime food selection modification program and a regular exercise program. You will need willpower, patience, and persistence. If you really try, it will work. The best tip, though, is to keep the weight (fat) off, rather than let it go and try to control it once it has crept up on you. Remember from Chapter 6 that only one person in 200 is able to keep the weight off after a successful weight loss program. The very few who succeed are those who implement lifetime changes in food selection and physical activity habits. As more people become educated and apply these two basic principles, the rate of success will increase.

29. **Are vitamin and mineral supplements necessary?**

Research has demonstrated that even when a person consumes as few as 1,200 calories per day, as long as the diet contains the recommended servings from the four basic food groups, the person does not need any additional vitamin supplements. Water-soluble vitamins cannot be stored for long periods of time, and high intakes are readily excreted from the body. Fat-soluble vitamins are stored in fatty tissues. Therefore, daily intake of these vitamins is not as crucial. Furthermore, excessive amounts of vitamins A and D can be detrimental to your health. Mineral requirements, with the possible exception of iron in women, are provided in sufficient quantities in a normal balanced diet. If you feel that your diet is not balanced, you need to determine which nutrients are missing before you start taking supplements (see the diet analysis in Appendix E). Better yet, you should use the vitamin and mineral charts given in Chapter 6 and increase the intake of those foods high in nutrients deficient in your diet.

30. **Do athletes or individuals who train for long periods of time need a special diet?**

Many people have felt that highly trained individuals need a special diet in order to be successful in their sport. The simple truth is that unless the diet is deficient in basic nutrients, there are no special, secret, or magic diets that will help a person perform better or develop faster as a result of what they are eating. Athletes' diets do not have to be any different from the regular recommended diet (50 to 60 percent carbohydrates, 20 to 30 percent fat, and 15 to 20 percent protein). As long as the diet is balanced, that is, it meets the daily servings from each of the four food groups, athletes do not need any additional supplements. Even weight trainers and body builders do not need any additional protein in excess of 20 percent of their total daily caloric intake. The only difference between a sedentary person and a highly trained one is in the total number of calories required on a daily basis. The trained person may consume more calories because of the increased energy expenditure as a result of intense physical training.

The only time that a normal diet should be modified is when an individual is going to participate in long-distance events lasting in excess of one hour (e.g., marathon, triathlon, and road cycling). Research has shown that athletic performance is significantly increased for these types of events by consuming a diet low in carbohydrates along with exhaustive physical training the fourth and fifth days prior to the event, followed by a diet high in carbohydrates (about 70 percent) and a progressive decrease in training intensity the last three days before the event.

31. **How detrimental are coffee and alcohol to good health?**

Caffeine and alcohol are drugs, and as such can produce several undesirable side effects. Caffeine doses in excess of 200 to 500 mg can produce an abnormally rapid heart rate, abnormal heart rhythms, increased blood pressure, birth defects, and increased body temperature. They can induce symptoms of anxiety, depression, nervousness, and dizziness, as well as increased secretion of gastric acids leading to stomach problems. The caffeine content of different drinks varies depending upon the product. For six ounces of coffee, the content varies from 65 mg for instant coffee to as high as 180 mg for drip coffee. Soft drinks, mainly colas, range in caffeine content from 30 mg to 60 mg per twelve-ounce can.

Among the detrimental effects caused by alcohol are liver damage (cirrhosis of the liver is among the fastest rising causes of death in the country), increased nutritional deficiencies, increased serum triglycerides, obesity, a disturbance in carbohydrate metabolism, and a decreased ability to use oxygen at the muscular level. However, one of the most significant ill effects of alcoholism is the breakdown of the family unit, which has an effect on the physical, emotional, and spiritual well-being of the person. Unfortunately, many times people start out as occasional social drinkers, and before they realize it, they have turned into alcoholics and are not willing to accept this fact.

Some attention has recently been given to studies that have shown higher HDL levels among individuals who drink the equivalent of six to eight ounces of alcohol per week. Because of this finding, newspaper headlines across the country read "moderate use of alcohol decreases risk for heart disease." Shortly thereafter, several investigators noted that HDL can be broken into separate components and that only the HDL-2 component (which is increased through aerobic exercise) offers protection against heart disease. Alcohol was found to increase the HDL-3 component only, which has not been shown to offer any protection against heart disease.

The negative effects of long-term caffeine and alcohol consumption, even in moderate amounts, are probably more detrimental to health and well-being than any short-term benefits derived from their consumption.

32. **Will exercise offset the detrimental effects of cigarette smoking?**

Physical exercise often motivates toward smoking cessation but does not offset any ill effects of smoking. If anything, smoking greatly decreases the ability of the blood to transport oxygen to working muscles. Oxygen is carried in the circulatory system by hemoglobin, the iron-containing pigment of the red blood cells. Carbon monoxide, a by-product of cigarette smoke, has 210 to 250 times greater affinity for hemoglobin over oxygen. Consequently, carbon monoxide combines much faster with hemoglobin, decreasing the oxygen-carrying capacity of the blood. Chronic smoking also increases airway resistance, requiring the respiratory muscles to work much harder and consume more oxygen just to ventilate a given amount of air. If you quit smoking, exercise does help increase the functional capacity of the pulmonary system.

33. How should I breathe during exercise?

During exercise, a greater amount of oxygen is required to produce the energy necessary to do the specific task. Therefore, you should allow your body to freely breathe through your mouth and nose. Do not attempt to regulate your own respiration by consciously altering the normal breathing pattern. The human body will automatically regulate ventilation during exercise. Any attempt on your part to modify this pattern will only result in a decreased efficiency of the cardiorespiratory system.

34. Can I exercise after donating blood?

The average amount taken when a person donates blood is about 500 ml (a half liter) out of a total volume of five liters. This volume is immediately replenished by reserve blood components stored in the body. Unless you are given special instructions not to exercise, there is no reason why you cannot continue with your regular program.

35. How fast are the benefits of exercise lost after a person stops exercising?

The length of time involved in losing the benefits of exercise varies among the different components of fitness and will also depend on the type of condition achieved prior to cessation. In regard to cardiovascular endurance, it has been estimated that four weeks of aerobic training are completely reversed in two consecutive weeks of physical inactivity. On the other hand, if you have been exercising regularly for months or years, two weeks of inactivity will not hurt you as much as someone who has only exercised for a few weeks. As a rule of thumb, after only forty-eight hours of aerobic inactivity, the cardiovascular system starts to lose some of its capacity. Flexibility can be maintained with two or three stretching sessions per week, and strength is easily maintained with just one maximal training session per week.

To maintain adequate fitness, it is recommended that you maintain a regular exercise program, even during periods of vacation. If you have to interrupt your program for reasons beyond your control, do not attempt to resume your training at the same level where you left off, but rather build up gradually again.

36. If weight training does not masculinize women, why do so many women body builders develop such heavy musculature?

In Chapter 3, you learned that the degree of masculinity and femininity is determined by genetic inheritance and not by the amount of physical activity. Individual variations among women in hormonal secretions of androgen, estrogen, progesterone, and testosterone cause some women to have a larger-than-average build, even without any type of physical training. Because of their larger-than-average build, many of these women often participate in sports where they can use their natural physical advantage.

Additionally, in the sport of body building the athletes follow intense training routines consisting of two or more hours of constant weight lifting with very short rest intervals between sets. Many times during the training routine, back-to-back exercises that require the use of the same muscle groups are performed. The objective of this type of training is to "pump" extra blood into the muscles, which makes the muscles appear much bigger than they really are in resting conditions. Based on the intensity and the length of the training session, the muscles can remain filled with blood, appearing measurably larger for several hours after completing the training session. Therefore, in real life, these women are not as muscular as they seem when they are "pumped up" for a contest.

In the sport of body building, a big point of controversy is the use of anabolic steroids and human growth hormones, even among women participants. Anabolic steroids are synthetic versions of the male sex hormone testosterone, which promotes muscle development and hypertrophy. The use of these hormones, however, can produce detrimental and undesirable side effects, which some women deem tolerable (e.g., hypertension, fluid retention, decreased breast size, deepening of the voice, facial whiskers, and body hair growth). The use of these steroids among women is definitely on the increase, and according to Dr. William Taylor, sportsmedicine physician in Florida, Dr. Robert Kerr, sportsmedicine physician in Southern California, and Carol Turner, body builder in Los Angeles, about 80 percent of women body builders have used steroids. Furthermore, several women's track-and-field coaches have indicated that as many as 95 percent of women athletes around the world in this sport will use anabolic steroids in order to remain competitive at the international level.

There is no doubt that women who take steroids will indeed build heavy musculature like men, and if taken long enough, will lead to masculinizing effects in all women. As a result, in the fall of 1985 the International Federation of Body Building instituted a mandatory steroid-testing program among women participating in the Miss Olympia contest.

When drugs are not used to promote development, increased health and femininity are the rule rather than the exception among women who participate in body building, strength training, or sports in general. The use of steroids will masculinize women and destroy the feminine charm that sports participation helps develop.

37. What can I do to improve my personal safety?

Accident prevention and personal safety are also part of a health enhancement program aimed at achieving total well-being. Proper nutrition, exercise, abstinence from cigarette smoking, and stress management are of little help if the person is involved in a disabling or fatal accident just because seatbelts were not used. Even though some factors in life are completely beyond our control, more often than not, personal safety and accident prevention are a matter of common sense. To improve your personal safety, you are encouraged to fill out one final questionnaire: the "Health Protection Plan for Environmental Hazards, Crime Prevention, and Personal Safety," which is contained in Appendix F. Many factors in life are affected by our actions, and by keeping in mind the recommendations given in this questionnaire, you can further improve your personal safety and well-being.

38. What is next now that I have completed the assignments in this book?

The objective of this book was to provide the information and experiences necessary to implement your personal fitness and wellness program. If you have read and successfully completed all of the assignments, including your regular exercise program, you should be convinced of the value of exercise and healthy lifestyle habits in the achievement of total well-being.

As you continue with your personal program, keep in mind that the greatest benefit of fitness and wellness is to improve the quality of your life. For most people who engage in a personal fitness and wellness program, this new quality of life is experienced after only a few weeks of training and practicing healthy lifestyle patterns. In some instances, however, especially for individuals who have led a poor lifestyle for a long time, it may take a few months before positive habits are established and feelings of well-being are experienced. But in the end, everyone who applies the principles of fitness and wellness will reap the desired benefits. Perhaps this new quality of life was best explained by Dr. George Sheehan, cardiologist and runner, when he wrote[9]:

> For every runner who tours the world running marathons, there are thousands who run to hear the leaves and listen to the rain, and look to the day when it is all suddenly as easy as a bird in flight. For them, sport is not a test but a therapy, not a trial but a reward, not a question but an answer.

The real challenge will come now that you are about to finish this course: a lifetime commitment to fitness and wellness. It is a lot easier to adhere to the program while in a structured setting. To make it easier, as you continue your program, remember to enjoy yourself and have fun along the way. Implement your program based on your interests and what you enjoy doing most. If such is the case, adhering to your new lifestyle will not be difficult. Hopefully, the activities that you have conducted over the last few weeks have helped you develop positive "addictions" that will carry on throughout life. If you have truly experienced the feelings expressed by Dr. Sheehan, you know that there is no looking back. But, if you have not been there, it is difficult to know what it is like. Improving the quality and most likely the longevity of your life is now in your hands. For some it may require persistence and commitment, but *only you can take control of your lifestyle and thereby reap the benefits of wellness.*

References

1. Allsen, P. E., J. M. Harrison, and B. Vance. *Fitness for Life: An Individualized Approach.* Dubuque, IA: Wm. C. Brown, 1984.
2. Arnheim, D. D. *Modern Principles of Athletic Training.* St. Louis, MO: Times Mirror/Mosby College Publishing, 1985.
3. Carroll, C. R. *Drugs in Modern Society.* Dubuque, IA: Wm. C. Brown, 1985.
4. Cooper, K. H. *The Aerobics Way.* New York: Mount Evans and Co., 1977.
5. Cooper, K. H. *The Aerobics Program for Total Well-Being.* New York: Mount Evans and Co., 1982.
6. Cureton, T. K. *The Physiological Effects of Exercise Programs Upon Adults.* Springfield, IL: Charles C. Thomas, Publisher, 1971.
7. Fox, E. L., and D. K. Mathews. *The Physiological Basis of Physical Education and Athletics.* Philadelphia: Saunders College Publishing, 1981.
8. Hoeger, W. W. K. *Ejericio, Salud y Vida [Exercise, Health and Life].* Caracas, Venezuela: Editorial Arte, 1980.
9. Human Relations Media. *What is Fitness?, Dynamics of Fitness: The Body in Action.* Pleasantville, NY: The Company, 1980.
10. McArdle, W. D., F. I. Katch, and V. L. Katch. *Exercise Physiology: Energy, Nutrition and Human Performance.* Philadelphia: Lea and Febiger, 1981.
11. Miller, R. W. "Osteoporosis, Calcium and Estrogens." *FDA Consumer.* Rockville, MD: U.S. Department of Health and Human Services, 1984.
12. "Osteoporosis: What Really Causes It?" *Nutrition Facts.* Tulsa, OK: Southwestern Metabolism and Diabetes Center, May 1985.
13. Paffenbarger, R. S., R. T. Hyde, A. L. Wing, and C. H. Steinmetz. "A Natural History of Athleticism and Cardiovascular Health." *JAMA* 252:491-495, 1984.
14. President's Council on Physical Fitness and Sports. "Physical Activity During Menstruation and Pregnancy." Series 8, No. 3. Washington, D.C., July 1978.
15. Remington, D., A. G. Fisher, and E. A. Parent. *How to Lower Your Fat Thermostat.* Provo, UT: Vitality House International, Inc., 1983.
16. Roen, P. B. "The Evening Meal and Atherosclerosis." *Journal of the American Geriatrics Society,* 1978.
17. Roy, S., and R. Irvin. *Sports Medicine: Prevention, Evaluation, Management, and Evaluation.* Englewood Cliffs, NJ: Prentice-Hall, Inc., 1983.
18. Strang Preventive Medicine Clinic. *Health Protection Plan for Environmental Hazards, Crime Prevention and Personal Safety.* New York: The Clinic, 1982.
19. Taylor, W. "Drugs and the Female Athlete." *Muscle and Fitness,* 104-107, 161-162, September 1985.
20. Teper, L. "The Straight Dope on Steroids and Women." *Muscle and Fitness,* 44-46, 164-171, January 1985.
21. Wells, C. L. *Women, Sport, and Performance: A Physiological Perspective.* Champaign, IL: Human Kinetics Publishers, Inc., 1985.

APPENDIX A

Physical Fitness and Wellness Profile

Fill out the enclosed profile as you obtain the results for each fitness and wellness component. After determining each component, discuss the objective and date of completion with your instructor.

Figure A.1. *Personal Fitness and Wellness Profile.*

Name: ______________________

Item	Pre-Assessment			Objective[a]	Post-Assessment		
	Date	Test Results	Classification		Date	Test Results	Classification
Cardiovascular Endurance							
Muscular Strength							
Muscular Flexibility							
Body Composition							
Cardiovascular Risk							
Cancer Risk: Lung							
Colon-Rectum							
Skin							
Breast[b]							
Cervical[b]							
Endometrial[b]							
Stress: Life Exp. Survey							
Vulnerability							
Smoking[c]							

Instructor Signature: ______________ Student Signature: ______________ Date: ________

[a]Indicate specific objective and date of completion. [b]Women only. [c]For test results indicate type and amount smoked, for classification indicate smoker, ex-smoker, non-smoker.

APPENDIX B

Muscular Strength Training Programs

A. STRENGTH-TRAINING EXERCISES WITHOUT WEIGHTS: Exercises 1 through 9.

For a complete body workout, use the following exercises: 1 (or 2), 3, 4, 5, 6, 7 (or 8), and 9.

B. STRENGTH-TRAINING EXERCISES WITH WEIGHTS: Exercises 10 through 24.

For a complete workout, use at least exercises 10 through 17, or you may substitute the following: 20 for 10; 18 or 19 for 11; 22 or 23 for 13; 21 for 15; and 24 for 17.

Photography for the exercises on strength training with weights courtesy of:

Universal Gym Equipment, Inc.
930 27th Avenue, S.W.
Cedar Rapids, Iowa

Many of these exercises can also be performed with free weights, but for safety reasons it is recommended that they be conducted on equipment as shown in these photographs. The exercises can be performed on single machines as illustrated in this Appendix or on a Universal Multi-Station Conditioning Machine, as shown in Figure B.2.

Refer to Chapter 3 for instructions on how to set up your strength-training program, including the resistance, number of repetitions, sets, and frequency of training.

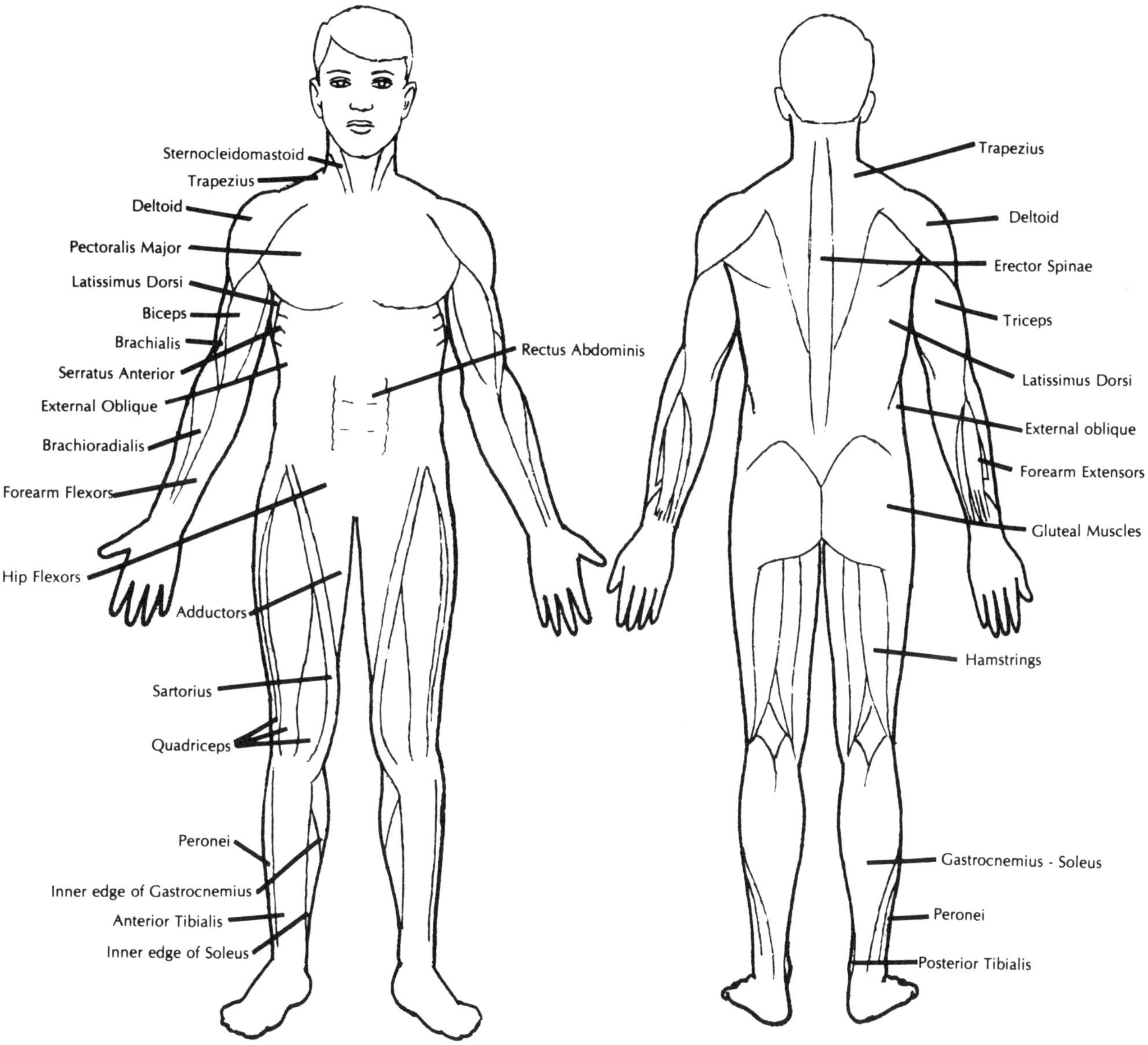

Figure B.1. *Major muscle groups of the human body.*

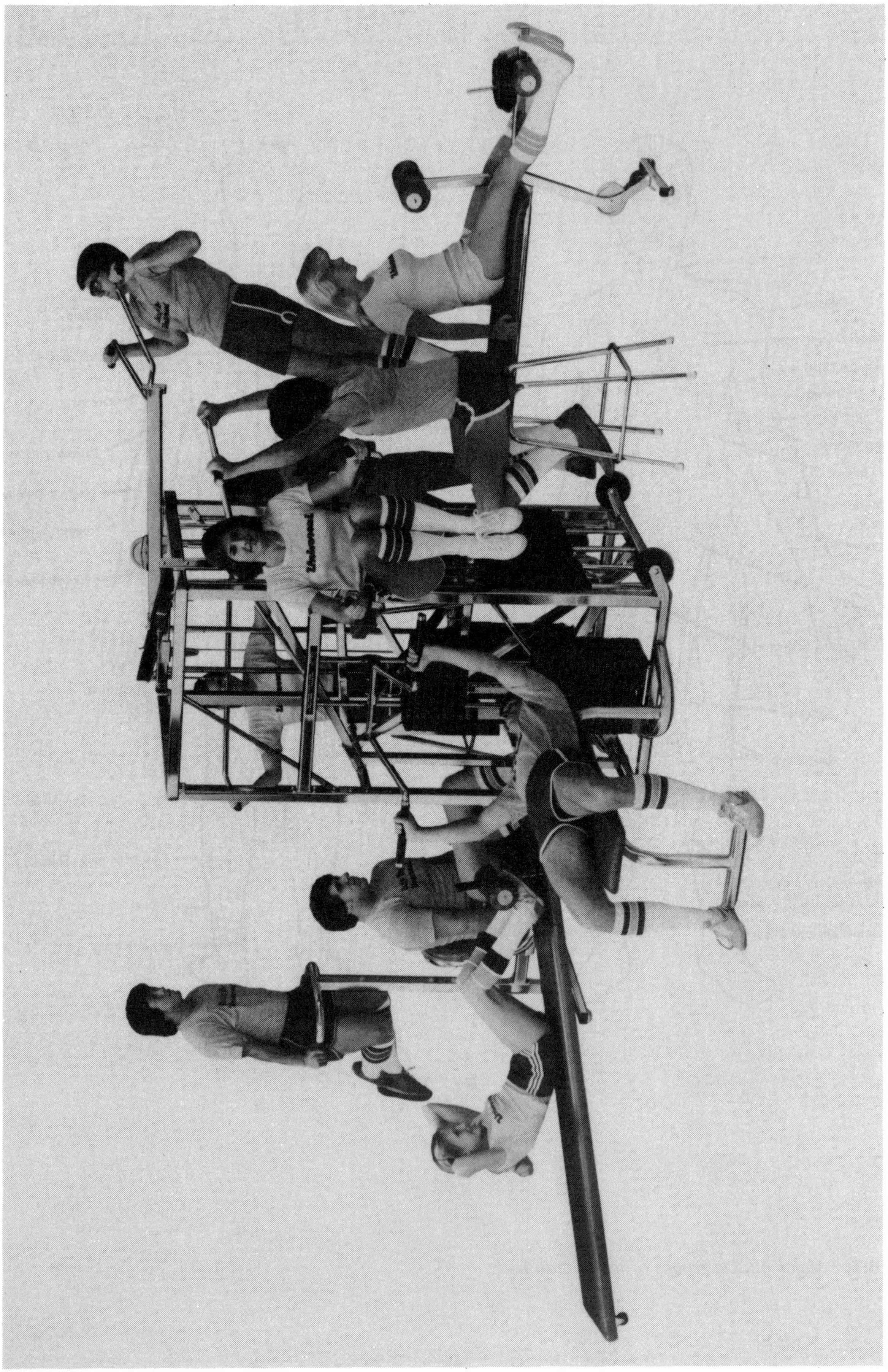

Figure B.2. *Universal Multi-Station Conditioning Machine (courtesy of Universal Gym Equipment, Inc., 930 27th Ave., S.W., Cedar Rapids, Iowa).*

Strength Training Exercises Without Weights

Exercise 1: STEP-UP

Action: Step up and down using a box (or chair or fireplace) approximately twelve to fifteen inches high. Conduct one set using the same leg each time you go up and then conduct a second set using the other leg. You could also alternate legs on each step-up cycle. You may increase the resistance by holding a child or some other object in your arms (hold the child or object close to the body to avoid increased strain on the lower back).

Muscles Developed: Gluteal muscles, quadriceps, gastrocnemius, and soleus.

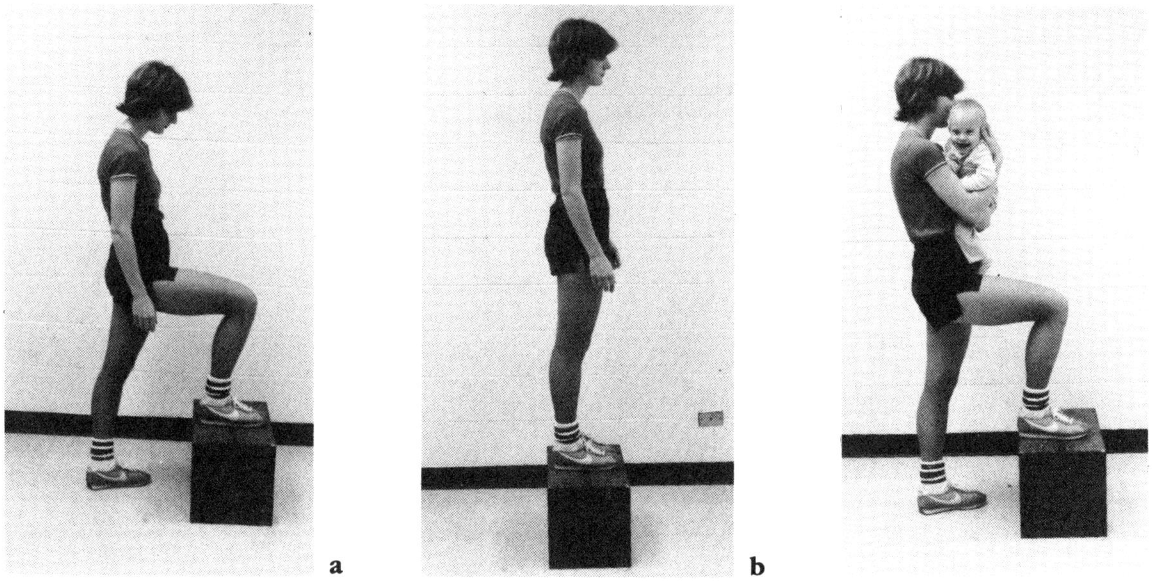

a b c

Exercise 2: HIGH JUMPER

Action: Start with the knees bent at approximately 150 degrees and jump as high as you can, raising both arms simultaneously.

Muscles Developed: Gluteal muscles, quadriceps, gastrocnemius, and soleus.

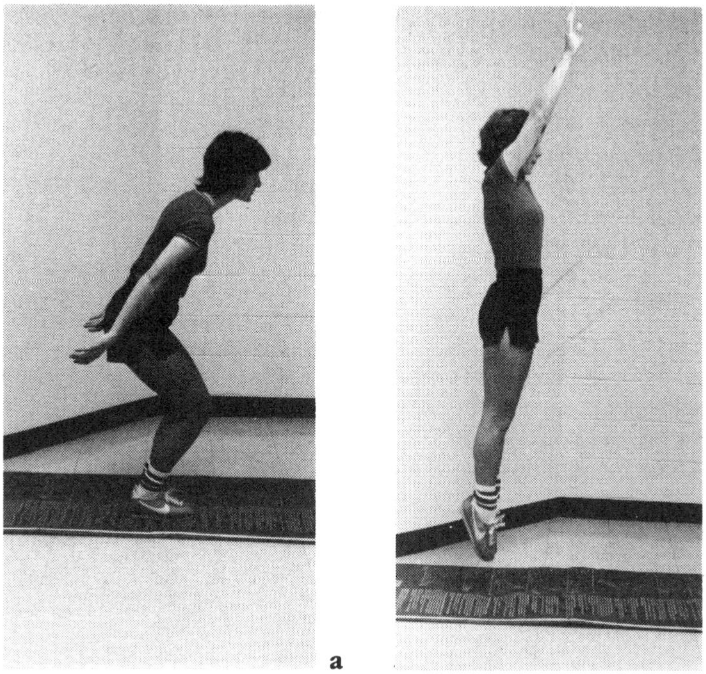

a b

Exercise 3: PUSH-UP

Action: Maintaining your body as straight as possible, flex the elbows, lowering the body until you almost touch the floor, then raise yourself back up to the starting position. If you are unable to perform the push-up as indicated, you can decrease the resistance by supporting the lower body with the knees rather than the feet (*see* illustration c) or using an incline plane and supporting your hands at a higher point than the floor (*see* illustration d). If you wish to increase the resistance, have someone else add resistance to your shoulders as you are coming back up (*see* illustration e).

Muscles Developed: Triceps, deltoid, pectoralis major, erector spinae, and abdominals.

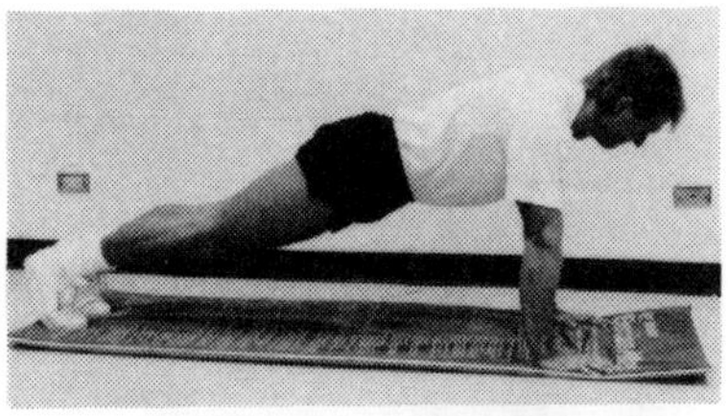

a

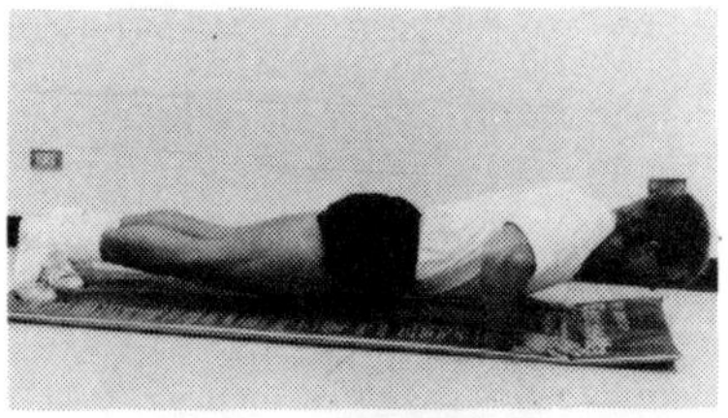

b

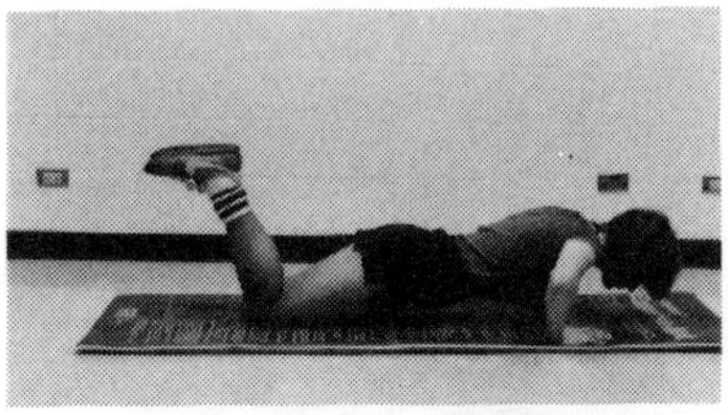

c

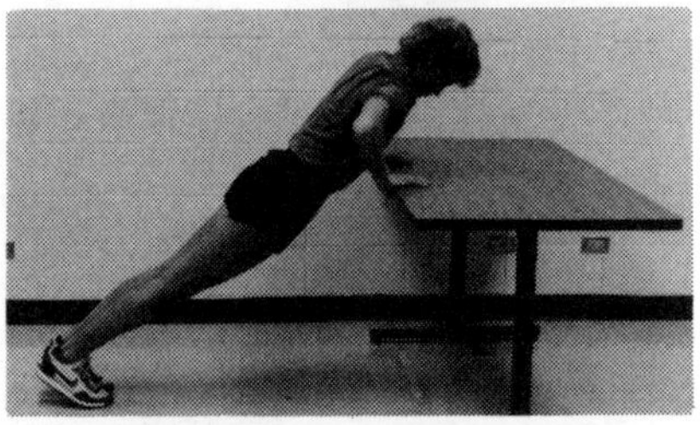

d

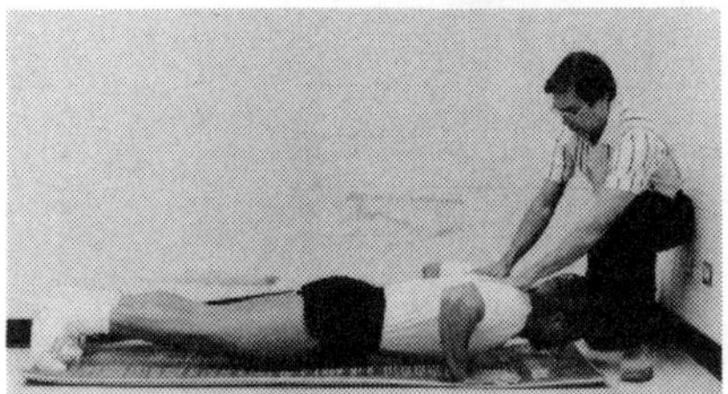

e

Exercise 4: SIT-UP

Action: Start with your head and shoulders off the floor, arms crossed on your chest, and knees slightly bent (the greater the flexion of the knee, the more difficult the sit-up). Now curl all the way up, then return to the starting position without letting the head or shoulders touch the floor, or allowing the hips to come off the floor. If you allow the hips to raise off the floor and the head and shoulders to touch the floor (*see* illustration c), you will most likely "swing up" on the next sit-up, which minimizes the work of the abdominal muscles. If you cannot curl up with the arms on the chest, place the hands by the side of the hips or even help yourself up by holding on to your thighs (illustrations d and e). Do not perform the sit-up exercise with your legs completely extended, as this will cause strain on the lower back.

Muscles Developed: Abdominal muscles and hip flexors.

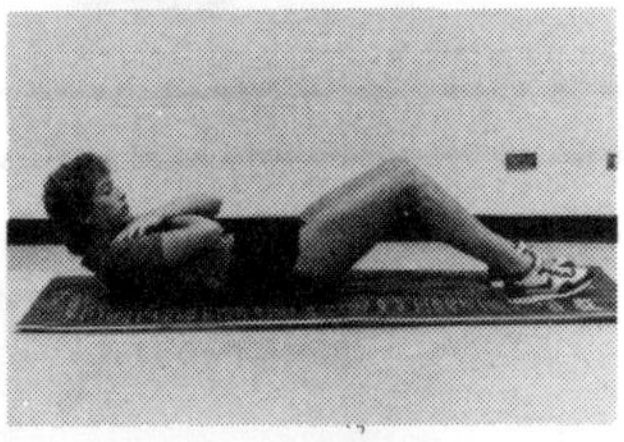

a

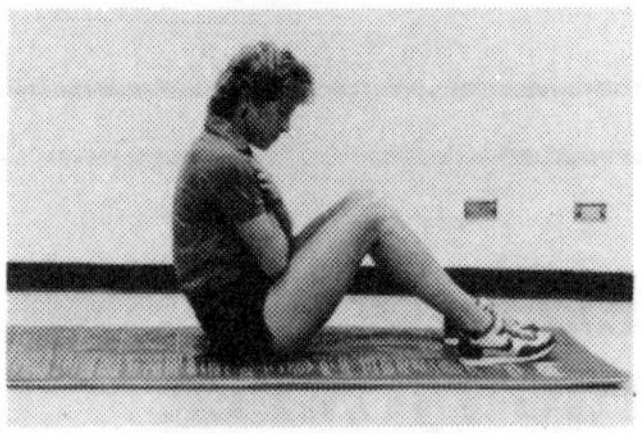

b

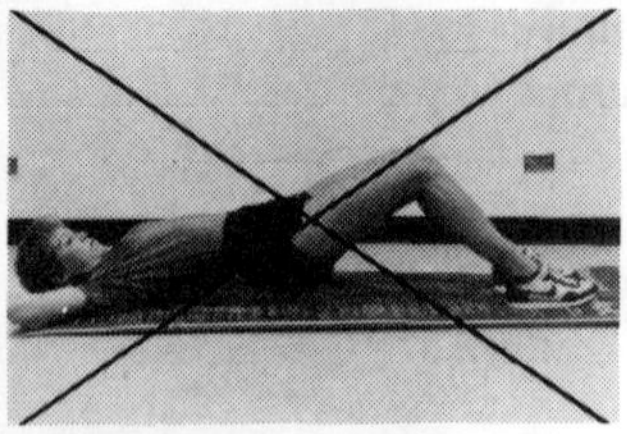

c

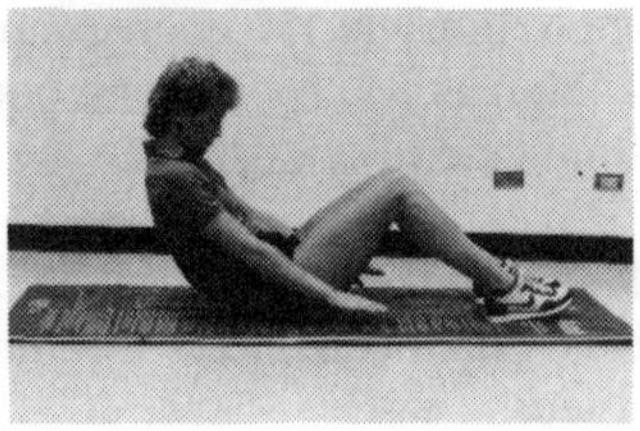

d

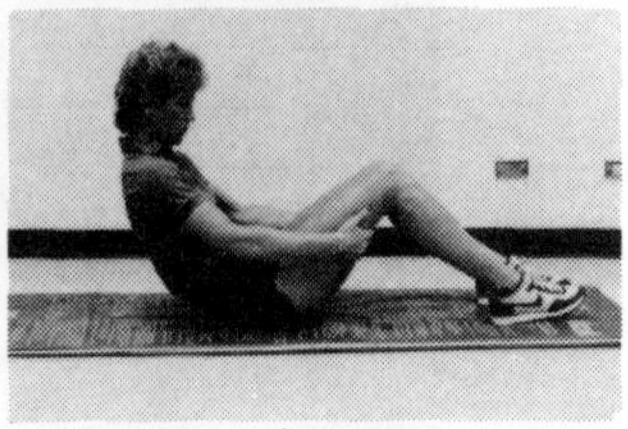

e

Exercise 5: LEG CURL

Action: Start with the foot about three inches off the floor and have someone else hold on to the back of your foot and apply enough resistance so that you can just barely bring the leg up to ninety degrees. Then return to starting position. Perform the exercise for both legs.

Muscles Developed: Hamstrings.

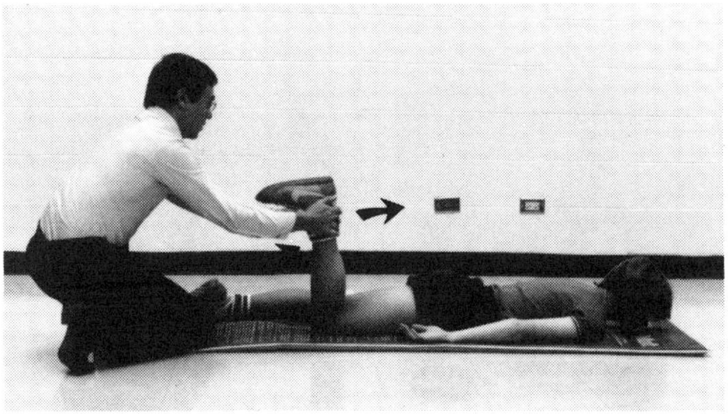

Exercise 6: MODIFIED DIP

Action: Place your hands and feet on opposite chairs with knees slightly bent (make sure that the chairs are well stabilized). Dip down at least to a ninety-degree angle at the elbow joint, then return to the initial position. To increase the resistance, have someone else hold you down by the shoulders on the way up (*see* illustration c).

Muscles Developed: Triceps, deltoid, and pectoralis major.

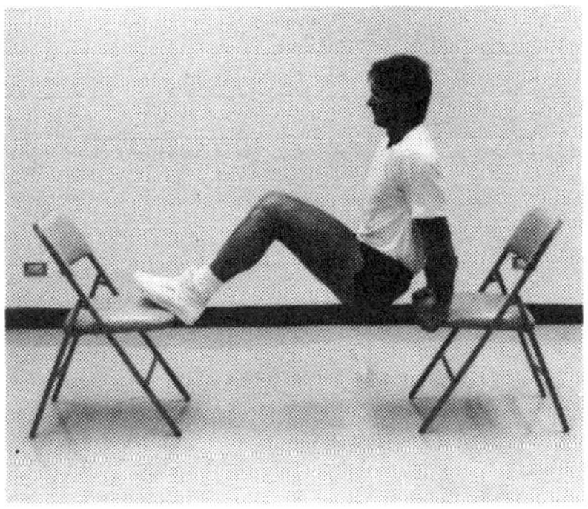

a

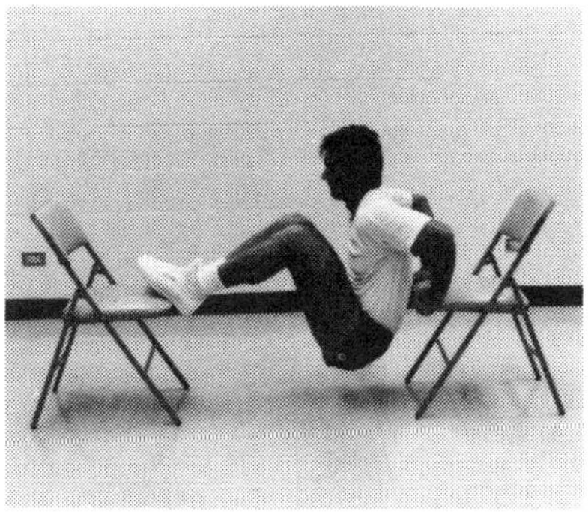

b

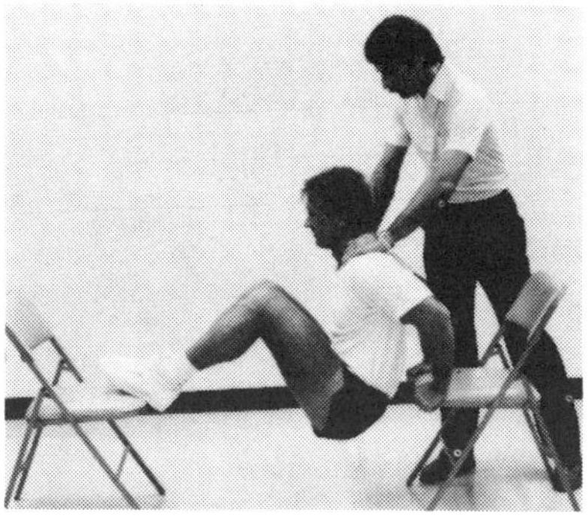

c

Exercise 7: PULL-UP

Action: Suspend yourself from a bar with a pronated grip (thumbs in). Pull your body up until your chin is above the bar, then lower the body slowly to the starting position. If you are unable to perform the pull-up as described, either have a partner hold your feet to push off and facilitate the movement upward (illustrations c and d), or use a lower bar and support your feet on the floor (illustration e).

Muscles Developed: Biceps, brachioradialis, brachialis, trapezius, and latissimus dorsi.

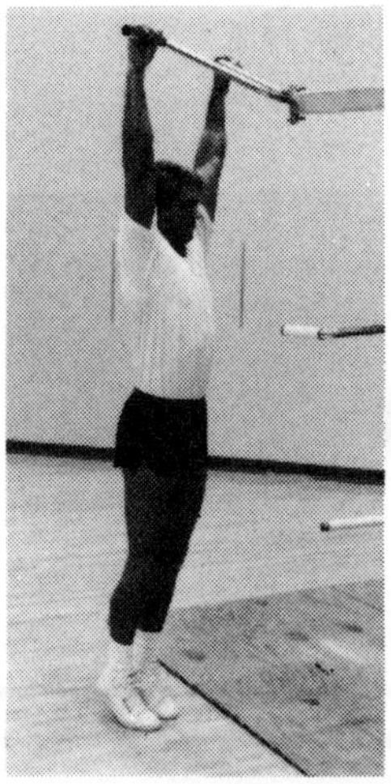
a

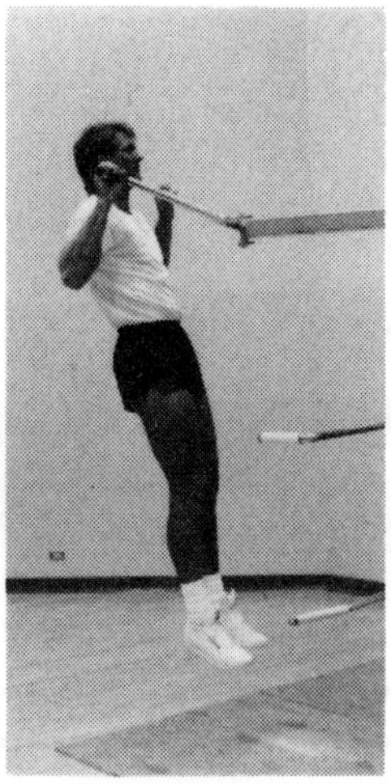
b

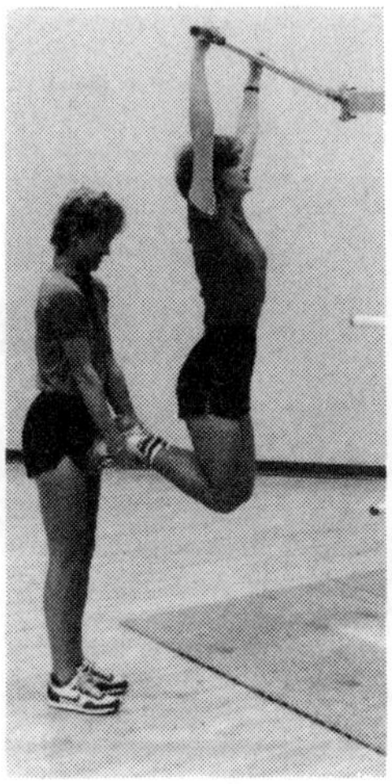
c

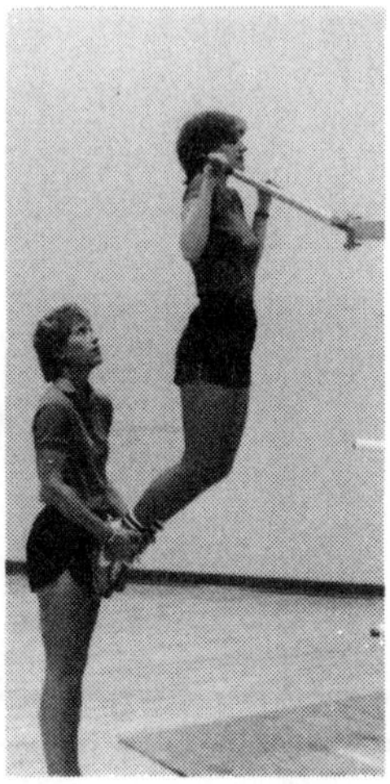
d

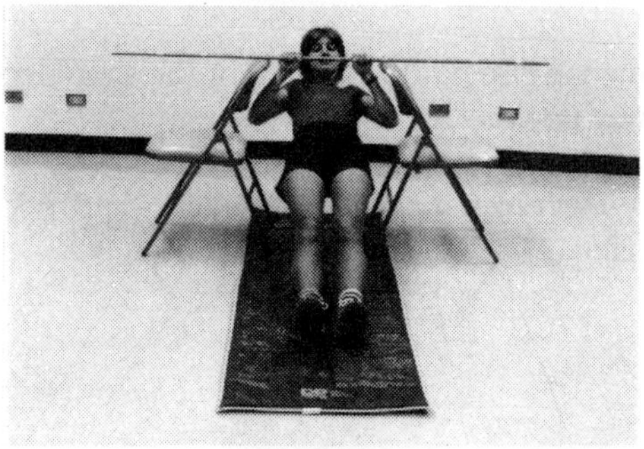
e

Exercise 8: ARM CURL

Action: Using a palms-up grip, start with the arm completely extended, and with the aid of a bucket filled (as needed) with sand or rocks, curl up as far as possible, then return to the initial position. Repeat the exercise with the other arm.

Muscles Developed: Biceps, brachioradialis, and brachialis.

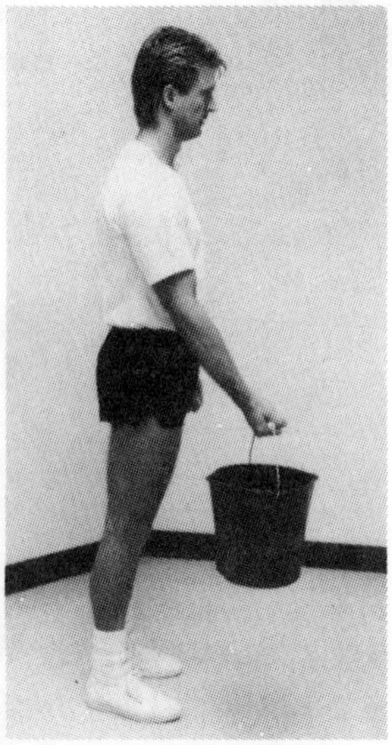
a

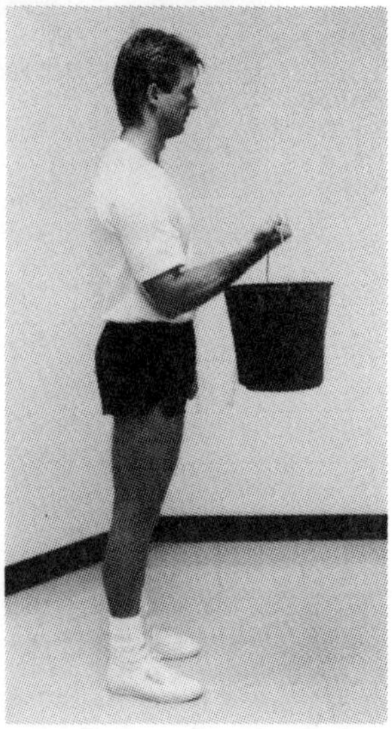
b

Exercise 9: HEEL RAISE

Action: From a standing position with feet flat on the floor, raise and lower your body weight by moving at the ankle joint only (for added resistance, have someone else hold your shoulders down as you perform the exercise).

Muscles Developed: Gastrocnemius and soleus.

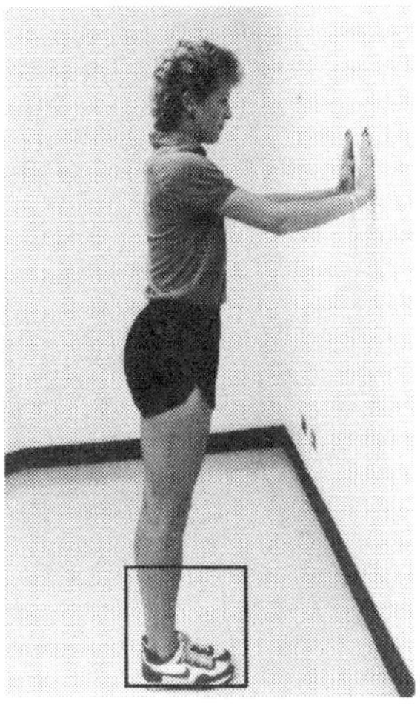

a

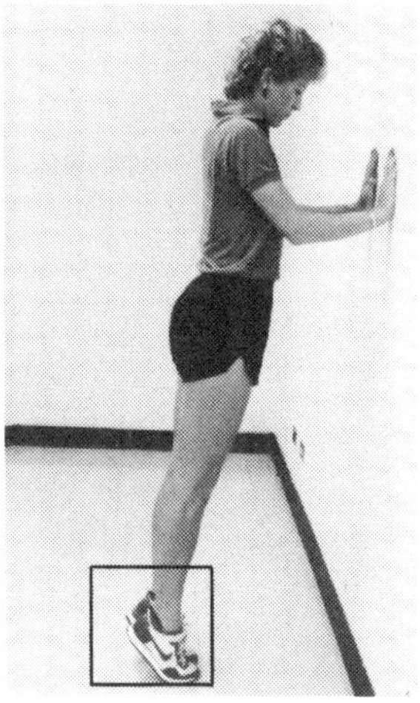

b

Strength Training Exercises With Weights

Exercise 10: ARM CURL

Action: Use a supinated or palms-up grip, and start with the arms almost completely extended. Now curl up as far as possible, then return to the starting position.

Muscles Developed: Biceps, brachioradialis, and brachialis.

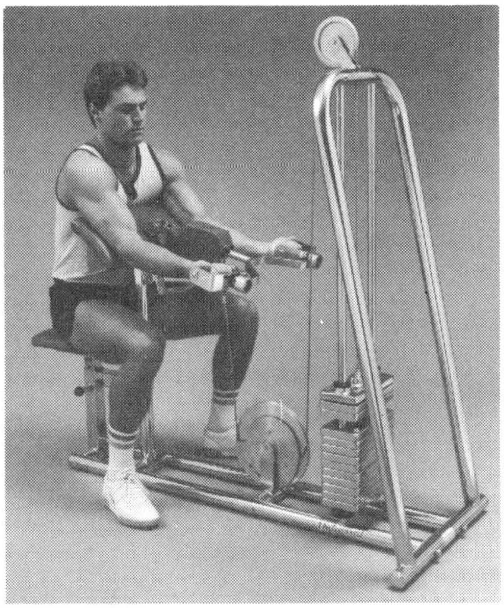

a

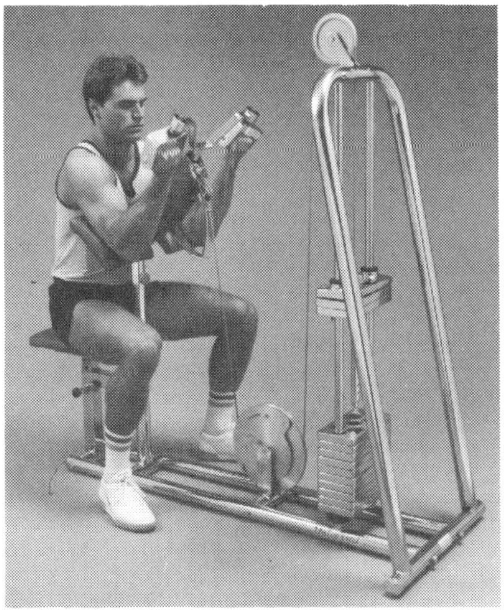

b

Exercise 11: LEG PRESS

Action: From a sitting position with the knees flexed at about ninety degrees and both feet on the footrest, fully extend the legs, then return slowly to the starting position.

Muscles Developed: Quadriceps and gluteal muscles.

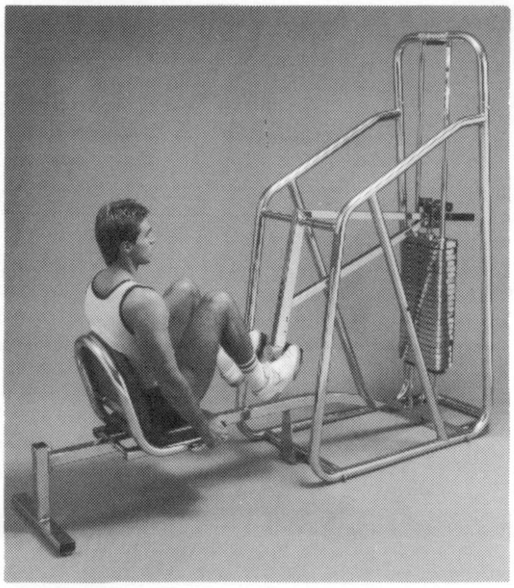

a

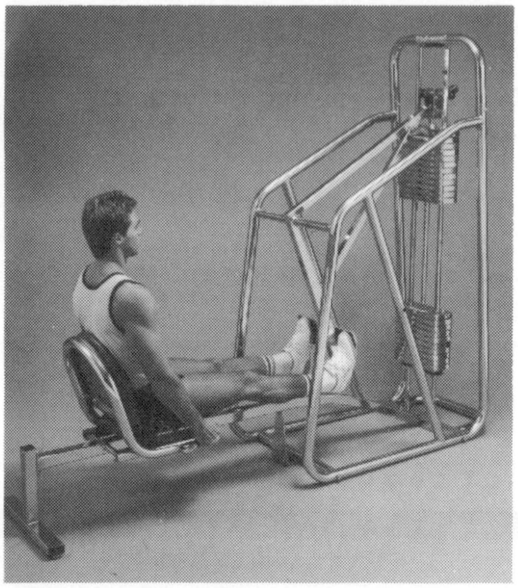

b

Exercise 12: SIT-UP

Action: Using either a horizontal or inclined board, stabilize your feet and flex the knees to about 100 to 120 degrees. Start with the head and shoulders off the board, curl all the way up, then return to the starting position without letting the head and shoulders touch the board (do not swing up, but rather curl up). You may curl straight up or use a twisting motion (twisting as you first start to come up), alternating on each sit-up.

Muscles Developed: Abdominals and hip flexors.

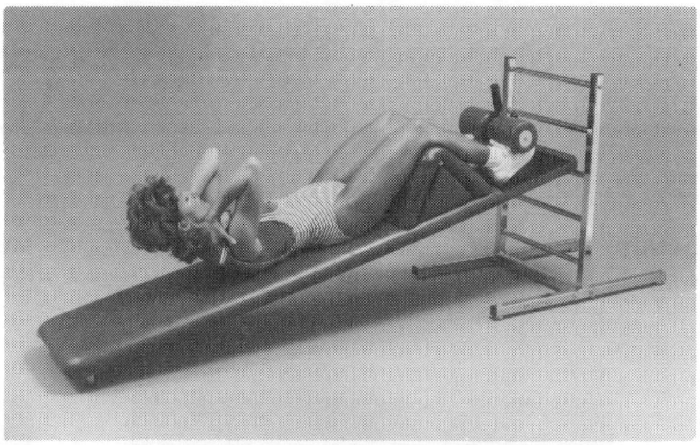

a

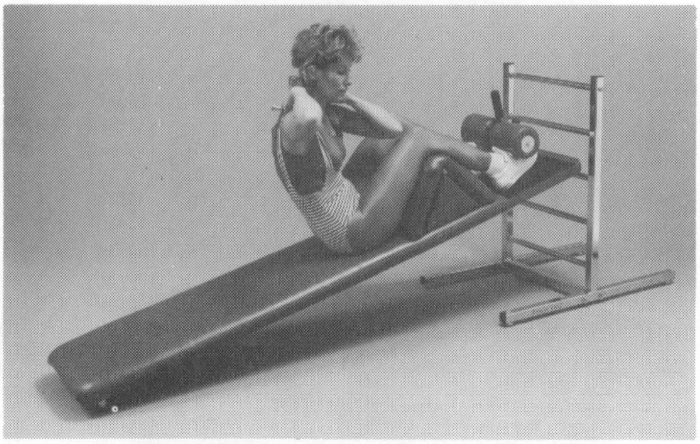

b

Exercise 13: BENCH PRESS

Action: Lie down on the bench with the head toward the weight stack, feet flat on the floor, and the bench press bar above the chest. Press upward until the arms are completely extended, then return to the starting position. Do not arch the back during the exercise.

Muscles Developed: Pectoralis major, triceps, and deltoid.

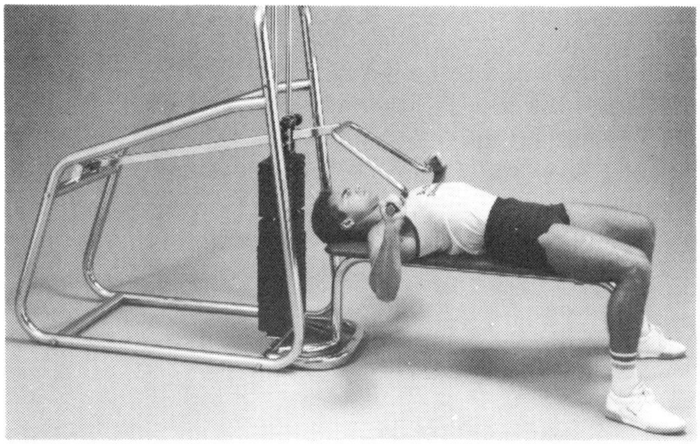
a

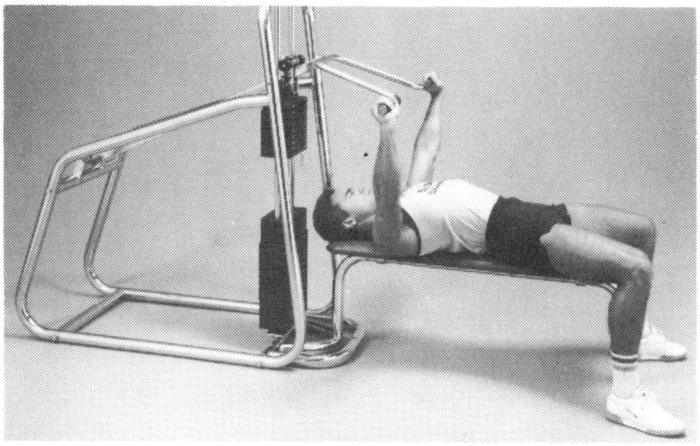
b

Exercise 14: LEG CURL

Action: Lie with the face down on the bench and legs straight with the back of the feet against the bar. Curl up to at least 90 degrees and return to the original position.

Muscles Developed: Hamstrings.

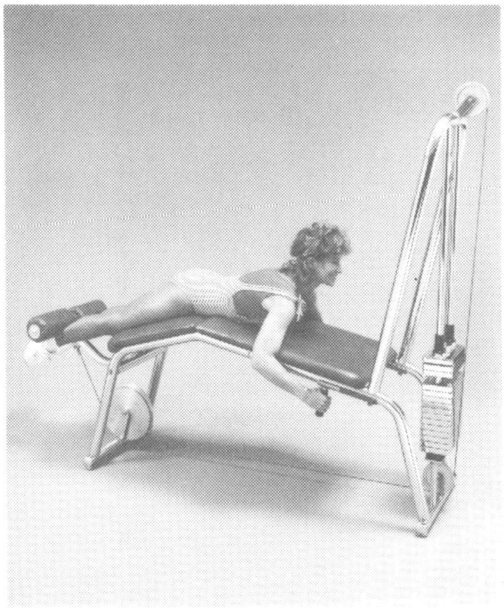
a

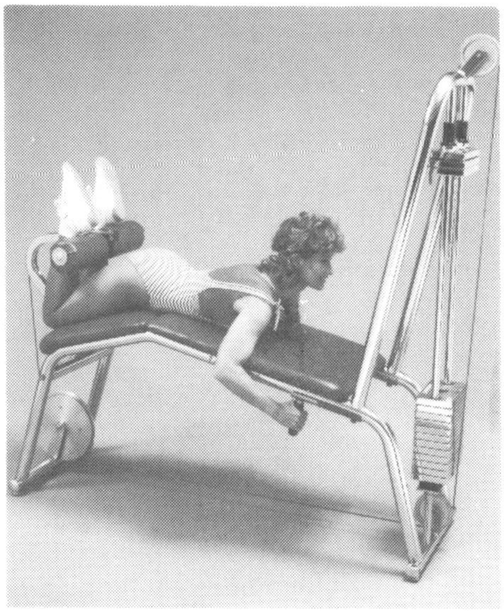
b

Exercise 15: LATERAL PULL-DOWN

Action: Start from a sitting position and hold the exercise bar with a wide grip. Pull the bar down until it touches the base of the neck, then return to the starting position (if a heavy resistance is used, stabilization of the body may be required by either using equipment as shown in the illustration or having someone else hold you down by the waist or shoulders).

Muscles Developed: Latissimus dorsi, pectoralis major, and biceps.

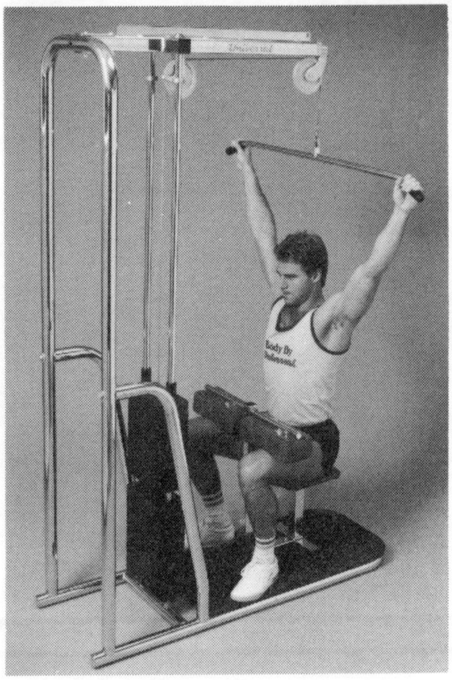
a

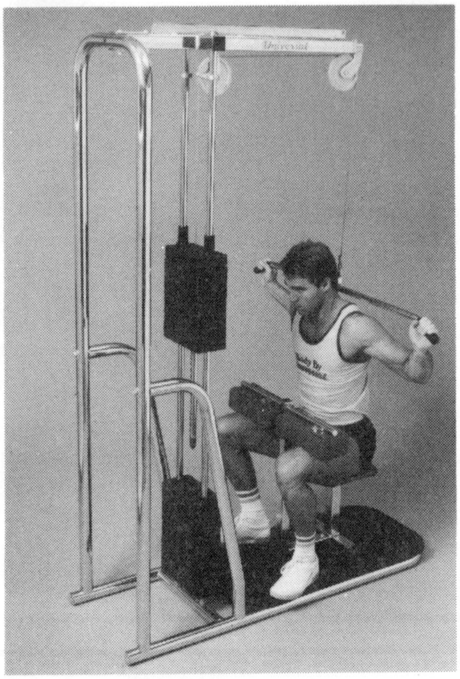
b

Exercise 16: HEEL RAISE

Action: Start with your feet either flat on the floor or the front of the feet on an elevated block, then raise and lower yourself by moving at the ankle joint only. If additional resistance is needed, you can use the squat machine, which is illustrated in Exercise 18.

Muscles Developed: Gastrocnemius and soleus.

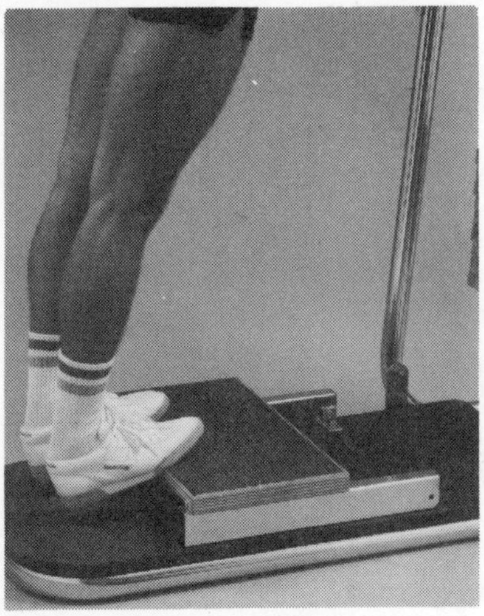
a

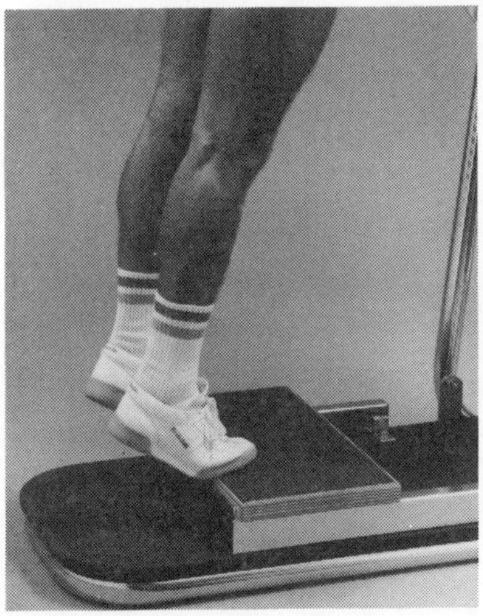
b

Exercise 17: TRICEP EXTENSION

Action: Using a palms-down grip, grasp the bar slightly closer than shoulder width, and start with the elbows almost completely bent. Fully extend the arms, then return to starting position.

Muscle Developed: Triceps.

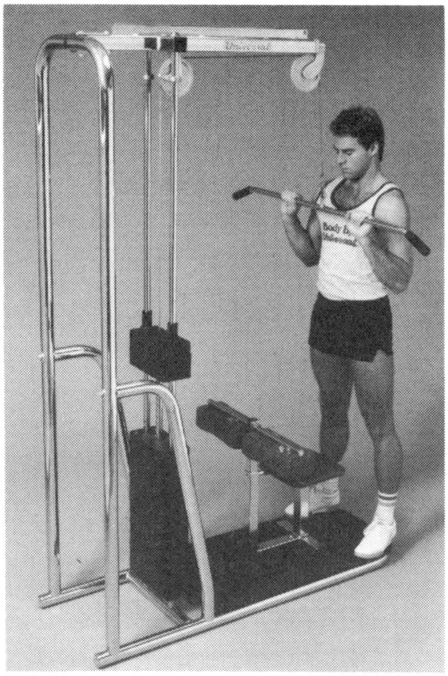

a

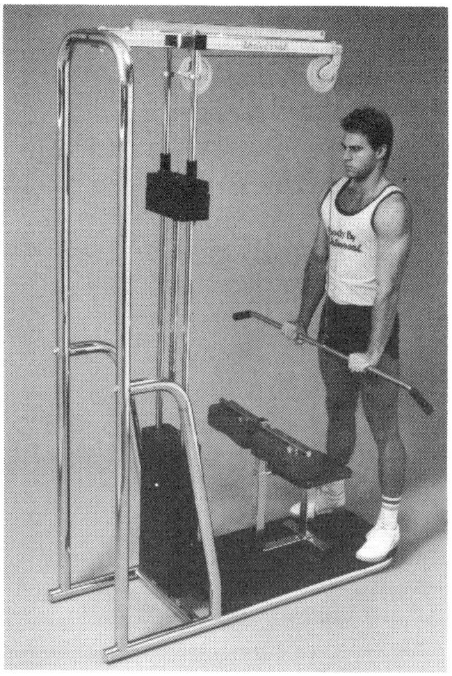

b

Exercise 18: SQUAT

Action: Start with the knees bent at about 120 degrees and shoulders under the padded bars. Completely extend the legs, then return to the original position.

Muscles Developed: Quadriceps, gluteal muscles, hamstrings, gastrocnemius, soleus, and erector spinae.

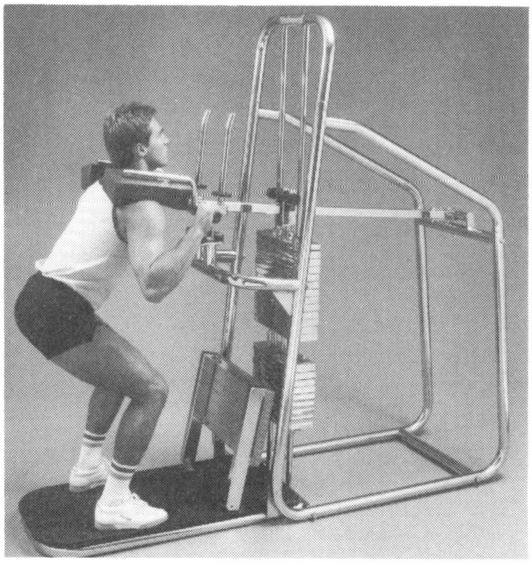

a

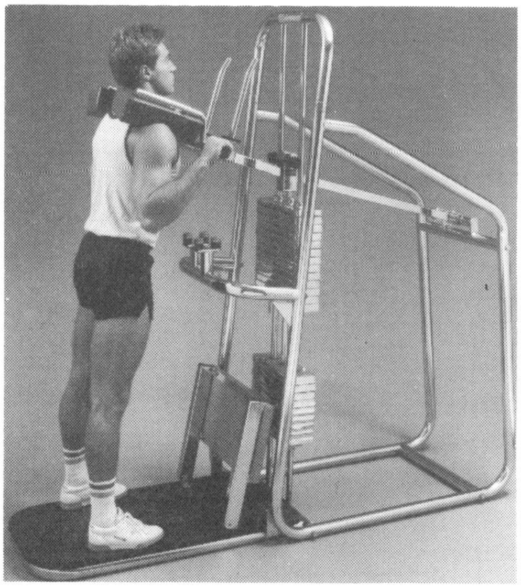

b

Exercise 19: QUADRICEPS LIFT Or LEG EXTENSION

Action: Sit in an upright position with feet under the padded bar. Extend the legs until they are completely straight, then return to the starting position.

Muscles Developed: Quadriceps.

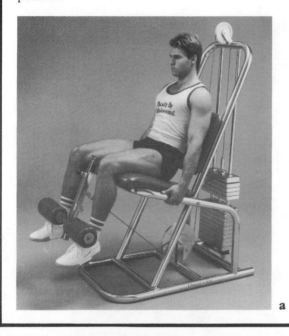

a

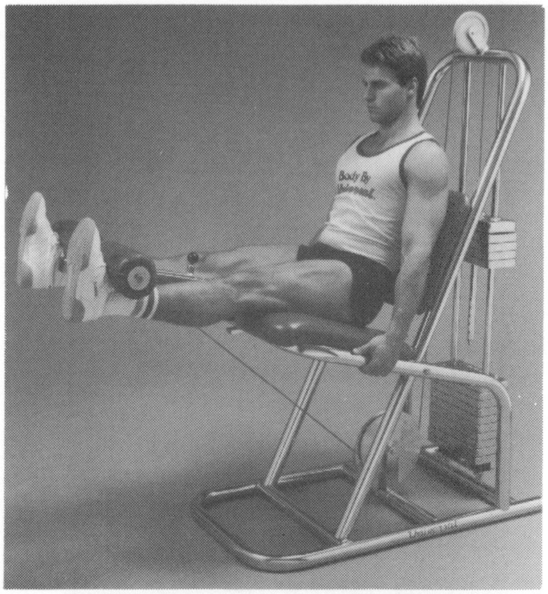

b

Exercise 20: UPRIGHT ROWING

Action: Start with the arms extended and grip the handles with the palms down. Pull all the way up to the chin, then return to the starting position.

Muscles Developed: Biceps, brachioradialis, brachialis, deltoid, and trapezius.

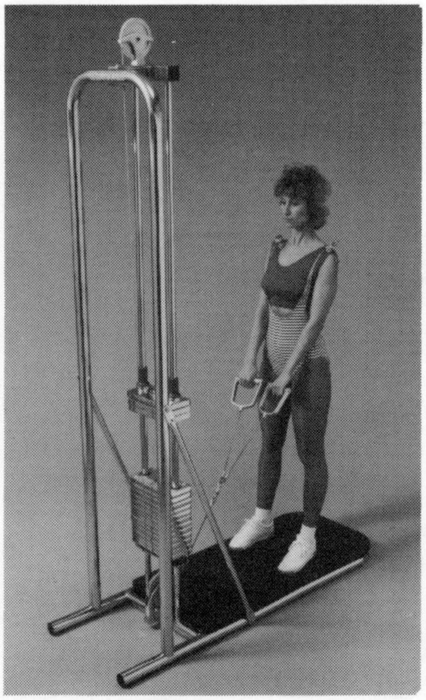

a

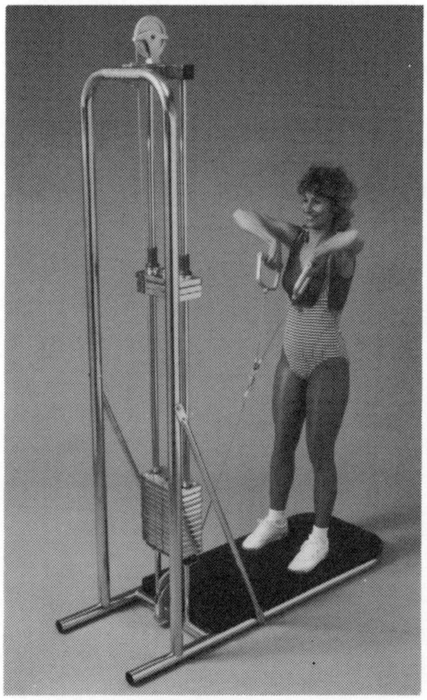

b

Exercise 21: BENT-ARM PULLOVER

Action: Sit back into the chair and grasp the bar behind your head. Pull the bar over your head all the way down to your abdomen and slowly return to the original position.

Muscles Developed: Latissimus dorsi, pectoral muscles, deltoid, and serratus anterior.

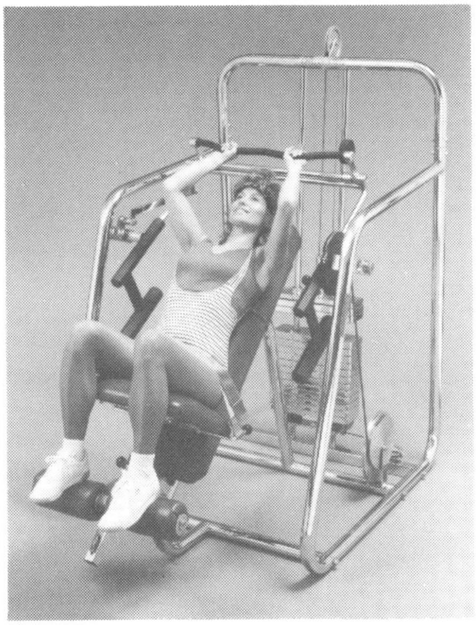

a

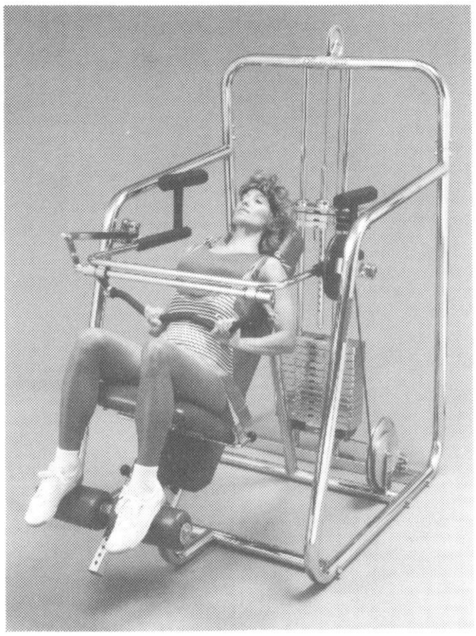

b

Exercise 22: CHEST PRESS

Action: Start with the arms to the side and elbows bent at ninety degrees. Press your arms forward until the padded bars touch in front of your chest, then return to the starting position.

Muscles Developed: Pectoralis major and deltoid.

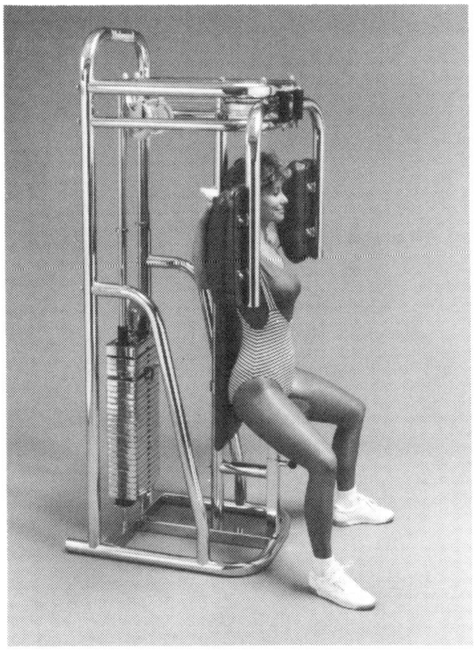

a

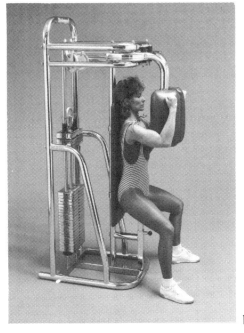

b

Exercise 23: SEATED OVERHEAD PRESS

Action: Sit in an upright position and grasp the bar wider than shoulder width. Press the bar all the way up until the arms are fully extended, then return to the initial position.

Muscles Developed: Triceps, deltoid, and pectoralis major.

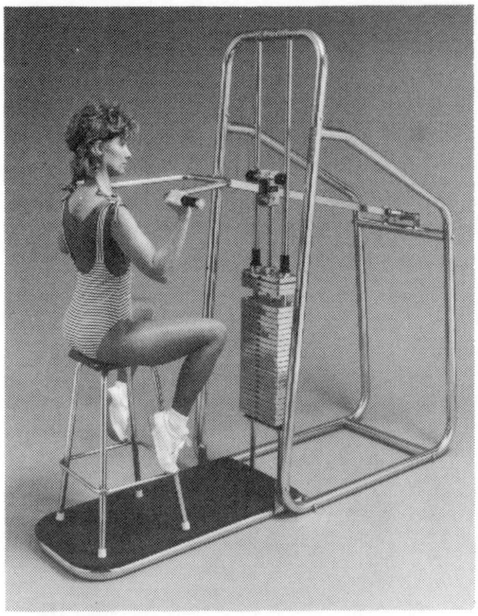
a

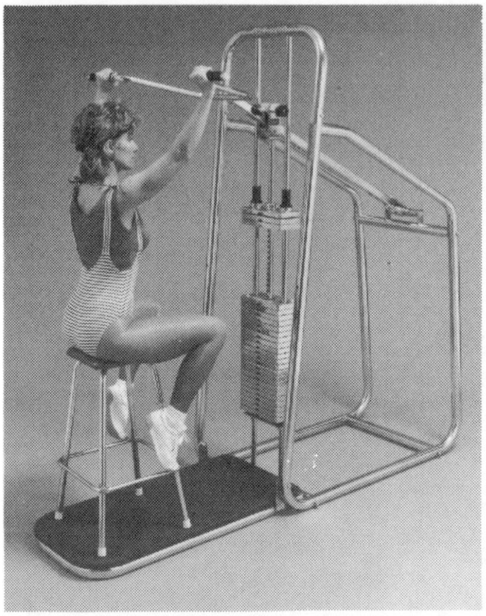
b

Exercise 24: DIP

Action: Start with your arms fully extended, knees bent, and feet crossed. Dip down at least to a ninety-degree angle at the elbow joint, then return to the initial position.

Muscles Developed: Triceps, deltoid, and pectoralis major.

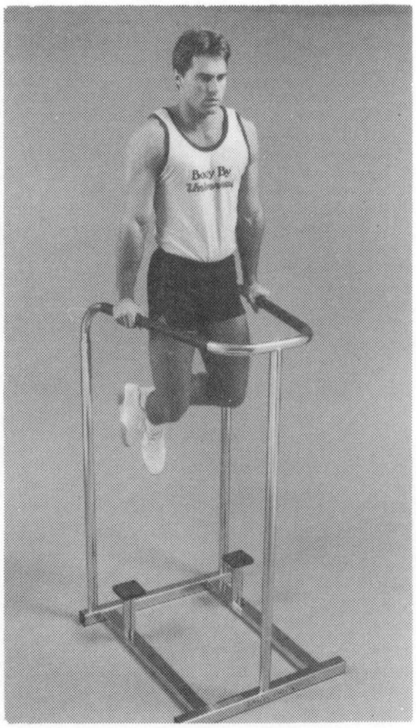

a

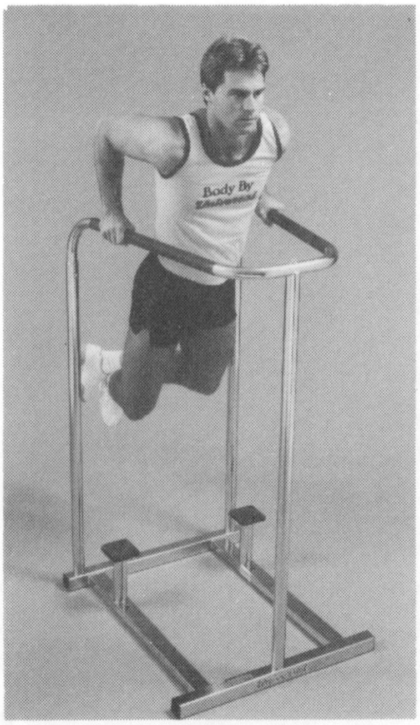

b

APPENDIX C

Flexibility Exercises

*Refer to Chapter 4 for instructions on how to set up and conduct your flexibility program, including the length of stretch, repetitions to be performed, and frequency of training.

Exercise 1: LATERAL HEAD TILT

Action: Slowly and gently tilt the head laterally. Repeat several times to each side.

Areas Stretched: Neck flexors and extensors and ligaments of the cervical spine.

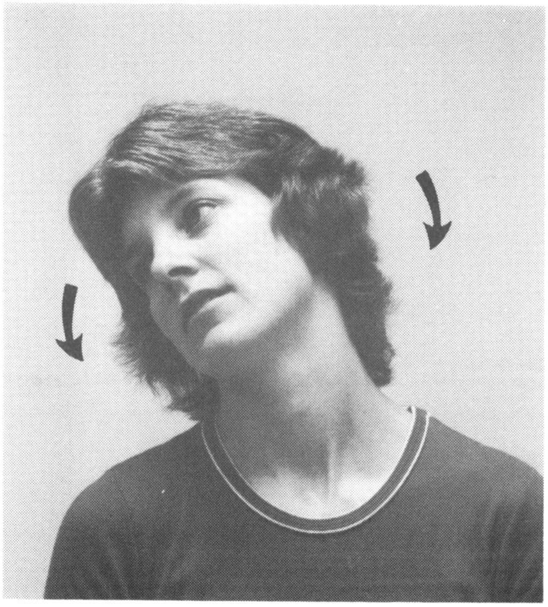

Exercise 2: ARM CIRCLES

Action: Gently circle your arms all the way around. Conduct the exercise in both directions.

Areas Stretched: Shoulder muscles and ligaments.

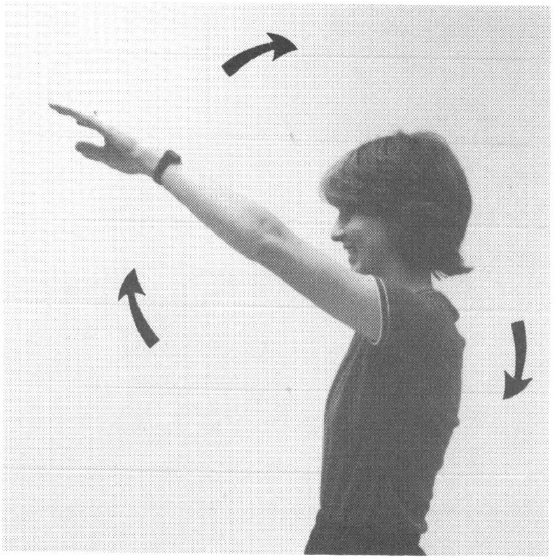

Exercise 3: SIDE STRETCH

Action: Stand straight up, feet separated to shoulder width, and place your hands behind your neck, interlocking the fingers. Now move the upper body to one side and hold the final stretch for a few seconds. Repeat on the other side.

Areas Stretched: Muscles and ligaments in the pelvic region.

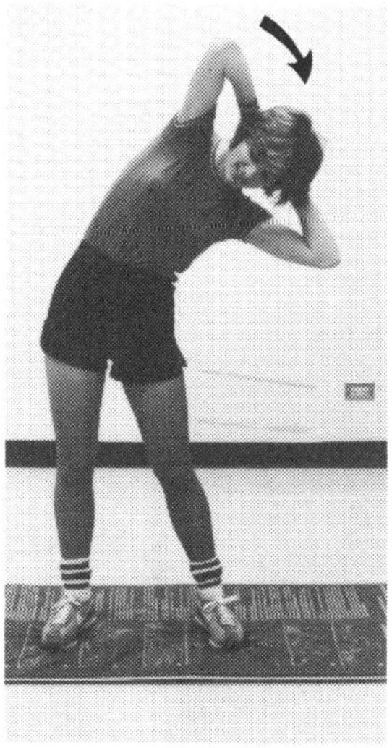

Exercise 4: TRUNK ROTATION STRETCH

Action: Place your arms slightly away from your body and rotate the trunk as far as possible, holding the final position for several seconds. Conduct the exercise for both the right and left sides of the body. You can also perform this exercise by standing about two feet away from the wall (back toward the wall), and then rotate the trunk, placing the hands against the wall.

Areas Stretched: Hip, abdominal, chest, back, neck, and shoulder muscles. Hip and spinal ligaments.

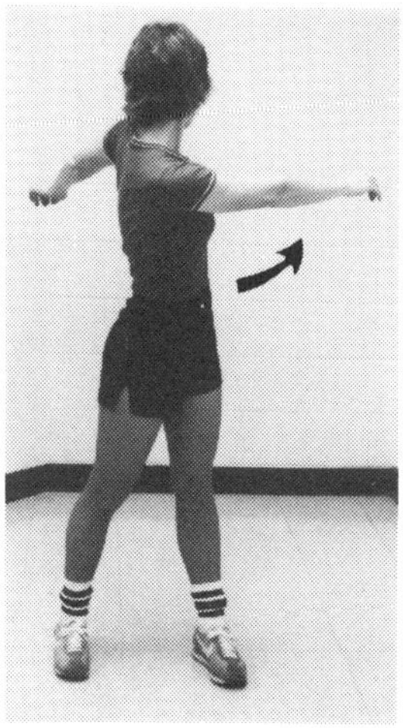

Exercise 5: CHEST STRETCH

Action: Kneel down behind a chair and place both hands on the back of the chair. Gradually push your chest downward and hold for a few seconds.

Areas Stretched: Chest (pectoral) muscles and shoulder ligaments.

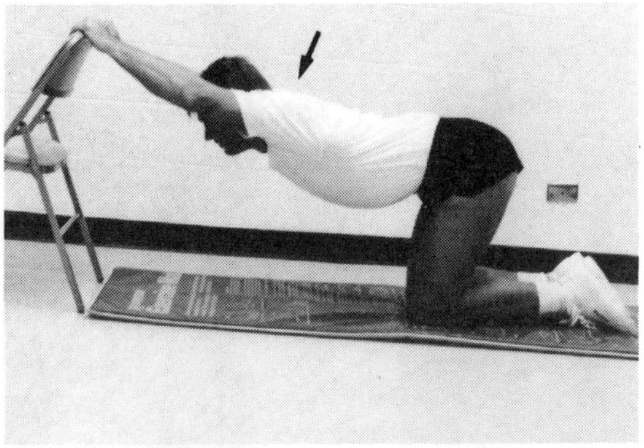

Exercise 6: SHOULDER HYPEREXTENSION STRETCH

Action: Place your hands on a table behind your back, then move your feet forward about a yard. Slowly lower your body as far as possible and hold this position for a few seconds.

Areas Stretched: Deltoid and pectoral muscles, and ligaments of the shoulder joint.

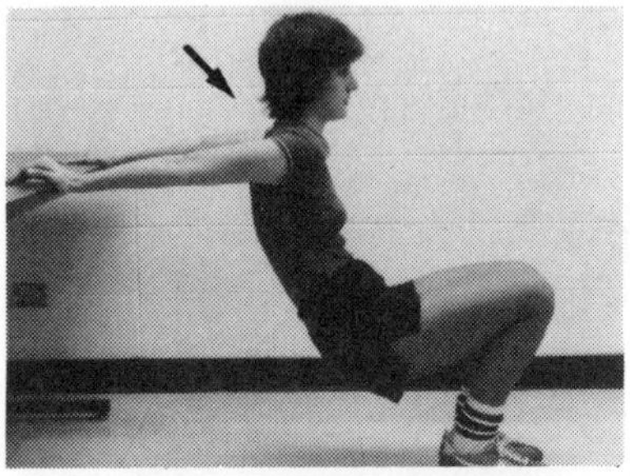

Exercise 7: SHOULDER ROTATION STRETCH

Action: With the aid of an elastic band, place the band behind your back and grasp the two ends using a reverse (thumbs-out) grip. Slowly bring the elastic band over your head, keeping the elbows straight. Repeat several times (bring the hands closer together for additional stretch).

Areas Stretched: Deltoid, latissimus dorsi, and pectoral muscles. Shoulder ligaments.

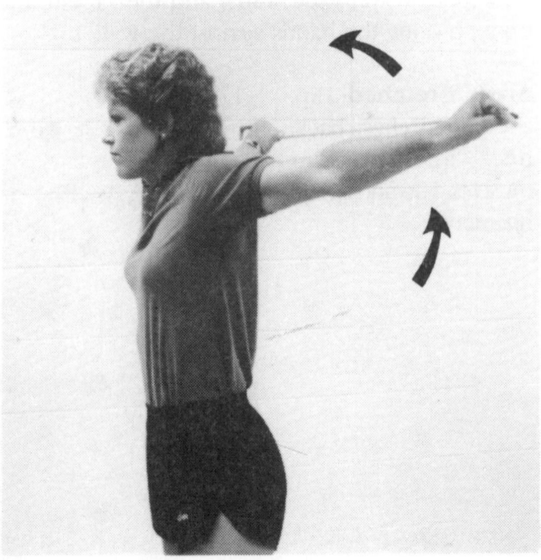

Exercise 8: QUAD STRETCH

Exercise 8: QUAD STRETCH

Action: Stand straight up and support yourself against a wall. Bring up one foot, flexing the knee. Grasp the front of the ankle and pull the ankle toward the gluteal region. Hold for several seconds. Repeat with the other leg.

Areas Stretched: Quadriceps muscle, and knee and ankle ligaments.

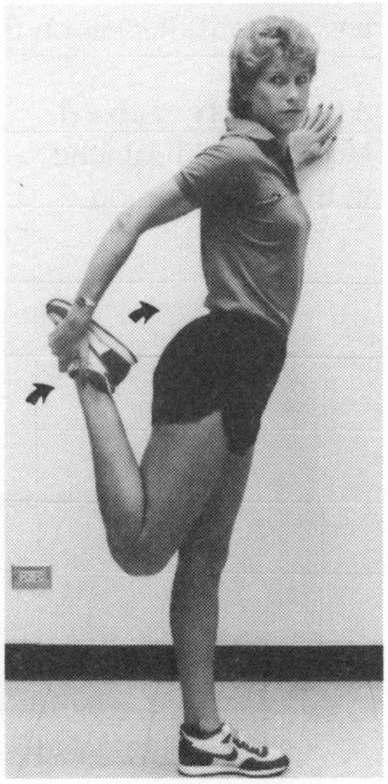

Exercise 9: HEEL CORD STRETCH

Action: Stand against the wall or at the edge of a step and stretch the heel downward, alternating legs. Hold the stretched position for a few seconds.

Areas Stretched: Heel cord (Achilles tendon), gastrocnemius, and soleus muscles.

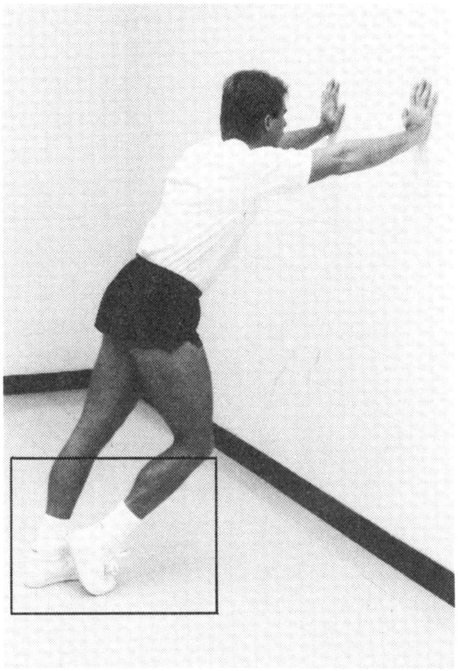

a

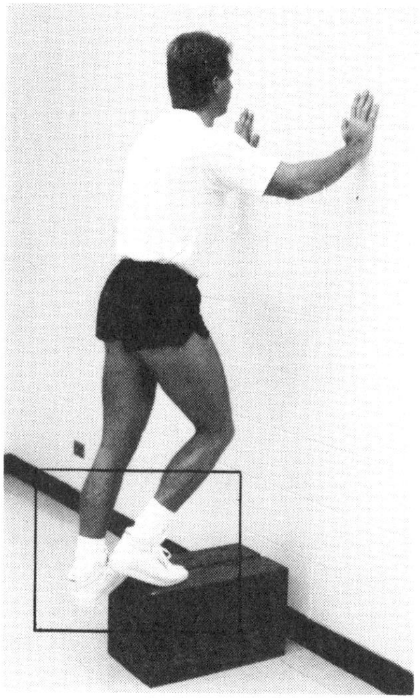

b

Exercise 10: ADDUCTOR STRETCH

Action: Stand with your feet about twice shoulder width and place your hands slightly above the knee. Flex one knee and slowly go down as far as possible, holding the final position for a few seconds. Repeat with the other leg.

Areas Stretched: Hip adductor muscles.

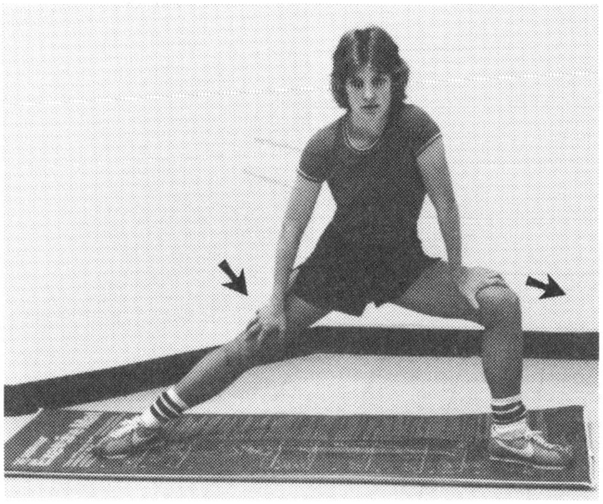

Exercise 11: SITTING ADDUCTOR STRETCH

Action: Sit on the floor and bring your feet in close to you, allowing the soles of the feet to touch each other. Now place your forearms (or elbows) on the inner part of the thigh and push the legs downward, holding the final stretch for several seconds.

Areas Stretched: Hip adductor muscles.

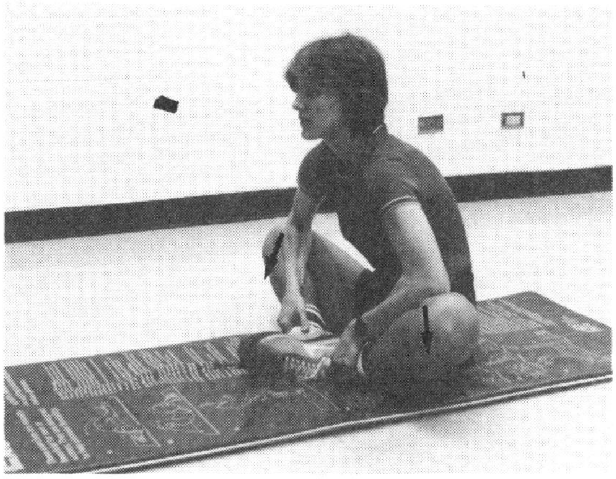

Exercise 12:
SIT AND REACH STRETCH

Action: Sit on the floor with legs together and gradually reach forward as far as possible. Hold the final position for a few seconds. This exercise may also be performed with the legs separated, reaching to each side as well as to the middle.

Areas Stretched: Hamstrings and lower back muscles, and lumbar spine ligaments.

Note: Additional stretching exercises for the lower back region are given in Appendix D.

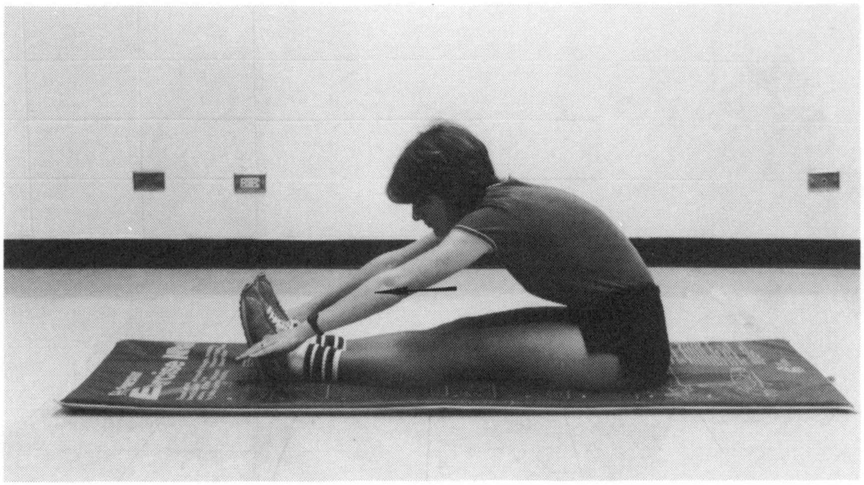

APPENDIX D

Exercises for the Prevention and Rehabilitation of Low Back Pain

Exercise 1: SINGLE-KNEE TO CHEST STRETCH

Action: Lie down flat on the floor. Bend one leg at approximately 100 degrees and gradually pull the opposite leg toward your chest. Hold the final stretch for a few seconds. Switch legs and repeat the exercise.

Areas Stretched: Lower back and hamstring muscles, and lumbar spine ligaments.

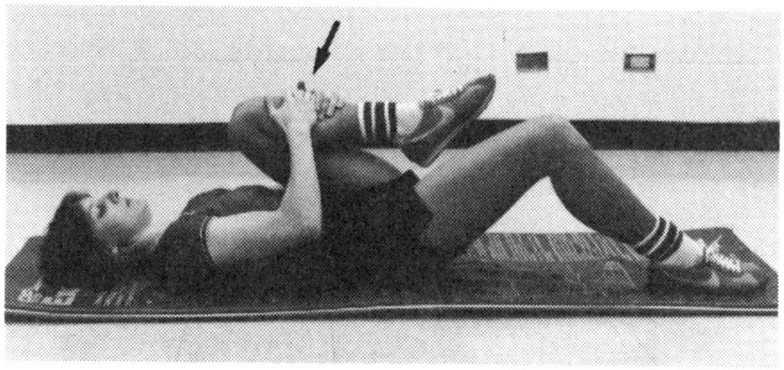

Exercise 2: DOUBLE-KNEE TO CHEST STRETCH

Action: Lie flat on the floor and then slowly curl up into a fetal position. Hold for a few seconds.

Areas Stretched: Upper and lower back and hamstring muscles. Spinal ligaments.

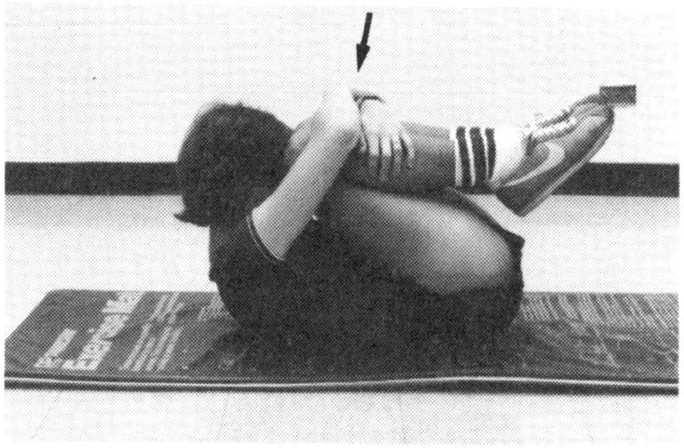

Exercise 3: UPPER AND LOWER BACK STRETCH

Action: Sit in a chair with feet separated greater than shoulder width. Place your arms to the inside of the thighs and bring your chest down toward the floor. At the same time, attempt to reach back as far as you can with your arms.

Areas Stretched: Upper and lower back muscles and ligaments.

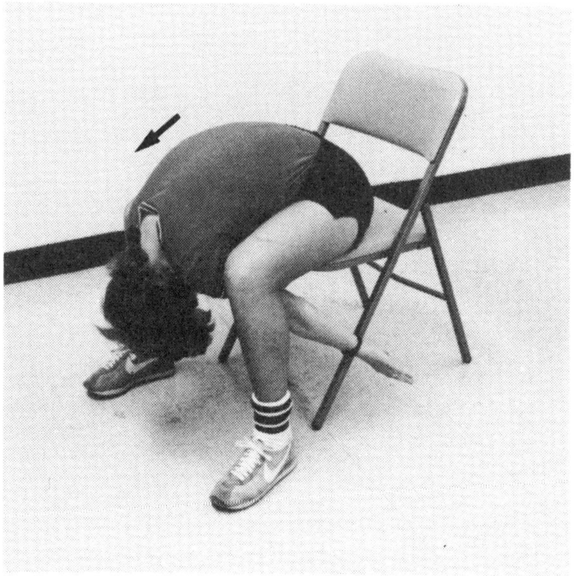

Exercise 4: SIT-AND-REACH STRETCH

(see Exercise 12 in Appendix C)

Exercise 5: PELVIC TILT

Action: Lie flat on the floor with the knees bent at about a 70-degree angle. Tilt the pelvis by tightening the abdominal muscles, flattening your back against the floor, and raising the lower gluteal area ever so slightly off the floor. Hold the final position for several seconds. The exercise can also be performed against a wall as shown in illustration c.

Areas Stretched:
Low back muscles and ligaments.

Areas Strengthened:
Abdominal and gluteal muscles.

Note: This is perhaps the most important exercise for the care of the lower back. It should be included as a part of your daily exercise routine and should be performed several times throughout the day when pain in the lower back is present as a result of muscle imbalance.

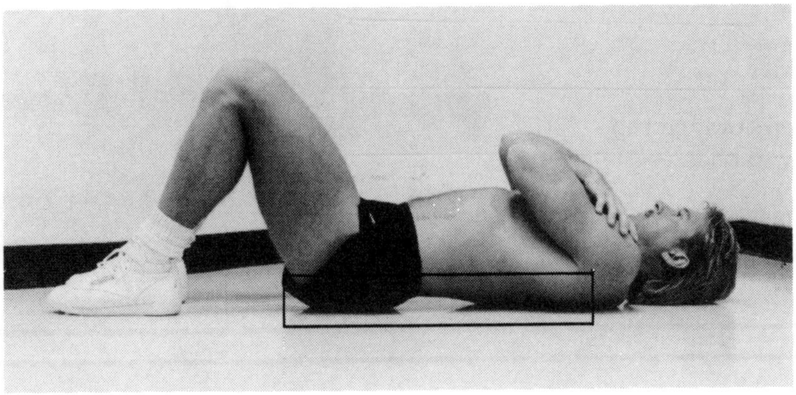

a

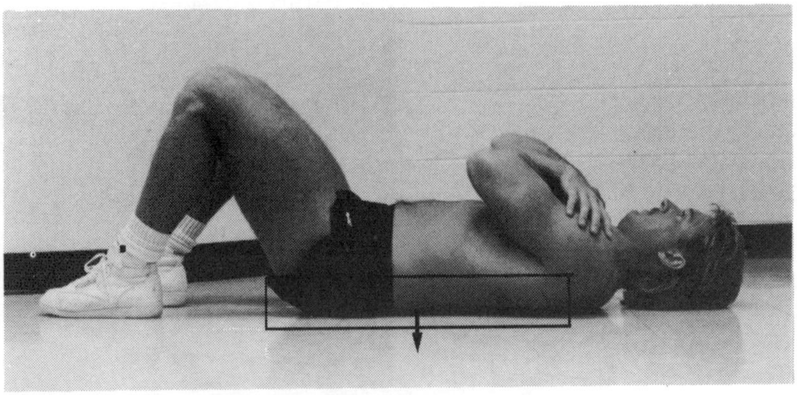

b

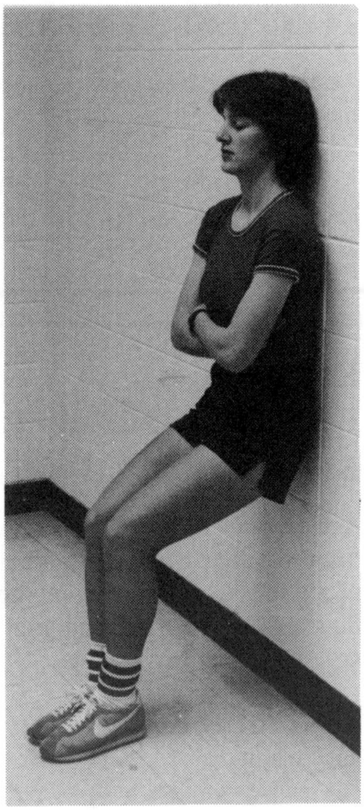

c

Exercise 6: SIT-UP (see Exercise 4 in Appendix B)

It is important that you do not stabilize your feet when performing this exercise, because doing so decreases the work of the abdominal muscles. Also, remember not to "swing up" but rather curl up as you perform the exercise.

APPENDIX E

Nutrition Analysis

- Nutritive Value of Selected Foods
- Dietary Analysis Forms

Code	Food	Amount	Weight gm	Calories	Protein gm	Fat gm	Sat. Fat gm	Cholesterol mg	Carbohydrate gm	Calcium mg	Iron mg	Sodium mg	Vit A I.U.	Vit B_1 mg	Vit B_2 mg	Niacin mg	Vit C mg
001.	Almonds, shelled	1/4 c	36	213	6.6	19	1.4	0	9	83	1.7	2	0	0.09	0.33	1.3	0
002.	Apple, raw, unpared	1 med	150	80	0.3	1	0	0	20	10	0.4	1	120	0.04	0.03	0.1	6
003.	Apple juice, canned or bottled	1/2 c	124	59	0.1	0	0	0	15	8	0.7	1	0	0.01	0.03	0.1	1
004.	Apple pie	1 piece (3½″)	118	302	2.6	13	3.5	120	45	9	0.4	355	40	0.02	0.02	0.5	1
005.	Applesauce, canned, sweetened	1/2 c	128	116	0.3	0	0	0	31	5	0.7	3	50	0.02	0.01	0	2
006.	Apricots, raw	3 (12 per lb)	114	55	1.1	0	0	0	14	18	0.5	1	2,890	0.06	0.04	0.6	11
007.	Apricots, canned, heavy syrup	3 halves; 1¾ tbsp liq.	85	73	0.5	0	0	0	19	9	0.3	1	1,480	0.02	0.02	0.3	3
008.	Apricots, dried, sulfured, uncooked	10 med halves	35	91	1.8	0	0	0	23	23	1.9	9	3,820	0	0.06	1.2	4
009.	Asparagus, cooked green spears	4 med	60	12	1.3	0	0	0	2	13	0.4	1	540	0.10	0.11	0.8	16
010.	Avocado, raw	1/8 med	120	185	2.4	19	3.2	0	7	11	0.6	4	310	0.12	0.22	1.7	15
011.	Bacon, cooked, drained	2 slices	15	86	3.8	8	2.7	30	1	2	0.5	153	0	0.08	0.05	0.8	0
012.	Banana, raw	1 sm (7¼″)	140	81	1.0	0	0	0	21	8	0.7	1	180	0.05	0.06	0.7	10
013.	Beans, green snap, cooked	1/2 c	65	16	1.0	0	0	0	3	32	0.4	4	340	0.05	0.06	0.3	8
014.	Beans, lentils	1/4 c	50	53	3.9	0	0	0	10	12	1.0	0	10	0.03	0.04	0.4	0
015.	Beans, lima (Fordhook), froz., cooked	1/2 c	85	84	6	0	0	0	17	40	2.1	1	240	0.15	0.08	1.1	15
016.	Beans, red kidney, cooked	1 c	185	218	14.4	1	0	0	40	70	4.4	6	10	0.20	0.11	1.3	0
017.	Bean sprouts, mung, raw	1/2 c	52	18	2.0	0	0	0	4	10	0.7	3	10	0.07	0.07	0.4	10
018.	Beef-chuck, cooked, trimmed, choice	3 oz.	85	212	25	12	7.8	80	0	11	3.1	43	20	0.05	0.19	3.8	0
019.	Beef, corned canned	3 oz.	85	163	21	10	8	70	0	22	5.0	802	0	0.02	0.27	3.9	0
020.	Beef, ground, lean	3 oz.	85	186	23.3	10	5	81	0	10	3.0	57	20	0.08	0.20	5.1	0
021.	Beef, round steak, cooked, trimmed	3 oz.	85	222	24.3	13	6	77	0	10	3.0	60	20	0.07	0.20	4.8	0
022.	Beef, rump roast	3 oz.	85	177	24.7	8	11	80	0	10	3.1	61	10	0.06	0.19	4.4	0
023.	Beef, sirloin, cooked	3 oz.	85	329	19.6	27	13	77	0	9	2.5	48	50	0.05	0.15	4.0	0
024.	Beer	12 fl. oz.	360	151	1.1	0	0	0	14	18	0	25	0	0.01	0.11	2.2	0
025.	Beets, red, canned, drained	1/2 c	80	32	0.8	0	0	0	8	15	0.6	164	15	0.01	0.02	0.1	2
026.	Beet greens, cooked	1/2 c	73	13	1.3	0	0	0	2	72	1.4	55	3,700	0.05	0.11	0.2	11
027.	Biscuits, baking powder, made from mix	1 med	35	114	2.5	6	1.1	0	18	60	0.8	272	0	0.06	0.06	0.7	0
028.	Blueberries, fresh cultivated	1/2 c	73	45	0.5	0	0	0	11	10	0.8	1	75	0.02	0.05	0.4	10
029.	Bologna	1 slice (1 oz.)	28	86	3.4	8	3	15	0	2	0.5	369	0	0.05	0.06	0.7	0
030.	Bouillon, broth	1 cube	4	5	.8	0	0	0	0	0	0	960	0	0	0	0	0
031.	Bran Cereal	1/2 c	30	72	3.8	1	0	0	22	25	3	247	2,000	1.0	0.80	3.0	20
032.	Bread, Corn	1 slice	78	161	5.8	6	0.1	0	23	94	0.9	490	120	0.10	0.15	0.5	1
033.	Bread, French enriched	1 slice	35	102	3.2	1	0.2	0	19	15	0.8	203	0	0.10	0.08	0.9	0
034.	Bread, rye (American)	1 slice	25	61	2.3	0	0	0	13	19	0.4	139	0	0.05	0.02	0.4	0
035.	Bread, white enriched	1 slice	25	68	2.2	1	0.2	0	13	21	0.6	127	0	0.06	0.05	0.6	0

(Continued)

Code	Food	Amount	Weight gm	Calories	Protein gm	Fat gm	Sat. Fat gm	Cholesterol mg	Carbohydrate gm	Calcium mg	Iron mg	Sodium mg	Vit A I.U.	Vit B_1 mg	Vit B_2 mg	Niacin mg	Vit C mg
036.	Bread, whole wheat	1 slice	25	61	2.6	1	0.6	0	12	25	0.8	132	0	0.06	0.03	0.7	0
037.	Broccoli, raw	1 sm stalk	114	38	4.1	0	0	0	7	117	1.3	17	2,835	0.10	0.23	0.9	125
038.	Broccoli, cooked drained	1 sm stalk	140	36	4.3	0	0	0	6	123	1.1	14	3,500	0.13	0.28	1.1	126
039.	Brussels sprouts, froz., cooked drained	1/2 c	78	28	3.2	0	0	0	5	25	0.8	8	405	0.06	0.11	0.5	63
040.	Bulgur, wheat	1 c	135	227	8.4	1	0	0	47	27	1.8	809	0	0.07	0.04	3.2	0
041.	Burrito, combination, Taco Bell	1	175	404	21	16	0	0	43	91	3.7	300	1,666	0.34	0.31	4.6	15
042.	Butter	1 tsp	5	36	0	4	0.4	12	0	1	0	46	160	0	0	0	0
043.	Buttermilk, cultured	1 c	245	88	8.8	0	1.3	5	12	296	0.1	319	10	0.10	0.44	0.2	2
044.	Cabbage, raw chopped	1/2 c	45	11	0.6	0	0	0	3	22	0.2	9	60	0.03	0.03	0.2	21
045.	Cabbage, boiled, drained wedge	1/2 c	85	16	0.9	0	0	0	3	36	0.3	10	100	0.02	0.02	0.1	21
046.	Cake, angel food, plain	1 piece	60	161	4.3	0	0	0	36	5	0.1	170	0	0.01	0.08	0.1	0
047.	Cake, devil's food, iced	1 piece	99	365	4.5	16	5	68	55	69	1.0	233	160	0.02	0.10	0.2	0
048.	Candy, hard	1 oz.	28	109	0	0	0	0	28	6	0.5	9	0	0	0	0	0
049.	Cantaloupe	1/4 melon 5" diam.	239	35	2.0	0	0	0	10	20	0.8	17	4,620	0.06	0.04	0.6	45
050.	Caramel (candy, plain or choc.)	1 oz.	28	113	1.1	3	1.6	0	22	42	0.4	64	0	0.01	0.05	0.1	0
051.	Carrots, raw	1 carrot 7½" long	81	30	0.8	0	0	0	7	27	0.5	34	7,930	0.04	0.04	0.4	6
052.	Carrots, cooked, drained	1/2 c	73	23	0.7	0	0	0	5	24	0.5	10	7,615	0.04	0.04	0.4	5
053.	Cauliflower, cooked, drained	1/2 c	63	14	1.5	0	0	0	3	13	0.5	6	40	0.06	0.05	0.4	35
054.	Celery, green, raw, long	1 outer stalk 8"	40	7	0.4	0	0	0	2	16	0.1	50	110	0.01	0.01	0.1	4
055.	Cheese, American	1 oz. slice	28	100	6	8	5.6	27	0	188	0.1	307	343	0.01	0.10	0	0
056.	Cheese, blue	1 oz.	28	100	6	8	5.3	25	1	89	0.1	510	204	0.01	0.11	0.3	0
057.	Cheese, cheddar	1 oz.	28	114	7	9	6	30	0	204	0.2	171	300	0.01	0.11	0	0
058.	Cheese, cottage, creamed	½ cup	105	112	14	5	6.4	15	3	99	0.3	241	180	0.03	0.26	0.1	0
059.	Cheese, creamed	1 oz.	28	99	6	8	3	31	1	167	0.3	71	320	0.02	0.14	0	0
060.	Cheese, souffle	1 portion	110	240	10.9	19	9.5	189	7	221	1.1	400	880	0.06	0.26	0.2	0
061.	Cheesecake	1 piece (3½")	85	257	4.6	16	9.0	150	24	48	0.4	189	216	0.03	0.11	0.4	4
062.	Cherries	10	75	47	0.9	0	0	0	12	15	0.3	8	450	0.20	0.24	1.6	41
063.	Cherry Pie	1 piece (3½")	118	308	3.1	13	5.0	137	45	17	0.4	355	40	0.02	0.02	0.5	1
064.	Chicken, drumstick Kentucky Fried	1	54	136	14	8	2.2	73	2	20	0.9	320	30	0.04	0.12	2.7	0
065.	Chicken, wing, Kentucky Fried	1	45	151	11	10	2.9	70	4	0	0.6	300	0	0.03	0.07	0	0
066.	Chicken, roast, light meat without skin	3 oz.	85	141	27	3	0.4	45	0	10	1.2	54	51	0.03	0.09	9.9	0
067.	Chicken, roast, dark meat without skin	3 oz.	85	149	24	5	0.8	50	0	11	1.5	54	127	0.06	0.19	4.7	0
068.	Chocolate, milk	1 oz.	28	147	2	9	3.6	5	16	65	0.3	27	80	0.02	0.10	0.1	0
069.	Clam, canned drained	3 oz.	85	83	13	2	0.2	50	2	46	3.5	750	93	0.01	0.09	0.9	9
070.	Cocoa, plain, dry	1 tbsp	5	14	0.9	1	0	0	3	7	0.6	0	0	0.01	0.02	0.1	0
071.	Coconut, shredded, packed	1/2 c	65	225	2.3	23	20	0	6	8	1.1	165	0	0.03	0.01	0.3	2

072.	Cod, cooked	3 oz.	85	144	24.3	4	1.5	60	0	27	0.9	63	150	0.06	0.09	2.7	0
073.	Cola	12 oz.	369	144	0	0	0	0	37	27	0	30	0	0	0	0	0
074.	Coffee	3/4 cup	180	1	0	0	0	0	0	1	0.2	2	0	0	0	0.1	0
075.	Coleslaw	1 c	120	173	1.6	17	1	5	6	53	0.5	144	190	0.06	0.06	0.4	35
076.	Collards, leaves without stems, cooked, drained	1/2 c	95	32	3.4	1	2	0	5	178	0.8	28	7,410	0.01	0.19	1.2	72
077.	Cookies, chocolate chip homemade	2 2¼" diam.	20	103	1	6	1.7	14	12	7	0.4	70	20	0.02	0.02	0.2	0
078.	Cookies, vanilla	5 1¾" diam.	20	93	1	3	0.8	10	15	8	0.1	50	25	0	0.01	0	0
079.	Corn, boiled on cob	1 ear 5" long	140	70	2.5	1	0	0	16	2	0.5	1	310	0.09	0.08	1.1	7
080.	Corn, canned, drained	1/2 c	83	70	2.2	1	0	0	16	4	0.4	195	290	0.03	0.04	0.8	4
081.	Cornflakes	1 c	25	97	2.0	0	0	0	21	3	0.6	251	180	0.29	0.55	2.9	9
082.	Cornmeal, degermed, yellow, enriched cooked	1/2 c	120	60	1.3	0	0	0	13	1	0.5	264	70	0.07	0.05	0.6	0
083.	Crackers, graham	2 squares	14	55	1.1	1	0.3	0	10	6	0.2	95	0	0.01	0.03	0.2	0
084.	Crackers, saltines	4 squares	11	48	1.0	1	0.3	0	8	2	0.1	123	0	0	0	0.1	0
085.	Cream, light coffee or table	1 tbsp	15	20	0.5	2	0.5	5	1	16	0	7	70	0	0.02	0	0
086.	Cream, heavy whipping	1 tbsp	15	53	0.3	6	1.3	12	1	11	0	5	230	0	0.02	0	0
087.	Croissants (Sara Lee)	1 roll	18	59	1.6	2	0.3	0	8	22	0.6	105	0	0.14	0.09	0.8	0
088.	Cucumbers, raw pared	9 sm slices	28	4	0.3	0	0	0	1	7	0.3	2	70	0.01	0.01	0.1	3
089.	Dates hydrated	5	46	110	0.9	0	0	0	29	24	1.2	1	20	0.04	0.04	0.9	0
090.	Doughnuts, plain	1	42	164	1.9	8	2	19	22	17	0.6	210	30	0.07	0.07	0.5	0
091.	Eggs, hard cooked	1 large	50	72	6	5	1.8	250	1	24	1.0	54	520	0.05	0.13	0	0
092.	Eggs, White	1 large	33	17	3.6	0	0	0	0	3	0	48	0	0	0.09	0	0
093.	Farina, enriched, quick cooking, cooked	1/2 c	123	51	1.6	0	0	0	11	5	6	176	0	0.06	0.03	0.5	0
094.	Figs, dried	1 large	21	60	1.0	0	0	0	15	26	0.6	1	20	0.16	0.17	3.9	0
095.	Filet of Fish, McDonald's	1	131	402	15	23	7.9	43	34	105	1.8	709	152	0.28	0.28	3.9	4
096.	Flounder	3 oz.	85	171	25.5	7	1	60	0	21	1.2	201	0	0.06	0.06	2.1	3
097.	Flour, all purpose enriched	1 c	125	455	13	1	0	0	95	20	3.6	3	0	0.55	0.33	4.4	0
098.	Flour, whole wheat	1 c	120	400	16	2	0	0	85	49	4.0	4	0	0.66	0.14	5.2	0
099.	Frankfurters, cooked	1	57	176	7	16	5.6	45	1	4	1.1	627	0	0.09	0.11	1.5	0
100.	Fruit cocktail	1 c	245	91	1	0	0	0	24	22	1.0	12	370	0.05	0.02	1.2	5
101.	Ginger ale	12 oz.	366	113	0	0	0	0	29	0	0	45	0	0	0	0	0
102.	Grapefruit, raw white	1/2 med	301	56	1	0	0	0	15	22	0.5	1	10	0.05	0.03	0.3	52
103.	Grapefruit, juice unsweetened canned	1/2 c	124	50	0.6	0	0	0	12	11	0.2	2	10	0.05	0.03	0.3	46
104.	Grapes, raw seedless European	10 grapes	50	34	0.3	0	0	0	9	6	0.2	2	50	0.03	0.03	0.2	2
105.	Grape juice, unsweetened bottled	1/2 c	127	84	0.3	0	0	0	21	14	0.4	3	0	0.05	0.03	0.3	0
106.	Haddock, fried (dipped in egg, milk, bread crumbs)	3 oz.	85	141	17	5	1	54	5	33	0.9	150	0	0.03	0.06	2.7	3
107.	Halibut, broiled with butter or margarine	3 oz.	85	144	21	6	2.1	55	0	15	0.6	114	570	0.03	0.06	7.2	1
108.	Hamburger, McDonald's	1	99	257	13	9	3.7	26	30	63	3.0	526	231	0.23	0.23	5.1	2

(Continued)

Code	Food	Amount	Weight gm	Calories	Protein gm	Fat gm	Sat. Fat gm	Cholesterol mg	Carbohydrate gm	Calcium mg	Iron mg	Sodium mg	Vit A I.U.	Vit B_1 mg	Vit B_2 mg	Niacin mg	Vit C mg
109.	Ham (cured pork) baked, trimmed	3 oz.	85	318	20	26	9.4	77	0	9	2.6	48	0	0.43	0.20	3.8	0
110.	Honey	1 tbsp	21	64	0	0	0	0	17	1	0.1	1	0	0	0.01	0.1	0
111.	Ice cream, vanilla	1/2 c	67	135	3	7	4.4	27	14	97	0.1	42	295	0.03	0.14	0.1	1
112.	Ice cream cone, Dairy Queen	medium	142	230	6	7	4.6	15	35	200	0	150	300	0.09	0.26	0	0
113.	Ice milk, vanilla	1/2 c	61	100	3	3	1.8	13	15	102	0.1	45	140	0.04	0.15	0.1	1
114.	Jelly	1 tbsp	18	49	0	0	0	0	13	4	0.3	3	0	0	0.01	0	1
115.	Kale, fresh cooked, drained	1/2 c	55	22	2.5	0	0	0	3	103	0.9	24	4,565	0.06	0.10	0.9	51
116	Lamb leg, roast, trimmed	3 oz.	85	237	22	16	7.3	60	0	9	1.4	53	0	0.13	0.23	4.7	0
117.	Lemon juice, fresh	1 tbsp	15	4	0.1	0	0	0	1	1	0	0	0	0	0	0	7
118.	Lentils, cooked	1/2 c	100	106	8	0	0	0	19	25	2.1	0	20	0.07	0.06	0.6	0
119.	Lettuce, crisp head	1 c sm chunks	75	10	0.7	0	0	0	2	15	0.4	7	250	0.05	0.05	0.2	5
120.	Lettuce, cos or romaine	1 c chopped	55	10	0.7	0	0	0	2	37	0.8	5	1,050	0.08	0.04	0.2	10
121.	Liver, beef, fried	1 slice 3 oz.	85	195	22	9	2.5	345	5	9	7.5	156	45,390	0.22	3.56	14.0	23
122.	Liverwurst, fresh	1 slice 1 oz.	28	87	5	7	3.5	50	1	3	1.5	0	1,800	0.06	0.37	1.6	0
123.	Lobster	1 c	145	138	27	2	1	293	0	94	1.2	305	0	0.15	0.10	0	0
124.	Macaroni, enriched cooked	1/2 c	70	78	2.4	0	0	0	16	6	0.7	1	0	0.10	0.06	0.8	0
125.	Macaroni and cheese	1/2 c	100	215	8.2	11	4	21	20	181	0.9	543	430	0.10	0.20	0.9	0
126.	Margarine	1 tsp	5	34	0	4	0.7	2	0	1	0	46	160	0	0	0	0
127.	Matzo	1 piece	30	117	3.0	0	0	0	25	*	*	0	*	*	*	*	*
128.	Mayonnaise	1 tsp	5	36	0	4	.7	3	0	1	0	28	13	0	0	0	0
129.	Milk, evaporated whole	1/2 c	126	172	9	10	5.8	40	13	329	0.2	149	405	0.05	0.43	0.2	2
130.	Milk, lowfat (2% fat)	1 c	246	145	10	5	3.1	5	15	352	0.1	150	200	0.10	0.52	0.2	2
131.	Milk shake, vanilla (McDonald's)	1	289	323	10	8	5.1	29	52	346	0.2	250	346	0.12	0.66	0.6	3
132.	Milk skim	1 c	245	88	9	0	0.3	5	12	296	0.1	126	10	0.09	0.44	0.2	2
133.	Milk, whole (3.5% fat)	1 c	244	159	9	9	5.1	34	12	288	0.1	120	350	0.07	0.40	0.2	2
134.	Molasses, medium	1 tbsp	20	50	0	0	0	0	13	33	0.9	3	0	0.01	0.01	0	0
135.	Mushrooms, fresh cultivated	1/2 c sliced	35	12	1.0	0	0	0	2	4	0.5	4	0	0.04	0.12	2.4	1
136.	Mustard greens, cooked drained	1/2 c	70	16	1.7	0	0	0	3	96	1.2	13	4,060	0.05	0.10	0.4	33
137.	Noodles, egg, enriched cooked	1/2 c	80	100	3.3	1	0	0	19	8	0.7	2	55	0.11	0.07	1.0	0
138.	Nuts, Brazil	1 oz. (6-8 nuts)	28	185	4.1	19	4.8	0	3	53	1.0	0	0	0.27	0.03	0.5	0
139.	Nuts, pecans	1 oz.	28	195	2.6	20	1.4	0	4	21	0.7	0	40	0.24	0.04	0.3	1
140.	Nuts, walnuts	1 oz. (14 halves)	28	185	4.2	18	1	0	5	28	0.9	1	10	0.09	0.4	0.3	1
141.	Oatmeal, quick, cooked	1/2 c	120	66	2.4	1	0.2	0	12	11	0.7	262	0	0.10	0.03	0.1	0
142.	Oil, soybean	1 tsp.	5	44	0	5	2	0	0	0	0	0	0	0	0	0	0
143.	Okra, cooked drained	1/2 c	80	23	1.6	0	0	0	5	74	0.4	2	390	0.11	0.15	0.7	16
144.	Olives, black ripe	10 extra large	55	61	0.5	7	1	0	1	40	0.8	385	30	0	0	0	0
145.	Onions, mature cooked, drained	1/2 c sliced	105	31	1.3	0	0	0	7	25	0.4	8	40	0.03	0.03	0.2	8
146.	Onion rings (Brazier) Dairy Queen	1 serving	85	360	6	17	6	15	33	20	0.4	125	0	0.09	0	0.4	2

147. Orange, raw (medium skin)	1 med	180	64	1.3	0	0	0	16	54	0.5	1	260	0.13	0.05	0.5	66
148. Orange juice, froz. reconstituted	1/2 c	125	61	0.9	0	0	0	15	13	0.1	1	270	0.12	0.02	0.5	60
149. Oysters, raw Eastern	1/2 c (6-9 med)	120	79	10	2	1.3	60	4	113	6.6	145	370	0.17	0.22	3.0	0
150. Pancakes	1 6" diam x ½" thick	73	169	5.2	5	1	36	25	74	0.9	310	90	0.12	0.16	0.9	0
151. Papaya, raw	½ med	227	60	0.9	0	0	0	15	31	0.5	5	2,660	0.06	0.06	0.5	85
152. Parsnips, cooked	1 large 9" long	160	106	2.4	1	0	0	24	72	1.0	13	50	0.11	0.13	0.2	16
153. Peaches, raw, peeled	1 2¾" diam.	175	58	0.9	0	0	0	15	14	0.8	2	2,030	0.03	0.08	1.5	11
154. Peaches, canned, heavy syrup	1 half 2⅛ tbsp liq.	96	75	0.4	0	0	0	19	4	0.3	2	410	0.01	0.02	0.6	3
155. Peanut butter	2 tbsp	32	188	8	16	1	0	6	18	0.6	194	0	0.04	0.04	4.8	0
156. Peanuts, roasted	1 oz.	28	166	7	14	1	0	5	21	0.6	119	0	0.09	0.04	4.9	0
157. Pears, Bartlett, raw	1 pear	180	100	1.1	1	0	0	25	13	0.5	2	30	0.03	0.07	0.2	7
158. Pears, canned, heavy syrup	1 half 2¼ tbsp liq.	103	78	0.2	0	0	0	20	5	0.2	1	0	0.01	0.02	0.1	1
159. Pears, frozen, cooked drained	1/2 c	80	55	4.1	0	0	0	10	15	1.5	92	480	0.22	0.07	1.4	11
160. Peas, early, canned, drained	1/2 c	85	75	4.0	0	0	0	14	22	1.6	200	585	0.08	0.05	0.7	7
161. Peppers, sweet, raw, 3" diam.	1 pepper 3¼"x3"	200	36	2.0	0	0	0	8	15	1.1	21	690	0.13	0.13	0.8	210
162. Pickles, dill	1 large 4" long	135	15	0.9	0	0	0	3	35	1.4	1,928	140	0	0.03	0	8
163. Pickles, sweet	1 large 3" long	35	51	0.2	0	0	0	13	4	0.4	0	30	0	0.01	0	2
164. Pineapple, raw	1/2 c diced	78	41	0.3	0	0	0	11	13	0.4	1	55	0.07	0.03	0.2	13
165. Pineapple, canned, heavy syrup	1/2 c	128	95	0.4	0	0	0	25	14	0.4	2	65	0.10	0.03	0.3	9
166. Pizza, Cheese, Thin 'n Crispy, Pizza Hut	1/2 10" pie	*	450	25	15	7	125	54	450	4.5	1,200	750	0.30	0.51	5.0	1
167. Pizza, Cheese, Thick 'n Chewy, Pizza Hut	1/2 10" pie	*	560	34	14	6	110	71	500	5.4	1,100	1,000	0.68	0.68	7.0	1
168. Plums, Japanese and hybrid, raw	1 plum 2⅛" diam.	70	32	0.3	0	0	0	8	8	0.3	1	160	0.02	0.02	0.3	4
169. Popcorn, popped, plain, large kernel	1 c	6	12	0.8	0	0	0	5	1	0.2	0	0	0	0.01	0.1	0
170. Pork, roast, trimmed	2 slices 3 oz.	85	179	24	8	2.2	65	0	11	3.1	863	0	0.55	0.22	4.3	0
171. Pork, sausage, cooked	1 sm link	17	72	2.8	6	2.1	13	1	0	0.3	221	0	0	0	0	0
172. Potato, baked in skin	1 potato 2 1/3x4¼"	202	145	4.0	0	0	0	33	14	1.1	6	0	0.15	0.07	2.7	31
173. Potato chips	10 chips	20	114	1.1	8	2.1	0	10	8	0.4	150	0	0.04	0.01	1.0	3
174. Potato, French fried long	10 strips 3½-4"	78	214	3.4	10	1.7	0	28	12	1.0	5	0	0.10	0.06	2.4	16
175. Potato, mashed, milk added	1/2 c	105	69	2.2	1	0.4	8	14	25	0.4	316	20	0.09	0.09	1.1	11
176. Prunes, dried "softenized" without pits	5 prunes	61	137	1.1	0	0	0	36	26	0.1	4	860	0.06	0.05	0.9	2
177. Prune juice, canned or bottled	1/2 c	128	99	0.5	0	0	0	24	18	5.3	3	0	0.02	0.02	0.5	3
178. Pumpkin Pie	1 (3½")	114	241	4.6	13	3	70	28	58	0.6	244	2,810	0.03	0.11	0.6	0
179. Raisins, unbleached, seedless	1 oz.	28	82	0.7	0	0	0	22	18	1.0	8	10	0.02	0.03	0.1	0
180. Rice, brown, cooked	1/2 c	96	116	2.5	1	0	0	25	12	0.5	275	0	0.09	0.02	1.3	0
181. Rice, white enriched, cooked	1/2 c	103	113	2.1	0	0	0	25	11	0.9	384	0	0.12	0.01	1.1	0
182. Salami, dry	1 oz.	28	128	7	11	1.6	24	0	4	1.0	349	0	0.10	0.07	1.5	0
183. Salmon, broiled with butter or margarine	3 oz.	85	156	23	6	2.2	53	0	0	0.9	99	150	0.15	0.06	8.4	0

(Continued)

Code	Food	Amount	Weight gm	Calories	Protein gm	Fat gm	Sat. Fat gm	Cholesterol mg	Carbohydrate gm	Calcium mg	Iron mg	Sodium mg	Vit A I.U.	Vit B_1 mg	Vit B_2 mg	Niacin mg	Vit C mg
184.	Salmon, canned Chinook	3 oz.	85	179	16.6	12	0.8	30	0	131	0.7	105	197	0.03	0.01	6.2	0
185.	Sardines, canned drained	1 oz.	28	58	7	3	1	20	0	124	0.8	233	60	0.01	0.06	1.5	0
186.	Sauerkraut, canned	1/2 c	118	21	1.2	0	0	0	5	43	0.6	878	60	0.04	0.05	0.3	17
187.	Shrimp, boiled	3 oz.	85	99	18	1	0.1	128	1	99	2.7	0	60	0	0.03	1.5	0
188.	Soup, cream of mushroom condensed, prepared with equal volume of milk	1 c	245	216	7	14	5.4	15	16	191	0.5	955	250	0.05	0.34	0.7	1
189.	Soup, split pea, condensed, prepared with equal volume of water	1 c	245	145	9	3	1.1	0	21	29	1.5	941	440	0.25	0.15	1.5	1
190.	Soup, tomato, condensed, prepared with equal volume of water	1 c	245	88	2.0	3	0.5	0	16	15	0.7	970	1,000	0.05	0.05	1.2	12
191.	Soup, vegetable beef, condensed, prepared with equal volume of water	1 c	245	78	5	2	0	0	10	12	0.7	1,046	2,700	0.05	0.05	1.0	0
192.	Spaghetti, in tomato sauce with cheese	1 c	250	260	8.8	9	2	10	37	80	2.3	955	1,080	0.25	0.18	2.3	13
193.	Spaghetti, with meatballs and tomato sauce	1 c	248	332	18.6	11.7	3	75	39	124	3.7	1,009	1,590	0.25	0.30	4.0	22
194.	Spareribs, cooked	3 oz.	85	377	17.8	33	12	73	0	8	2.2	31	0	0.37	0.18	2.9	0
195.	Spinach, raw, chopped	1 c	55	14	1.8	0	0	0	2	51	1.7	39	4,460	0.06	0.11	0.3	28
196.	Spinach, canned, drained	1/2 c	103	25	2.3	1	0	0	4	121	2.6	242	8,200	0.02	0.12	0.3	15
197.	Spinach, froz., cooked, drained	1/2 c	103	24	3.1	0	0	0	4	116	2.2	54	8,100	0.07	0.16	0.4	20
198.	Squash, summer, cooked	1/2 c	90	13	0.8	0	0	0	3	23	0.4	1	350	0.05	0.07	0.7	9
199.	Squash, winter, baked mashed	1/2 c	103	70	1.9	0	0	0	18	41	1.0	1	6,560	0.05	0.14	0.7	8
200.	Strawberries, raw	1 c	149	55	1.0	1	0	0	13	31	1.5	1	90	0.04	0.10	0.9	88
201.	Sundae, choc. Dairy Queen	medium	184	300	6	7	4.9	79	53	200	1.1	175	300	0.06	0.26	0	0
202.	Sugar, white granulated	1 tsp	4	15	0	0	0	0	4	0	0	0	0	0	0	0	0
203.	Sweet potato, baked	1 potato 5″ long	146	161	2.4	1	0	0	37	46	1.0	14	9,230	0.10	0.08	0.8	25
204.	Syrup (maple)	1 tbsp	20	50	0	0	0	0	13	33	0.2	3	0	0	0	0	0
205.	Taco, Taco Bell	1	83	186	15	8	0	0	14	120	2.4	79	120	0.09	0.16	2.9	0
206.	Tangerine	1 med 2⅜″ diam.	116	39	0.7	0	0	0	10	34	0.3	2	360	0.05	0.02	0.1	27
207.	Tea, brewed	1/4 c	180	0	0	0	0	0	0	0	0	0	0	0	0	0	0
208.	Tomato sauce (catsup)	1 tbsp	15	16	0.3	0	0	0	4	3	0.1	156	105	0.01	0.01	0.2	2
209.	Tomatoes, raw	1 tomato 3½ oz.	100	20	1.0	0	0	0	4	12	0.5	3	820	0.05	0.04	0.6	21
210.	Tomatoes, canned	1/2 c	121	26	1.2	0	0	0	5	7	0.6	157	1,085	0.06	0.04	0.9	21
211.	Tortillas, corn, lime	1 6″ diam.	30	63	1.5	1	0	0	14	60	0.9	0	6	0.04	0.02	0.3	0
212.	Tuna, canned, oil pack, drained	3 oz.	85	167	25	7	1.7	60	0	7	1.6	0	70	0.04	0.10	10.1	0
213.	Tuna, canned, water pack, solids and liquid	3½ oz.	99	126	27.7	1	0	55	0	16	1.6	41	0	0	0.10	13.2	0
214.	Turkey, roast (light and dark mixed)	3 oz.	85	162	27	5	1.5	73	0	7	1.5	111	0	0.04	0.15	6.5	0

215. Turnip, cooked, drained	1/2 c cubed	78	18	0.6	0	0	0	4	27	0.3	27	0	0.03	0.04	0.3	17
216. Turnip greens, cooked drained	1/2 c	73	19	2.1	0	0	0	3	98	1.3	14	5,695	0.04	0.08	0.4	16
217. Veal, cooked loin	3 oz.	85	199	22	11	4	90	0	9	2.7	55	0	0.06	0.21	4.6	0
218. Vegetables, mixed, cooked	1 c	182	116	5.8	0	0	0	24	46	2.4	348	4,505	0.22	0.13	2.0	15
219. Watermelon	1 c diced	160	42	0.8	0	0	0	10	11	0.8	2	940	0.05	0.05	0.3	11
220. Wheat germ, plain toasted	1 tbsp	6	23	1.8	1	0	0	3	3	0.5	0	10	0.11	0.05	0.3	1
221. Whiskey, gin, rum, vodka 90 proof	1/2 11 oz (jigger)	42	110	0	0	0	0	0	0	0	0	0		0	0	0
222. Whole wheat cereal, cooked	1/2 c	123	55	2.2	0	0	0	12	9	0.06	260	0	0.08	0.03	0.8	0
223. Whole wheat flakes, ready-to-eat	1 c	30	106	3.1	1	0	0	24	12	2	310	1,410	0.35	0.42	3.5	11
224. Whopper, Burger King	1	*	606	29	32	10.5	100	51	37	6.0	909	641	0.02	0.03	5.2	13
225. Wine, dry table 12% alc.	3½ fl. oz.	102	87	0.1	0	0	0	4	9	0.4	5	0	0	0.01	0.1	0
226. Wine, red dry 18.8% alc.	2 fl. oz.	59	81	0.1	0	0	0	5	5	0	4	0	0.01	0.02	0.2	0
227. Yeast, brewers	1 tbsp	8	23	3.1	0	0	0	3	17	1.4	10	0	1.25	0.34	3.0	0
228. Yogurt, plain low fat	1 8-oz. container	226	113	7.7	4	2.3	15	12	271	0.1	115	150	0.09	0.41	0.2	2

Adapted from:

Nutritive Value of American Foods in Common Units. Agriculture Handbook No. 456. U.S. Dept. of Agriculture. Washington, D.C. November 1975.

Young, E. A., E. H. Brennan, and G. L. Irving, Guest Eds. Perspectives on Fast Foods. Public Health Currents, 19(1), 1979, Published by Ross Laboratories, Columbus, OH.

Dennison, D. The Dine System: the Nutrition Plan For Better Health. C. V. Mosby Comp. St. Louis, Mo., 1982.

Pennington, S. A. T. and H. N. Church. Food Values of Portions Commonly Used. Harper and Row Publishers, New York, 1985.

Kullman, D. A. ABC Milligram Cholesterol Diet Guide. Merit Publications, Inc. North Miami Beach, Florida 1978.

Figure E.1. *Dietary Analysis.*

Date: ______________

Foods	Amount	Calories	Protein (gm)	Fat (total) (gm)	Sat. Fat (gm)	Chol-esterol (mg)	Carbo-hydrates (gm)	Cal-cium (mg)	Iron (mg)	Sodium (mg)	Vit. A (I.U.)	Vit. B_1 (mg)	Vit B_2 (mg)	Nia-cin (mg)	Vit. C (mg)
Totals															

Figure E.1. *Dietary Analysis.*

Date: ______________

Foods	Amount	Calories	Protein (gm)	Fat (total) (gm)	Sat. Fat (gm)	Chol-esterol (mg)	Carbo-hydrates (gm)	Cal-cium (mg)	Iron (mg)	Sodium (mg)	Vit. A (I.U.)	Vit. B_1 (mg)	Vit B_2 (mg)	Nia-cin (mg)	Vit. C (mg)
Totals															

Figure E.1. *Dietary Analysis.*

Date: ________

Foods	Amount	Calories	Protein (gm)	Fat (total) (gm)	Sat. Fat (gm)	Chol-esterol (mg)	Carbo-hydrates (gm)	Cal-cium (mg)	Iron (mg)	Sodium (mg)	Vit. A (I.U.)	Vit. B_1 (mg)	Vit B_2 (mg)	Nia-cin (mg)	Vit. C (mg)
Totals															

Figure E.2. *Three-Day Nutritional Analysis.*

Day	Calories	Protein (gm)	Fat (gm)	Sat. Fat (gm)	Chol-esterol (mg)	Carbo-hydrates (gm)	Calcium (mg)	Iron (mg)	Sodium (mg)	Vit. A. (I.U.)	Vit. B1 (mg)	Vit. B2 (mg)	Niacin (mg)	Vit. C (mg)
One														
Two														
Three														
Totals														
Average[a]														
Percentages[b]														

Recommended Daily Dietary Allowances

Men 15-18 yrs.	See below[c],*	< 20%*	< 30%*	See below[d],*	< 300*	50% >*	1,200	18	3,000*	5,000	1.4	1.7	18	60
Men 19-22 yrs.		< 20%	< 30%		< 300	50% >	800	10	3,000	5,000	1.5	1.7	19	60
Men 23-50 yrs.		< 20%	< 30%		< 300	50% >	800	10	3,000	5,000	1.4	1.6	18	60
Women 15-18 yrs.		< 20%	< 30%		< 300	50% >	1,200	18	3,000	4,000	1.1	1.3	14	60
Women 19-22 yrs.		< 20%	< 30%		< 300	50% >	800	18	3,000	4,000	1.1	1.3	14	60
Women 23-50 yrs.		< 20%	< 30%		< 300	50% >	800	18	3,000	4,000	1.0	1.2	13	60
Pregnant		25%	< 30%		< 300	50% >	400	See below[e]	3,000	5,000	0.4	0.3	2	20
Lactating		22%	< 30%		< 300	50% >	400		3,000	5,000	0.5	0.5	5	40

[a]Divide totals by 3 or number of days assessed.

[b]Percentages: Protein and Carbohydrates = multiply avg. by 4 and divide by avg. calories, Fat = multiply avg. by 9 and divide by avg. calories, Saturated Fat = divided avg. grams of saturated fat by avg. grams of fat.

*Amounts based on recommendations by nutrition experts.

[c]Use Figure 6.5 for all categories.

[d]Less than 50% of total fat for all categories.

[e]Add 30 to 60 mg of supplemental iron during and 3 months after pregnancy.

APPENDIX F

Health Protection Plan For Environmental Hazards, Crime Prevention, and Personal Safety

*Questionnaire published by the Preventive Medicine/Strang Clinic. New York, 1982. Reproduced with permission.

Personal Environment

In addition to environmental problems in the community at large there are also important problems in our own immediate environment that affect our health, well-being, and comfort. These are problems we can control and improve ourselves. The following self-assessment relates to environmental hazards dealing with water, wastes, noise and air pollution in our everyday lives. All "no" answers are a cue to ACTION.

Concerning AIR POLLUTION, do you...?	YES	NO
...Know the optimal conditions for temperature, humidity and air movement in your home?	○	○
...Change the air filters once a year in your air conditioners or forced air heating systems?	○	○
...Are your work areas ventilated so that fumes and dusts do not accumulate?	○	○
...Do your throat or nasal passages feel moist and clear in the morning (not dry or stuffy)?	○	○
...Know what to do when the weather report says the quality of the air is unsatisfactory?	○	○
...Know what a "killer smog" is?	○	○
...If you smoke, do you avoid smoking in a bedroom or areas where children play?	○	○

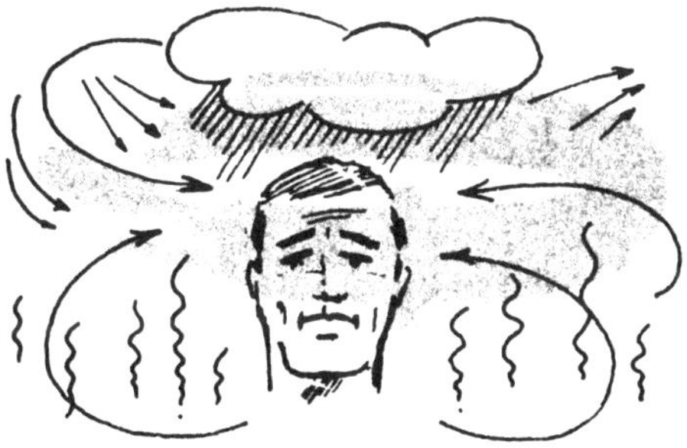

RISK FACTORS:

- *Bronchitis, asthma, emphysema, and heart disease are all aggravated by air pollution.*
- *Chronic exposure to dusts of metal or wood are risk factors for cancer of the respiratory passages.*
- *Children of cigarette smokers have a higher than usual incidence of respiratory infections.*
- *Many so-called allergies of the sinuses and upper respiratory tract are really due to air pollution.*

AWARENESS COUNTS:

- **The optimal air comfort levels are 66-68°F temperature, 30-40% humidity, and air movement at 20-50 feet per minute. Lower humidity will lead to dryness of the respiratory passages, increase skin evaporation and make your home feel colder than it is.**
- **When the air quality is reported as "unsatisfactory" people with heart and lung disease should stay indoors.**
- **"Killer smog" refers to trapped air which cannot rise, with no available dispersing breeze, which accumulates industrial, auto and heating combustion products into a suffocating density. This may be fatal to those with cardiopulmonary disease, and uncomfortable for everyone.**

Concerning WATER...?	YES	NO
...Have you checked your home drinking water in the last year for clarity, color and taste?	○	○
...If you shake up a glass of tap water does it remain clear (not foamy or frothy)?	○	○
...Do you have a screen filter on your water tap?	○	○
...Do you check restaurant water and ice for clarity and cleanliness?	○	○
...Do you know the common water-borne diseases?	○	○
...Do you know what kind of water purification tablets are best for traveling?	○	○
...Do you take care when traveling in developing countries or in unsettled areas to drink bottled water, or coffee, tea, or soup made with boiling water, and to avoid ice cubes?	○	○
...Do you think all wilderness water is safe?	○	○
...Do you know what source of water is almost always safe to drink?	○	○

Concerning WASTE...?	YES	NO
...Do you place ordinary kitchen waste in plastic bags for disposal?	○	○
...Do you know what kinds of wastes require special handling?	○	○
...Are your garbage cans free from bad odors?	○	○
...Is your sink or toilet bowl free from bad odors or back up of waste water in your drain?	○	○
...If you live in a home with a septic tank do you know its location?	○	○
...Do you know the last time the septic tank was cleaned?	○	○

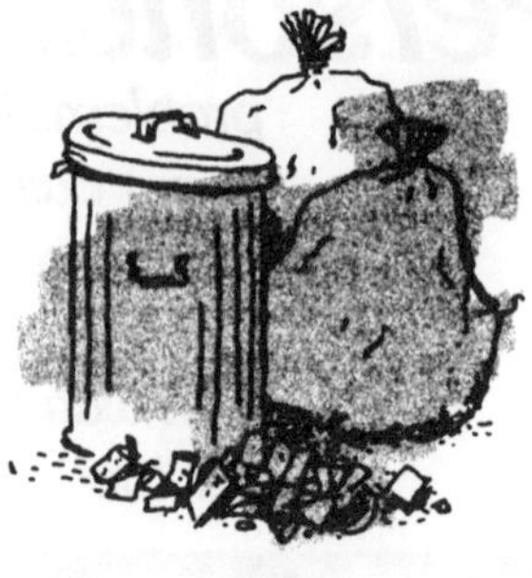

RISK FACTORS: WATER AND WASTE

- *Diseases associated with water and waste include: typhoid fever, cholera, hepatitis, poliomyelitis, E. coli dysentery and amoebic dysentery.*
- *Very hard water containing large amounts of magnesium can cause diarrhea in children. It is difficult to wash with, and will cause deposits in water pipes.*
- *Chlorine is commonly used for water purification. An excess is harmful since it may be converted into chloroform, a toxic chemical.*
- *The presence of water supplies in proximity to industrial plants is a cause for concern since there are many instances of toxic chemicals leaking into local water supplies in this country.*

AWARENESS COUNTS: WATER

- **All water taps should have screen filters to trap particulate material which may accidentally enter the water supply. These should be removed and cleaned regularly.**
- **Frothy water is due to detergents leaking into the water supply and this can cause intestinal upsets.**
- **Cloudy water may be due only to rusty pipes and while it may stain kitchen utensils it is not harmful; but turbid water with an odor may be due to seepage of sewage or industrial wastes into the water supply and this can be dangerous to health. Every state has a water supply agency that can give you information on the condition of your local water supply. However, if your water comes from a well, no one is checking it for purity. You must take the initiative and find out from the state agency how this can be done.**
- **The best type of water purification tablets is the iodine-releasing variety rather than the chlorine type. These are obtainable from your local pharmacy. Use these only if traveling in an area where bottled water is not available.**
- **Not all wilderness water is pure. It may come from springs which have toxic chemicals, or be contaminated by animal use upstream. If purified water is not available, the safest water to drink is rain water. (Make sure it is stored in a clean container.)**

AWARENESS COUNTS: WASTE

- **Plastic bags for disposal of ordinary wastes have the advantage of keeping your garbage containers, indoor and outdoor, clean and free of odors. This helps prevent fly, roach, and rodent infestation, and the accidental contamination of food.**
- **Aerosol cans, solvents, and fuels should not be placed in plastic bags, and should not be disposed of with household wastes because of the hazards of fire and explosion; your local waste disposal service should be contacted regarding special handling.**
- **Bad odors or backup of waste water into your sink, tub, or toilet is a serious matter since this is untreated sewage and poses a health hazard. There may be an obstruction in the sewage system; check with your plumber first. If you have a septic tank, it may have to be cleaned. The frequency of cleaning of septic tanks depends on size and use. Three to four years of regular use is an average duration of time before cleaning is necessary.**
- **It's important to know the location of your septic tank and also those of your neighbors in relationship to your well water supply. There should be a distance of 100 feet between the septic tank and well. Your board of health can give you additional information about specific conditions in your area.**

Concerning NOISE...?	YES	NO
...Do you know how to tell if you are in an environment which could damage your hearing?	○	○
...Do you know that permanent hearing loss can occur with a single exposure to a painfully loud noise?	○	○
...Are you aware of the other effects on your health that noise can have other than hearing loss?	○	○
...Do you know the accidents that can occur due to noise causing "warning concealment"?	○	○
...Are you aware of "slow reaction time" as a noise associated danger?	○	○
... Do you know what age group is especially susceptible to noise induced hearing loss?	○	○

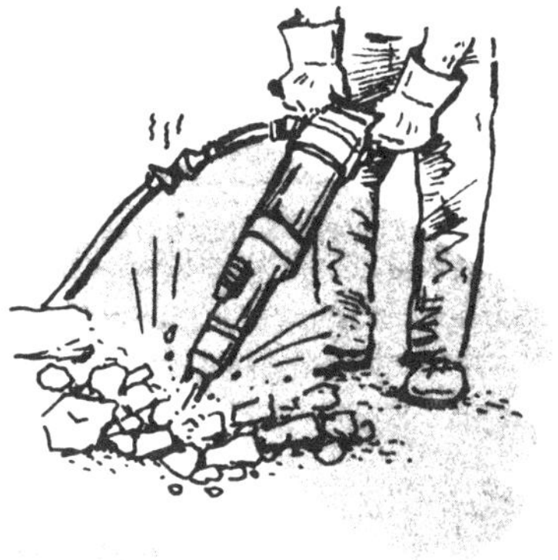

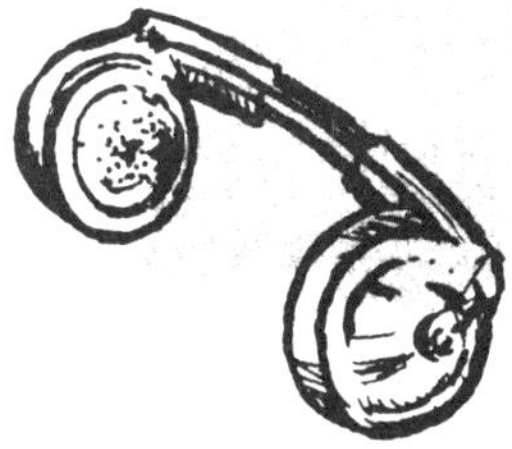

RISK FACTORS:

NOISE

- *Noise hazards can lead not only to permanent hearing damage, but it has been established that noise can cause personality disorders, increase aggressive behavior and have an aggravating effect on headaches, hypertension, and peptic ulcers. It also lowers work efficiency and interferes with sleep patterns.*

AWARENESS COUNTS:

- ***If you are in a noisy environment several hours a day where you have to raise your voice to be heard, you are in an area of potential danger for hearing loss. Noise that is painfully loud, such as pneumatic hammers or amplified rock music, has the greatest potential to damage hearing.***
- ***The age group in which there is particular susceptibility to hearing loss is adolescence.***
- ***It is particularly important to sleep in a quiet environment; use rugs, drapes, double windows, and finally ear plugs if necessary, to obliterate disturbing sound. (Cotton makes a poor plug unless saturated with wax or vaseline. Sponge plastic ear plugs are better.)***
- ***Pleasant background music can sometimes be used to mask disturbing sounds. However, background noise can conceal safety warnings, or lead to slow reaction time and thus contribute to accidents.***

FOLLOW-THROUGH

For information on all environmental hazards, write to:

The U.S. Environmental Protection Agency
Office of Public Affairs (A-107) Washington, D.C. 20460

For information about noise hazards, write to:

The National Information Center for Quiet
P.O. Box 57171 Washington, D.C. 20037

Crime Prevention

Through your own efforts, you can learn to reduce the opportunity and temptation for the criminal by accepting the responsibility to do everything possible for the protection of your personal well being and property. All "no" answers are a cue to ACTION.

To protect yourself, do you...?	YES	NO
...Always us a peephole or chain lock to identify your visitor?	○	○
...Watch out for suspicious people or cars in your neighborhood?	○	○
...Make an effort to get better acquainted with your neighbors, especially if you live in a large apartment building?	○	○
...Avoid resisting the orders of a robber or purse snatcher?	○	○
...List only your last name and initials in the phone directory and on the mailbox?	○	○
...Always lock your doors during the day, even if you are at home?	○	○
...Leave lights on doors you will be using when you return after dark?	○	○
...Always have your key in your hand when you return home so you can open the door immediately?	○	○

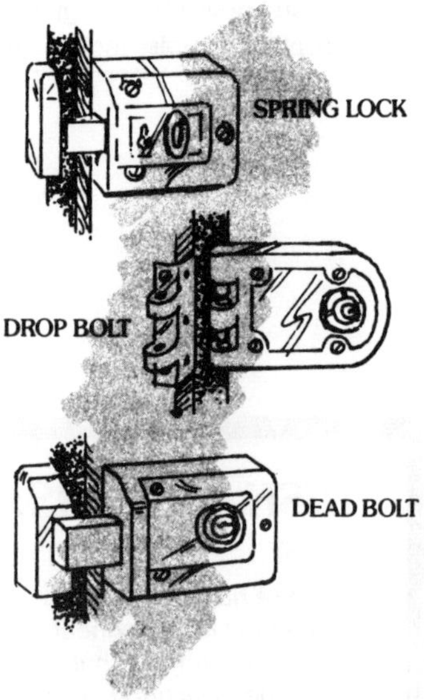

RISK FACTORS:

PROTECTING YOURSELF

- *Women alone and the elderly are at highest risk at being victims of crime.*
- *People who are disabled are more vulnerable to crime.*
- *Certain areas of every large city are high crime areas and should be avoided if possible.*

AWARENESS COUNTS:

- **List only your last name and initial in the phone directory and on the mailbox, particularly if you are a woman living alone.**
- **Always have your key ready when you return home.**
- **Always ask a visitor to identify himself before you let him in.**
- **Use automatic timers to turn on lights, radio, etc.**
- **If a window or lock has been forced or broken while you were out, use a neighbor's phone to call the police and wait outside until they arrive.**
- **Be cautious of unidentified phone callers. Hang up immediately if the caller will not identify himself.**
- **When traveling about at night, try to have a companion with you.**
- **Remember to ask for identification *before* you let repairmen, meter readers, or any other stranger into your home.**

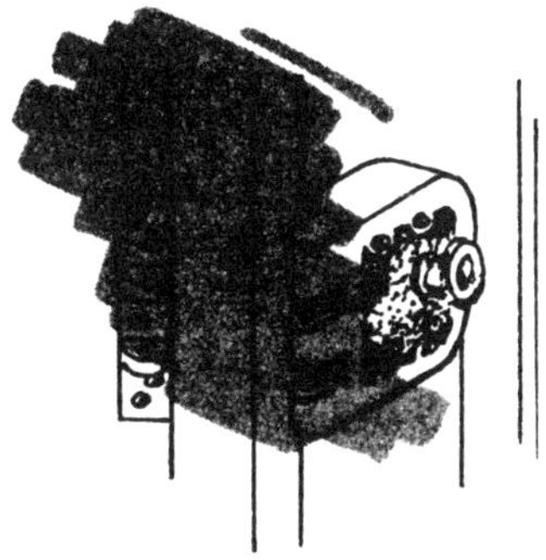

VERTICAL BOLT

To protect yourself, do you...?	YES	NO
...Make specal plans for your home when you are away on vacation?	○	○
...Avoid leaving a key under the doormat or in any accessible area?	○	○
...Have you made sure that your door (s) have sturdy locks?	○	○
...Check all windows and doors regularly for security?	○	○
...Stop newspaper and milk deliveries when you go on vacation?	○	○
...Keep especially valuable items in a safety deposit box away from home?	○	○

RISK FACTORS:

PROTECTING YOUR HOME

- Those at higher risk of home crime are people who leave their homes unattended for long periods of time and those who are nighttime travellers.
- Most crime takes place under cover of darkness.
- Letting mail and newspapers accumulate at your door announces the vulnerability of your home.

AWARENESS COUNTS:

- **Keep your doors locked at all times.**
- **Have lights on an automatic timer while you are away.**
- **An alarm system is a useful crime deterrent.**
- **Make sure windows are secured.**
- **Make sure doorways and hallways are well lighted.**
- **Leave a radio on (a radio uses little electricity and gives the impression that your home is occupied).**

About Locks: Doors should be equipped with either a drop-bolt or dead-bolt lock. Do not use spring locks on any outside door. Spring locks work simply by closing the door and can be easily opened with a plastic card. Drop-bolt or dead-bolt locks can only be unlocked with a key.

FOLLOW-THROUGH

Check with your local police department about joining the Operation Identification Program. You are provided with a sticker to display on your home and your valuable property is engraved with a non-removable code number. The police have a registered list of this property and statistics show that burglars avoid such homes because marked items are difficult to dispose of. Many police departments have crime prevention units and will give you personal advice.

Many states make available the Federal Crime Insurance Program – it provides federal crime insurance against burglary and robbery losses – rates depend upon the crime rate in the area where your home is located. For more information write to:

Federal Crime Insurance, P.O. Box 11033
Washington, D.C. 20014 Toll Free (800) 638-8780

Review your homeowner's insurance coverage to make sure you have adequate coverage.

Personal Safety

While not all accidents are preventable, many are. Failure to take simple precautionary measures increases the risk of an avoidable accident. See if you can identify safety problem areas. All "yes" answers are a cue to Action.

Concerning PERSONAL SAFETY,	**YES**	**NO**
...Have you had any accidents in the past years which could have been prevented?	○	○
...If yes, where did this occur? at home?	○	○
in your automobile?	○	○
at work?	○	○
To ensure your SAFETY AT HOME,	**YES**	**NO**
...Do you fail to go through your dwelling, room by room, deliberately looking for safety hazards once a year?	○	○
...Does your dwelling have fewer than two means of escape in the event of an emergency?	○	○
...If you smoke, do you ever smoke in bed?	○	○
...Do you fail to keep a first aid kit, smoke alarm and fire extinguisher at home?	○	○
...Are there loose electrical wiring or fixtures around your home?	○	○
...Are carpets put down without non-skid backings?	○	○
...Are poisons and pills in areas within reach of pre-school children?	○	○
In the BATHROOM, do you fail to...	**YES**	**NO**
...Check the temperature of bath or shower water with your hand first?	○	○
...Make sure electrical appliances are never used near water?	○	○
...Use non-skid paste-ons or rubber mats for bathtub and shower surfaces?	○	○

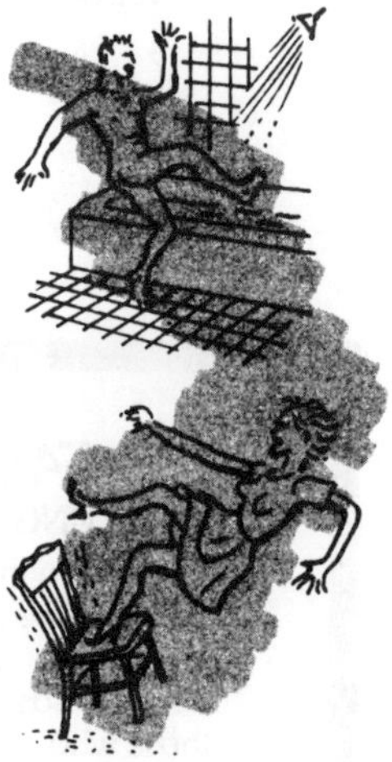

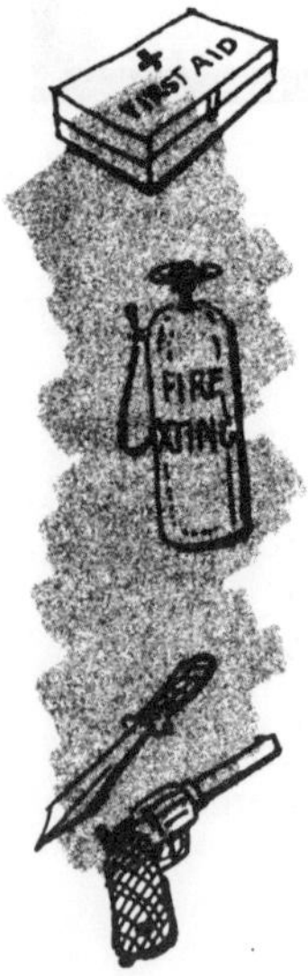

In the KITCHEN, do you fail to...	**YES**	**NO**
...Store knives with points away from the hand, or in special holders?	○	○
...Keep curtains away from the cooking range?	○	○
...Keep electrical appliances away from water?	○	○
...Keep floors clean of grease and dirt?	○	○
...Are you currently exposed to any of the material listed below?	○	○
dust (such as wood, leather, heavy metals, dyestuff)?	○	○
petroleum products?	○	○
radiation?	○	○
solvents?	○	○
...If yes to any of the above...was your exposure usually indoors?	○	○
...Did your exposure occur for an equivalent of at least one eight hour day per week for a period of five years?	○	○
...If yes to dust, chemicals or petroleum products, was your skin or clothing regularly contacted by these materials?	○	○
To ensure your SAFETY IN YOUR AUTOMOBILE, do you...?	**YES**	**NO**
...Neglect to <u>always</u> fasten your seat belts?	○	○
...Ever drink alcoholic beverages before driving?	○	○
...Drive even when you are sleepy?	○	○
...Drive more than <u>40%</u> of the time in the dark?	○	○
...Have you received more than <u>one</u> moving traffic violation this past year?	○	○
...Have you had more than <u>one</u> accident this past year?	○	○

RISK FACTORS: PERSONAL SAFETY

- *Accidents are the leading cause of death among those under 44 years old.*
- *Accidents are the fourth most common cause of death in this country ranking behind heart disease, cancer and stroke.*

AWARENESS COUNTS:

- It is especially important that potential problem areas at home, on the road, and at work be identified so that you can create a relatively accident free environment. Improving your accident-prone behavior is the only way to decrease your risk of accidents.
- Your home or apartment should be regularly checked for safety hazards: ■ Slippery stairways ■ Unfastened carpets ■ Faulty fixtures or outlets ■ Store poisons, firearms in safe place ■ Have safety guard rails on upper level windows ■ Place smoke detectors in strategic areas ■ Have emergency numbers posted by the phone ■ Fire strikes more than 1,500 homes every day.
- Automobile accidents take more lives each year than any other type of accident or illness. Many of these can be prevented: ■ Make sure your car is in safe running condition, especially brakes and tires ■ Wear seat belts at <u>all</u> times. ■ Never drive while drinking. ■ Never drive while sleepy. ■ Always lock your car.

To ensure your SAFETY AT WORK,	YES	NO
...Does your place of work fail to have regular safety checks?	○	○
...Does your place of work fail to have regular emergency drills such as fire drills?	○	○
...Does your place of work fail to have a current fire emergency plan?	○	○
...Does your place of work fail to have rules governing the use of machinery and protective equipment?	○	○

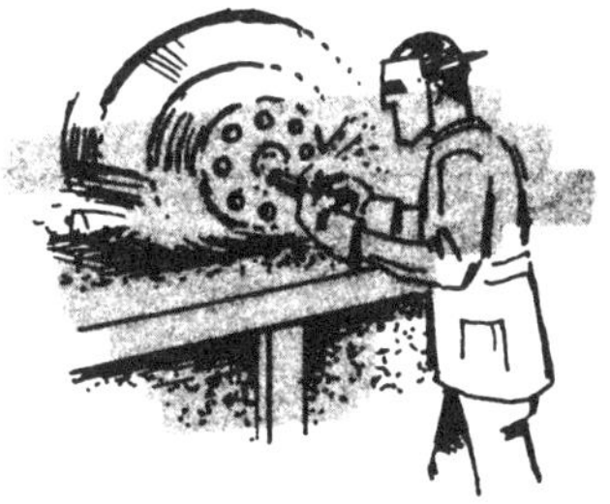

...Have you ever worked at a job where you were exposed to: asbestos? ○○ chemicals? ○○ coal dust? ○○

RISK FACTORS:

SAFETY AT WORK

- *13,000 accidental deaths per year occur on the job and over 2 million people are disabled or injured.*
- *Almost 30 billion dollars per year and about 25 million work days are lost due to accidents at work.*

AWARENESS COUNTS:

- Know where fire extinguishers are located.
- Is there a fire emergency plan in your office?
- Know the mandatory safety standards which apply to your business or industry.
- Use all protective clothing required.
- Know the names and hazards of <u>all</u> materials you are exposed to.

FOLLOW-THROUGH

For information regarding safety procedures and requirements <u>on the job</u> write to:
The U.S. Department of Labor, Washington, D.C. 20212
Or get in touch with the Department of Labor office in your region. Or write to:
The National Institute for Occupational Safety and Health, Post Office Building, Cincinnati, Ohio 45202
For information regarding the safety of consumer products, write to:
U.S. Consumer Product Safety Commission Office of Washington, D.C. 20207
For information regarding all kinds of accidents, write to:
The National Safety Council, 444 N. Michigan Avenue, Chicago, Illinois 60611

Preventive Medicine Institute/Strang Clinic 55 East 34 Street • New York, N.Y. 10016 • (212) 683-1000

Index